Symptoms in the Pharmacy

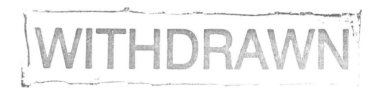

Symptoms in the Pharmacy

A Guide to the Management of Common Illness

ALISON BLENKINSOPP
BPharm, FRPharmS, PhD
Professor of the Practice of Pharmacy
School of Pharmacy
University of Bradford
UK

PAUL PAXTON
MB, ChB, DRCOG
Former GP, and GP Trainer, Cambridge UK

AND

JOHN BLENKINSOPP
MB, ChB, BPharm, MRPharmS
Chief Medical Officer, Avipero Ltd., UK

SEVENTH EDITION

WILEY Blackwell

This edition first published 2014 © 2014 John Wiley & Sons Ltd
© 2005, 2009 by Alison Blenkinsopp, Paul Paxton and John Blenkinsopp
© 1989, 1995, 1998, 2002 by Blackwell Publishing Ltd

Registered office: John Wiley & Sons, Ltd, The Atrium, Southern Gate, Chichester, West Sussex, PO19 8SQ, UK

Editorial offices: 9600 Garsington Road, Oxford, OX4 2DQ, UK
The Atrium, Southern Gate, Chichester, West Sussex, PO19 8SQ, UK
111 River Street, Hoboken, NJ 07030-5774, USA

For details of our global editorial offices, for customer services and for information about how to apply for permission to reuse the copyright material in this book please see our website at www.wiley.com/wiley-blackwell

Library of Congress Cataloging-in-Publication Data

Blenkinsopp, Alison, author.
  Symptoms in the pharmacy : a guide to the management of common illnesses / Alison Blenkinsopp, Paul Paxton, and John Blenkinsopp. – Seventh edition.
    p. ; cm.
  Includes bibliographical references and index.
  ISBN 978-1-118-66173-4 (pbk.)
  I. Paxton, Paul, author.   II. Blenkinsopp, John, author.   III. Title.
  [DNLM: 1. Drug Therapy–Handbooks.   2. Pharmaceutical Services–Handbooks.   3. Diagnosis–Handbooks.
4. Referral and Consultation–Handbooks.   QV 735]
  RS122.5
  615.5′8–dc23
                                                                                                2013037473

A catalogue record for this book is available from the British Library.

Wiley also publishes its books in a variety of electronic formats. Some content that appears in print may not be available in electronic books.

Cover design by Opta Design

Set in 10/12pt Sabon by Aptara Inc., New Delhi, India
Printed and bound in Malaysia by Vivar Printing Sdn Bhd

2   2016

Contents

Preface, vi

Introduction: How to Use This Book, 1

Respiratory Problems
Colds and flu, 19
Cough, 33
Sore throat, 45
Allergic rhinitis (hay fever), 53
Respiratory symptoms for direct referral, 62

Gastrointestinal Tract Problems
Mouth ulcers, 69
Heartburn, 76
Indigestion, 85
Nausea and vomiting, 95
Motion sickness and its prevention, 98
Constipation, 102
Diarrhoea, 112
Irritable bowel syndrome, 124
Haemorrhoids, 132

Skin Conditions
Eczema/dermatitis, 143
Acne, 153
Athlete's foot, 159
Cold sores, 167
Warts and verrucae, 172
Scabies, 178
Dandruff, 182
Psoriasis, 186

Painful Conditions
Headache, 193
Musculoskeletal problems, 210

Women's Health
Cystitis, 225
Dysmenorrhoea, 234
Menorrhagia, 243
Vaginal thrush, 246
Emergency hormonal contraception, 255
Common symptoms in pregnancy, 263

Men's Health
Benign prostatic hyperplasia, 269
Hair loss, 274

Eye and Ear Problems
Eye problems: the painful red eye, 281
Common ear problems, 289

Childhood Conditions
Illnesses affecting infants and children up to 16 years, 297
Colic, 303
Teething, 306
Napkin rash, 307
Head lice, 313
Threadworms (pinworms), 319
Oral thrush, 323

Insomnia
Difficulty sleeping, 331

Prevention of Heart Disease
Prevention of heart disease, 343

Appendix: Summary of Symptoms for Direct Referral, 359

Index, 361

Colour plates are found facing page 184 and 185.

Preface

This is the seventh edition of our book and appears 25 years after the first. Among the changes since the sixth edition is the move of more medicines from the prescription-only medicine (POM) category to the pharmacy (P) medicine category. New sections and case studies on orlistat and tranexamic acid are thus included. Important safety advice about the use of OTC medicines in chidren has been incorporated. We have updated and extended information about common infectious diseases to reflect changing patterns of illness.

There have also been further changes in the National Health Service (NHS). The importance of self-care continues to increase recognized and the public health role of community pharmacies has become more prominent. NHS-funded community pharmacy minor ailment schemes have spread to more areas in England as well as in Wales, Northern Ireland and Scotland. Under these schemes patients who are exempt from NHS prescription charges can obtain free treatment from the pharmacy. The schemes are well used, particularly for children's minor illness and we have further expanded our explanation of common childhood illnesses to enable the pharmacist to manage where appropriate, to reassure and refer when necessary.

A strength of this book has always been its evidence-based approach. The findings of new systematic reviews of published evidence together with evidence-based treatment guidelines have been incorporated and updated throughout. We have continued to introduce evidence on complementary therapies. We have strengthened our advice on working in partnership with patients.

As for previous editions we have received positive and constructive feedback and suggestions from pharmacists (undergraduate students, pre-registration trainees and practising pharmacists) and have tried to act on your suggestions. We have continued to add more accounts by patients to our case studies. We thank all the pharmacists who sent us comments and we hope you like the new edition.

We once again thank Kathryn Coates and her network of mums, who provided advice on childhood conditions and on women's health, and on the sort of concerns and queries that they hoped their pharmacists would answer.

Alison Blenkinsopp
Paul Paxton
John Blenkinsopp

Plates 1, 4, 6, 7, 8, 10, 11 and 13 from Robin Graham-Brown and Tony Burns. *Lecture Notes Dermatology*, 9th edition. Oxford: Blackwell Publishing, 2007. Reproduced with permission from the authors.

Introduction: How to Use This Book

Every working day, people come to the community pharmacy for advice about minor ailments. For the average community pharmacy a minimum of 10 such requests will be received each day; for some the figure is far higher. With increasing pressure on doctors' workload it is likely that the community pharmacy will be even more widely used as a first port of call for minor illness. Members of the public present to pharmacists and their staff in three ways:

- Requesting advice about symptoms
- Asking to purchase a named medicine
- Requiring general health advice (e.g. about dietary supplements)

The pharmacist's role in responding to symptoms and overseeing the sale of over the counter (OTC) medicines is substantial and requires a mix of knowledge and skills in the area of diseases and their treatment. In addition, pharmacists are responsible for ensuring that their staff provide appropriate advice and recommendations.

Research on the appropriateness of advice giving in community pharmacies has identified a set of criteria that pharmacists can use to consider their own pharmacy's approach;

- General communication skills.
- What information is gathered by pharmacy staff?
- How is the information gathered by the pharmacy staff?
- Issues to be considered by pharmacy staff before giving advice.
- Rational content of advice given by pharmacy staff.
- How is the advice given?
- Rational product choice made by pharmacy staff.
- Referral.

(Reproduced from Bissell P, Ward PR and Noyce PR. Appropriateness in measurement: application to advice giving in community pharmacies. *Social Science and Medicine* 2000; 51: 343–359, Copyright 2000, with permission from Elsevier).

Symptoms in the Pharmacy: A Guide to the Management of Common Illness, Seventh Edition.
Alison Blenkinsopp, Paul Paxton and John Blenkinsopp.
© 2014 John Wiley & Sons, Ltd. Published 2014 by John Wiley & Sons, Ltd.

Key skills are:

- Differentiation between minor and more serious symptoms
- Listening skills
- Questioning skills
- Treatment choices based on evidence of effectiveness
- The ability to pass these skills on by acting as a role model for other pharmacy staff

Working in partnership with patients

In this book we refer to the people seeking advice about symptoms as patients. It is important to recognise that many of these patients will in fact be healthy people. We use the word 'patient' because we feel that the terms 'customer' and 'client' do not capture the nature of consultations about ill health.

Pharmacists are skilled and knowledgeable about medicines and about the likely causes of illness. In the past the approach has been to see the pharmacist as expert and the patient as beneficiary of the pharmacist's information and advice. But patients are not blank sheets or empty vessels. They are experts in their own and their children's health. The patient:

- May have experienced the same or a similar condition in the past
- May have tried different treatments already
- Will have their own ideas about possible causes
- Will have views about different sorts of treatments
- May have preferences for certain treatment approaches

The pharmacist needs to take this into account in the consultation with the patient and to enable patients to participate by actively eliciting their views and preferences. Not all patients will want to engage in decision making about how to manage their symptoms but research shows that many do. Some will want the pharmacist to simply make a decision on their behalf. What the pharmacist needs to do is to find out what the patient wants.

Much lip service has been paid to the idea of partnership working with patients. The question is how to achieve this? Health care professionals can only truly learn about how to go about working in partnership by listening to what real patients have to say. The list below comes from a study of lay people's 'tips' on how consultations could be more successful. Although the study was concerned with medical consultations many of the tips are equally relevant to pharmacists' response to patients' symptoms.

How to make a consultation more successful from the patient's perspective – tips from lay people

- Introduce yourself with unknown patients
- Keep eye contact
- Take your time, don't show your hurry
- Avoid prejudice – keep an open mind
- Treat patients as human beings and not as a bundle of symptoms
- Pay attention to psychosocial issues
- Take the patient seriously
- Listen – don't interrupt the patient
- Show compassion; be empathic
- Be honest without being rude
- Avoid jargon, check if the patient understands
- Avoid interruptions
- Offer sources of trusted further information (leaflets, weblinks)

(Reproduced from Bensing J.M., Deveugele M., Moretti F., Fletcher I., van Vliet L., van Bogaert M., Rimondini M. How to make the medical consultation more successful from a patient's perspective? Tips for doctors and patients from lay people in the United Kingdom, Italy, Belgium and the Netherlands. *Patient Education and Counseling*: 2011, 84(3), 287–293. Copyright 2011 with permission from Elsevier).

Use these tips to reflect on your own consultations about minor illness both during and afterwards. Try to feel how the consultation is going from the patient's perspective.

Reading and listening to patients' accounts of their experience can provide valuable insights. Websites and blogs can give a window into common problems, questions, and help to see the patient perspective, and can also show how powerful social media can be in sharing experience and information (Netmums is a good example, www.netmums.com). Do not be patronizing about lay networks, why not contribute your own expertise?

Responding to a request for a named product

Where a request is made to purchase a named medicine, the approach needs to take into account that the person making the request might be an expert or a novice user. We define the expert user as someone who has used the medicine before for the same or a similar condition and is familiar with it. While pharmacists and their staff need to ensure that the requested medicine is appropriate, they also need to bear in mind the previous knowledge and experience of the purchaser.

Research shows that the majority of pharmacy customers do not mind being asked questions about their medicine purchase. An exception to this is those who wish to buy a medicine they have used before and would prefer not to be subjected to the same questions each time they ask for the product. There are two key points here for the pharmacist: firstly, it can be helpful to briefly explain why questions are needed, and secondly, fewer questions are normally needed where customers request a named medicine that they have used before.

A suggested sequence in response to a request for a named product

Ask whether the person has used the medicine before, and if the answer is yes, ask if any further information is needed. Quickly check on whether other medicines are being taken. If the person has not used the medicine before, more questions will be needed. One option is to follow the sequence for responding to requests for advice about symptoms (see below). It can be useful to ask how the person came to request this particular medicine, for example, have they seen an advertisement for it? Has it been recommended by a friend or family member?

Pharmacists will use their professional judgement in dealing with regular customers whom they know well and where the individual's medication history is known. The pharmacy patient medication records (PMRs) are a source of back-up information for regular customers. However, for new customers where such information is not known, more questions are likely to be needed.

Responding to a request for help with symptoms

1 Information gathering: By developing rapport and by listening and questioning to obtain information about symptoms, for example, to identify problems that require referral; what treatments (if any) have helped before; what medications are being taken regularly; what the patient's ideas, concerns and expectations are about their problem and possible treatment.
2 Decision making: Is referral for a medical opinion required?
3 Treatment: The selection of possible, appropriate and effective treatments (where needed), offering options to the patient and advising on use of treatment.
4 Outcome: Telling the patient what action to take if the symptoms do not improve.

Information gathering

Most information required to make a decision and recommend treatment can be gleaned from just listening to the patient. The process should start with open-type questions and perhaps an explanation of why it is necessary to ask personal questions. Some patients do not yet understand why the pharmacist needs to ask questions before recommending treatment. An example might be:

> Patient: Can you give me something for my piles?
> Pharmacist: I'm sure I can. To help me give the best advice, though, I'd like a bit more information from you, so I need to ask a few questions. Is that OK?
> Patient: That's fine.
> Pharmacist: Could you just tell me what sort of trouble you get with your piles?

Hopefully, this will lead to a description of most of the symptoms required for the pharmacist to make an assessment. Other forms of open questions could include the following: How does that affect you? What sort of problems does it cause you? By carefully listening and possibly reflecting on comments made by the patient, the pharmacist can obtain a more complete picture.

> Patient: Well, I get spells of bleeding and soreness. It's been going on for years.
> Pharmacist: You say years?
> Patient: Yes, on and off for 20 years since my last pregnancy. I've seen my doctor several times and had them injected, but it keeps coming back. My doctor said that I'd have to have an operation but I don't want one; can you give me some suppositories to stop them bleeding?
> Pharmacist: Bleeding...?
> Patient: Yes, every time I go to the toilet blood splashes around the bowl. It's bright red.

This form of listening can be helped by asking questions to clarify points: I'm not sure I quite understand when you say..., or I'm not quite clear what you meant by.... Another useful technique is to summarise the information so far: I'd just like to make sure I've got it right. You tell me you've had this problem since....

Once this form of information gathering has occurred there will be some facts still missing. It is now appropriate to move onto some direct questions.

> Pharmacist: How are your bowels.... Has there been any change?
> (This question is very important to exclude a more serious cause for the symptoms that would require referral.)
> Patient: No, they are fine, always regular.
> Pharmacist: Can you tell me what sort of treatments you have used in the past, and how effective they were?

Other questions could include what treatments have you tried so far this time? What sort of treatment were you hoping for today? What other medications are you taking at present? Do you have any allergies?

Decision making

Triaging is the term given to assessing the level of seriousness of a presenting condition and thus the most appropriate action. It has come to be associated with both prioritisation (e.g. as used in accident and emergency (A&E) departments) and clinical assessment. Community pharmacists have developed procedures for information gathering when responding to requests for advice that identify when the presenting problem can be managed within the pharmacy and when referral for medical advice is needed. The use of questioning to obtain the sorts of information needed is discussed below. Furthermore, in making this clinical assessment, pharmacists incorporate management of certain conditions and make recommendations about this.

The use of protocols and algorithms in the triaging process is common in many countries including the United Kingdom, with computerised decision-support systems increasingly used. It is possible that in the future computerised decision support may play a greater part in face-to-face consultations, perhaps including community pharmacies.

If the following information were obtained, then a referral would be required:

> *Pharmacist:* Could you tell me what sort of trouble you have had with your piles?
> *Patient:* Well, I get spells of bleeding and soreness. It's been going on for years, although seems worse this time....
> *Pharmacist:* When you say worse, what does that mean?
> *Patient:* Well... my bowels have been playing up and I've had some diarrhoea.... I have to go three or four times a day... and this has been going on for about 2 months.

For more information on when to refer see 'D: Danger symptoms' under the ASMETHOD pneumonic below.

Treatment

The pharmacist's background in pharmacology, therapeutics and pharmaceutics gives a sound base on which to make logical treatment choices based on the individual patient's need, together with the characteristics of the medicine concerned. In addition to the effectiveness of the active ingredients included in the product, the pharmacist will need to consider potential interactions, cautions, contraindications and adverse reaction profile of each constituent. Evidence-based practice requires pharmacists need to carefully think about the effectiveness of the treatments they recommend, combining this with their own and the patient's experience.

Concordance in the use of OTC medicines is important and the pharmacist will elicit the patient's preferences and discuss treatment options in this context. Some pharmacists have developed their own OTC formularies with preferred treatments that are recommended by pharmacists and their staff. In some areas these have been discussed with local general practitioners (GPs) and practice nurses to cover the referral of patients from the GP practice to the pharmacy.

PMRs can play an important part in supporting the process of responding to symptoms. Prior to the introduction of the new Community Pharmacy Contractual Framework (CPCF) in 2005 research showed that only one in four pharmacists recorded OTC treatment on the pharmacist's own PMR system. Yet such recording can complete the profile of medication, and review of concurrent drug therapy can identify potential drug interactions and adverse effects. In addition, such record keeping can make an important contribution to clinical governance. Improvements in IT systems in pharmacies will make routine record keeping more feasible. Keeping records for specific groups of patients, for example, older people, is one approach in the meantime.

The CPCF for England and Wales has contained, since 2005, a requirement to keep certain records of OTC advice and purchases:

> *For patients known to the pharmacy staff, records of advice given, products purchased or referrals made will be made on a patient's pharmacy record when the pharmacist deems it to be of clinical significance* (Essential service specification: Self Care).

Pharmacy computer systems do not all included this feature so most records have to be kept as hard copy, making it difficult for pharmacists to consult them as a clinical record in the future.

Effectiveness of treatments

Pharmacists and their staff should, wherever possible, base treatment recommendations on evidence. For more recently introduced medicines and for those that have moved from presription-only medicine (POM) to pharmacy (P) medicine, there is usually an adequate evidence base. For some medicines, particularly older ones, there may be little or no evidence. Here, pharmacists need to bear in mind that absence of evidence does not in itself signify absence of effectiveness. Current evidence of effectiveness is summarised in the relevant *British National Formulary* (BNF) monograph. The BNF can be found at www.bnf.org.uk. Useful websites for clinical guidelines are NHS Evidence (https://www.evidence.nhs.uk/) which includes NHS Clinical Knowledge Summaries (CKS), the Scottish Inter-Collegiate Guideline Network (SIGN) at www.sign.ac.uk and the National Institute for Health and Care Excellence at www.nice.org.uk. The website for NHS Choices at www.nhs.uk includes Symptom Checkers and management advice for minor ailments.

Key interactions between OTC treatments and other drugs are included in each section of this book. The BNF provides an alphabetical listing of drugs and interactions, together with an indication of clinical significance. In this book, generic drug names are italicised.

For symptoms discussed in this book, the section on 'Management' includes brief information about the efficacy, advantages and disadvantages of possible therapeutic options. Also included are useful points of information for patients about the optimum use of OTC treatments, under the heading 'Practical points'.

Outcome

Most of the symptoms dealt with by the community pharmacist will be of a minor and self-limiting nature and should resolve within a few days. However, sometimes this will not be the case and it is the pharmacist's responsibility to make sure that patients know what to do if they do not get better. Here, a defined timescale should be used, as suggested in the relevant sections of this book, so that when offering treatment the pharmacist can set a time beyond which the patient should seek medical advice if symptoms do not improve. The 'Treatment timescales' outlined in this book naturally vary according to the symptom and sometimes according to the patient's age, but are usually less than 1 week.

Pharmacists are likely to be increasingly involved in the management of long-term chronic or intermittent conditions. Here, monitoring of progress is important and a series of consultations is likely rather than just one.

Developing your consultation skills

Effective consultation skills are the key to finding out what the patient's needs are and deciding whether you can manage the symptoms or whether they might need to be referred to another practitioner. A useful framework for thinking about and improving your consultation skills is provided by Roger Neighbour's five 'checkpoints'.

A	Connecting	'Have we got a rapport?'	Rapport building skills
B	Summarising (clinical process)	'Can I demonstrate to the patient I have understood why she has come?'	Listening and eliciting skills (history taking and summarising to the patient)
C	Handing over	'Has the patient accepted the management plan we agreed?'	Concordance skills
D	Safety netting	'Have I anticipated all likely outcomes?'	Contingency plans
E	Housekeeping*	'Am I in good condition for the next patient?'	Taking care of yourself

*Housekeeping – This is where practitioners look to themselves and their response to the consultation. It may involve having a brief chat with a colleague, a coffee, or merely acknowledging to oneself the effect a particular consultation has had.

Structuring the consultation

Pharmacists need to develop a method of information seeking that works for them. There is no right and wrong here. Some pharmacists find that a mnemonic such as the two shown below can be useful, although care needs to be taken not to recite questions in rote fashion without considering their relevance to the individual case. Good listening will glean much of the information required. The mnemonic can be a prompt to ensure all relevant information has been obtained. Developing rapport is essential to obtain good information, and reading out a list of questions can be off-putting and counterproductive.

W – Who is the patient and what are the symptoms?
H – How long have the symptoms been present?
A – Action taken?
M – Medication being taken?

W: The pharmacist must first establish the identity of the patient: the person in the pharmacy might be there on someone else's behalf. The exact nature of the symptoms should be established: patients often self-diagnose illnesses and the pharmacist must not accept such a self-diagnosis at face value.

H: Duration of symptoms can be an important indicator of whether referral to the doctor might be required. In general, the longer the duration, the more likely is the possibility of a serious rather than a minor case. Most minor conditions are self-limiting and should clear up within a few days.

A: Any action taken by the patient should be established, including the use of any medication to treat the symptoms. About one in two patients will have tried at least one remedy before seeking the pharmacist's advice. Treatment may have consisted of OTC medicines bought from the pharmacy or elsewhere, other medicines prescribed by the doctor on this or a previous occasion or medicines borrowed from a friend or neighbour or found in the medicine cabinet. Homoeopathic or herbal remedies may have been used. The cultural traditions of people from different ethnic backgrounds include the use of various remedies that may not be considered medicines.

If the patient has used one or more apparently appropriate treatments without improvement, referral to the family doctor may be the best course of action.

M: The identity of any medicines taken regularly by the patient is important for two reasons: possible interactions and potential adverse reactions. Such medicines will usually be those prescribed by the doctor, but may also include OTC products. The pharmacist needs to know about all the medicines being taken by the patient because of the potential for interaction with any treatment that the pharmacist might recommend.

The community pharmacist has an increasingly important role in detecting adverse drug reactions, and consideration should be given to the possibility that the patient's symptoms might be an adverse effect caused by medication. For example, whether gastric symptoms such as indigestion might be due to a non-steroidal anti-inflammatory drug (NSAID) taken on prescription or a cough might be due to an angiotensin-converting enzyme (ACE) inhibitor being taken by the patient. Where the pharmacist suspects an adverse drug reaction to a prescribed medicine, the pharmacist should discuss with the doctor what actions should be taken (perhaps including a Yellow Card report to the Commission on Human Medicines (formerly Committee on Safety of Medicines), which can now be made by the pharmacist or patient) and the doctor may wish the patient to be referred so that treatment can be reviewed.

The second mnemonic, ASMETHOD, was developed by Derek Balon, a community pharmacist in London:

A – Age and appearance
S – Self or someone else
M – Medication
E – Extra medicines
T – Time persisting
H – History
O – Other symptoms
D – Danger symptoms.

Some of the areas covered by the ASMETHOD list have been discussed already. The others can now be considered.

A: Age and appearance

The appearance of the patient can be a useful indicator of whether a minor or more serious condition is involved. If the patient looks ill, for example, pale, clammy, flushed or grey, the pharmacist should consider referral to the doctor. As far as children are concerned, appearance is important, but in addition the pharmacist can ask the parent whether the child is generally well. A child who is cheerful and energetic is unlikely to have anything other than a minor problem, whereas one who is quiet and listless, or who is fractious, irritable and feverish, might require referral.

The age of the patient is important because the pharmacist will consider some symptoms as potentially more serious according to age. For example, acute diarrhoea in an otherwise healthy adult could reasonably be treated by the pharmacist. However, such symptoms in a baby could produce dehydration more quickly; elderly patients are also at a higher risk of becoming dehydrated. Oral thrush is common in babies, while less common in older children and adults; the pharmacist's decision about whether to treat or refer could therefore be influenced by age.

Age will play an important part in determining any treatment offered by the pharmacist. Some preparations are not recommended at all for children under 12 years, for example, loperamide. Hydrocortisone cream and ointment should not be recommended for children under 10 years; aspirin should not be used in children under 16 years; corticosteroid nasal sprays and omeprazole should not be recommended for those under 18 years. Others must be given in a reduced dose or as a paediatric formulation and the pharmacist will thus consider recommendations carefully.

Other OTC preparations have a minimum specified age, for example, 16 years for emergency hormonal contraception, 12 years for nicotine replacement therapy (NRT) and 18 years for treatments of vaginal thrush. Pharmacists are used to assessing patients' approximate age and would not routinely ask for proof of age here, unless there was a specific reason to do so.

S: Clarification as to who is the patient

M: Medication regularly taken, on prescription or OTC

E: Extra medication tried to treat the current symptoms

T: Time, that is, duration of symptoms

H: History

There are two aspects to the term 'history' in relation to responding to symptoms: first, the history of the symptom being presented, and second, previous medical history. For example, does the patient have diabetes, hypertension or asthma? PMRs should be used to record relevant existing conditions.

Questioning about the history of a condition may be useful; how and when the problem began, how it has progressed and so on. If the patient has had the problem before, previous episodes should be asked about to determine the action taken by the patient and its degree of success. In recurrent mouth ulcers, for example, do the current ulcers resemble the previous ones, was the doctor or dentist seen on previous occasions, was any treatment prescribed or OTC medicine purchased and, if so, did it work?

In asking about the history, the timing of particular symptoms can give valuable clues as to possible causes. The attacks of heartburn that occur after going to bed or on stooping or bending down are indeed likely to be due to reflux, whereas those that happen during exertion such as exercise or heavy work may not be.

History taking is particularly important when assessing skin disease. Pharmacists often think, erroneously, that recognition of the appearance of skin conditions is the most important factor in responding to such symptoms. In fact, many dermatologists would argue that history taking is more important because some skin conditions resemble each other in appearance. Furthermore, the appearance may be altered during the course of the condition. For example, the use of a topical corticosteroid inappropriately on infected or infested skin may substantially change the appearance; allergy to ingredients such as local anaesthetics may produce a problem in addition to the original complaint. The pharmacist must therefore know which creams, ointments or lotions have been applied.

O: Other symptoms

Patients generally tend to complain about the symptoms that concern them most. The pharmacist should always ask whether the patient has noticed any other symptoms or anything different from usual because, for various reasons, patients may not volunteer all the important information. Embarrassment may be one such reason, so patients experiencing rectal bleeding may only mention that they have piles or are constipated.

The importance or significance of symptoms may not be recognised by patients, for example, those who have constipation as a side-effect from a tricyclic antidepressant will probably not mention their dry mouth because they can see no link or connection between the two problems.

D: Danger symptoms

These are the symptoms or combinations of symptoms that should ring warning bells for pharmacists because immediate referral to the doctor is required. Blood in the sputum, vomit, urine or faeces would be examples of such symptoms, as would unexplained weight loss. Danger symptoms are included and discussed in each section of this book so that their significance can be understood by the pharmacist.

Decision making: risk assessment

In making decisions the pharmacist assesses the possible risk to the patient of different decision paths. The possible reasons for referral for further advice include:

- 'Danger' or 'red flag' signs or symptoms
- Incomplete information (e.g. an ear condition where the ear has not been examined)
- Duration or recurrence of symptoms

As a general rule, the following indicate a higher risk of a serious condition and should make the pharmacist consider referring the patient to the doctor:

- Long duration of symptoms
- Recurring or worsening problems
- Severe pain
- Failed medication (one or more appropriate medicines used already, without improvement)
- Suspected adverse drug reactions (to prescription or OTC medicine)
- Danger symptoms

For relevant sections of this book, the duration of symptoms beyond which the pharmacist should consider immediate referral is defined in the section 'When to refer'. In addition, for relevant sections a 'Treatment timescale' is included – this is the length of time for which the problem might be treated before the patient sees the doctor. Some community pharmacists now use referral forms as an additional means of conveying information to the doctor with the patient.

Discussions with local family doctors can assist the development of protocols and guidelines for referral, and we recommend that pharmacists take the opportunity to develop such guidelines with their medical and nursing colleagues in primary care. Joint discussions of this sort can lead to effective two-way referral systems and local agreements about preferred treatments.

Accidents and injuries

Pharmacists are often asked to offer advice about injuries, many of which are likely to be minor with no need for onward referral. The list below shows the types of injuries that would be classified as 'minor'.

- Cuts, grazes and bruising
- Wounds, including those that may need stitches
- Minor burns and scalds
- Foreign bodies in eye, nose or ear
- Tetanus immunisation after an injury
- Minor eye problems
- Insect bites or other animal bites
- Minor head injuries where there has been no loss of consciousness or vomiting
- Minor injuries to legs below the knee and arms below the elbow, where patients can bear the weight through their foot or move their fingers
- Minor nose bleeds

Pharmacists need to be familiar with the assessment and treatment of minor injuries in order to make a decision about when referral is needed. Referral to A&E may need to be considered in certain circumstances. The list below provides general guidance on when a person might need to immediately go to A&E.

- There has been a serious head injury with heavy bleeding.
- The person is, or has been, unconscious.
- There is a suspected broken bone or dislocation.
- The person is experiencing severe chest pain or is having trouble breathing.
- The person is experiencing severe stomach ache that cannot be treated by OTC remedies.
- There is severe bleeding from any part of the body.

At least 20% of attendances at A&E are for conditions that could have been managed in primary care and an estimated 8% could have been managed in the pharmacy. Given that each attendance at A&E costs the NHS around £60 pharmacies have an important role in educating patients about appropriate use of the service.

Privacy in the pharmacy

The vast majority of community pharmacies in England and Wales have a consultation area. Research shows that most pharmacy customers feel that the level of privacy available for a pharmacy consultation is now acceptable. There is some evidence of a gap between patients' and pharmacists' perceptions of privacy.

Pharmacists observe from their own experience that some patients are content to discuss even potentially sensitive subjects in the pharmacy. While this is true for some people, others are put off asking for advice because of insufficient privacy.

The pharmacist should always bear the question of privacy in mind and, where possible, seek to create an atmosphere of confidentiality if sensitive problems are to be discussed. Using professional judgement and personal experience, the pharmacist can look for signs of hesitancy or embarrassment on the patient's part and can suggest moving to a quieter part of the pharmacy or to the consultation area to continue the conversation.

Patient Group Directions and symptoms in the pharmacy

A Patient Group Direction (PGD) is a legal framework to allow the safe supply of a medicine for specific patients. PGDs are widely used in the NHS and in some areas community pharmacies are commissioned to provide a service which may include one or more PGDs, the most common being Stop Smoking services, the supply of emergency hormonal contraception, and the provision of in fluenza vaccinations. PGDs can also be used in private sector services. Pharmacies providing NHS or private PGDs are required to meet specific criteria for quality and safety of services. Such requirements usually include demonstration of competencies, and the keeping of certain records. The list below shows the range of PGDs that might be seen in community pharmacies.

Erectile dysfunction
Antimalarials
Influenza and hepatitis B vaccine
Meningitis Vaccine
Stop smoking (varenicline)
Hair loss
Emergency contraception
Salbutamol inhalers (for repeat supply)
Oral contraception
Cystitis treatment (trimethoprim)
Weight loss (orlistat 120 mg)

Working in partnership

With family doctors and nurse colleagues in primary care

Community pharmacists are the key gateway into the formal NHS through their filtering of symptoms, with referral to the family doctor when necessary. This filtering is more correctly termed triaging and will be increasingly important in maximising the skills and input of pharmacists and nurses.

Many community pharmacists are now working more closely with local GP practices and primary care organisations by participating in NHS minor ailment schemes. Roughly one quarter of the pharmacies in England provide this service. Nurses provide care in GP practice-based minor illness clinics, walk-in centres and other settings such as minor injuries units and A&E departments.

There is a great deal of scope for joint working in the area of OTC medicines. We suggest that pharmacists might consider the following steps:

• Agreeing guidelines for referral with local family doctors, perhaps including feedback from the GP to the pharmacist on the outcome of the referral. Two-way referrals with walk-in centres are also helpful.
• Using PMRs to keep information on OTC recommendations to patients.
• Keeping local family doctors and nurses informed about POM to P changes.
• Using referral forms when recommending that a patient see his or her doctor.
• Agreeing an OTC formulary with local GPs and practice nurses.
• Agreeing with local GPs the response to suspected adverse drug reactions.

Actions like these will help to improve communication, will increase GPs' and nurses' confidence in the contribution the pharmacist can make to patient care and will also support the pharmacist's integration into the primary care team.

Respiratory Problems

Colds and flu

The common cold comprises a mixture of viral upper respiratory tract infections (URTIs). Although colds are self-limiting, many people choose to buy over the counter (OTC) medicines for symptomatic relief. Some of the ingredients of OTC cold remedies may interact with prescribed therapy, occasionally with serious consequences. Therefore, careful attention needs to be given to taking a medication history and selecting an appropriate product.

What you need to know
Age (approximate)
Child, adult
Duration of symptoms
Runny/blocked nose
Summer cold
Sneezing/coughing
Generalised aches/headache
High temperature
Sore throat
Earache
Facial pain/frontal headache
Flu
Asthma
Previous history
Allergic rhinitis
Bronchitis
Heart disease
Present medication

Significance of questions and answers

Age

Establishing who the patient is – child or adult – will influence the pharmacist's decision about the necessity of referral to the doctor and

Symptoms in the Pharmacy: A Guide to the Management of Common Illness, Seventh Edition. Alison Blenkinsopp, Paul Paxton and John Blenkinsopp.
© 2014 John Wiley & Sons, Ltd. Published 2014 by John Wiley & Sons, Ltd.

choice of treatment. Children are more susceptible to URTI than are adults.

Duration

Patients may describe a rapid onset of symptoms or a gradual onset over several hours; the former is said to be more commonly true of flu, the latter of the common cold. Such guidelines are general rather than definitive. The symptoms of the common cold usually last for 7–14 days. Some symptoms, such as a cough, may persist after the worst of the cold is over.

Symptoms

Runny/blocked nose

Most patients will experience a runny nose (rhinorrhoea). This is initially a clear watery fluid, which is then followed by the production of thicker and more tenacious mucus (this may be purulent). Nasal congestion occurs because of dilatation of blood vessels, leading to swelling of the lining surfaces of the nose. This narrows the nasal passages that are further blocked by increased mucus production.

Summer colds

In summer colds, the main symptoms are nasal congestion, sneezing and irritant watery eyes; these are more likely to be due to allergic rhinitis (see p. 54).

Sneezing/coughing

Sneezing occurs because the nasal passages are irritated and congested. A cough may be present (see p. 197) either because the pharynx is irritated (producing a dry, tickly cough) or as a result of irritation of the bronchus caused by postnasal drip.

Aches and pains/headache

Headaches may be experienced because of inflammation and congestion of the nasal passages and sinuses. A persistent or worsening frontal headache (pain above or below the eyes) may be due to sinusitis (see below and p. 33). People with flu often report muscular and joint aches and this is more likely to occur with flu than with the common cold (see below).

High temperature

Those suffering from a cold often complain of feeling hot, but in general a high temperature will not be present. The presence of fever may be an indication that the patient has flu rather than a cold (see below).

Sore throat

The throat often feels dry and sore during a cold and may sometimes be the first sign that a cold is imminent (see p. 45).

Earache

Earache is a common complication of colds, especially in children. When nasal catarrh is present, the ear can feel blocked. This is due to blockage of the Eustachian tube, which is the tube connecting the middle ear to the back of the nasal cavity. Under normal circumstances, the middle ear is an air-containing compartment. However, if the Eustachian tube is blocked, the ear can no longer be cleared by swallowing and may feel uncomfortable and deaf. This situation often resolves spontaneously, but decongestants and inhalations can be helpful (see 'Management' below). Sometimes the situation worsens when the middle ear fills up with fluid. This is an ideal site for a secondary infection to settle. When this does occur, the ear becomes acutely painful and is called acute otitis media (AOM). AOM is a common infection in young children. The evidence for antibiotic use is conflicting with some trials showing benefit and others showing no benefit for taking antibiotics. In about 80% of children, AOM will resolve spontaneously in about 3 days without antibiotics. Antibiotics have also been shown to increase the risk of vomiting, diarrhoea and rash.

In summary, a painful ear can initially be managed by the pharmacist. There is evidence that both *paracetamol* and *ibuprofen* are effective treatments for AOM. However, if pain were to persist or be associated with an unwell child (e.g. high fever, very restless or listless, vomiting), then referral to the GP would be advisable.

Facial pain/frontal headache

Facial pain or frontal headache may signify sinusitis. Sinuses are air-containing spaces in the bony structures adjacent to the nose (maxillary sinuses) and above the eyes (frontal sinuses). In a cold, their lining surfaces become inflamed and swollen, producing catarrh. The secretions drain into the nasal cavity. If the drainage passage becomes blocked, fluid builds up in the sinus and can become secondarily (bacterially) infected. If this happens, persistent pain arises in the sinus areas. The maxillary sinuses are most commonly involved. A recent systematic review indicated only a small benefit from antibiotics even in sinusitis that had lasted for longer than 7 days infection. Antibiotics are, however, recommended if the symptoms of sinusitis: persist for more than 10 days; are severe with fever, facial pain, nasal discharge over 3–4 days; or when sinusitis symptoms develop following a recent cold which has started to settle.

Flu

Differentiating between colds and flu may be needed to make a decision about whether referral is needed. Patients in 'at-risk' groups might be considered for antiviral treatment. Flu is generally considered to be likely if:

- temperature is 38°C or higher (37.5°C in the elderly);
- a minimum of one respiratory symptom – cough, sore throat, nasal congestion or rhinorrhoea – is present; or
- a minimum of one constitutional symptom – headache, malaise, myalgia, sweats/chills, prostration – is present.

Flu often starts abruptly with sweats and chills, muscular aches and pains in the limbs, a dry sore throat, cough and high temperature. Someone with flu may be bedbound and unable to go about usual activities. There is often a period of generalised weakness and malaise following the worst of the symptoms. A dry cough may persist for some time.

True influenza is relatively uncommon compared to the large number of flu-like infections that occur. Influenza is generally more unpleasant, although both usually settle with no need for referral.

Flu can be complicated by secondary lung infection (pneumonia). Complications are much more likely to occur in the very young, the very old and those who have pre-existing heart disease, respiratory disease (asthma or chronic obstructive pulmonary disease (COPD)), kidney disease, a weak immune system or diabetes. Warning that complications are developing may be given by a severe or productive cough, persisting high fever, pleuritic-type chest pain (see p. 62) or delirium.

Asthma

Asthmatic attacks can be triggered by respiratory viral infections. Most asthma sufferers learn to start or increase their usual medication to prevent such an occurrence. However, if these measures fail, referral is recommended.

Previous history

People with a history of chronic bronchitis, also known as COPD may need referral. COPD should be considered in patients over the age of 35 who have a risk factor such as smoking, and who have shortness of breath on exercise, long-term cough, regular sputum production, and frequent winter 'bronchitis' or wheeze. Such patients may be advised to see their doctor if they have a bad cold or flu-like infection, as it often causes an exacerbation of their bronchitis. In this situation, the doctor is likely to increase the dose of inhaled anticholinergics and β-2 agonists and prescribe a course of antibiotics. Certain medications are best avoided in those with heart disease, hypertension and diabetes.

Present medication

The pharmacist must ascertain any medicines being taken by the patient. It is important to remember that interactions might occur with some of the constituents of commonly used OTC medicines.

If medication has already been tried for relief of cold symptoms with no improvement and if the remedies tried were appropriate and used for a sufficient amount of time, referral to the doctor might occasionally be needed. In most cases of colds and flu, however, OTC treatment will be appropriate.

When to refer

Earache not settling with analgesic (see above)

In the very young

In the very old

In those with heart or lung disease, for example, COPD, kidney disease, diabetes, compromised immune system

With persisting fever and productive cough

With delirium

With pleuritic-type chest pain

Asthma

Treatment timescale

Once the pharmacist has recommended treatment, patients should be advised to see their doctor in 10–14 days if the cold has not improved.

Management

The use of OTC medicines in the treatment of colds and flu is widespread, and such products are heavily advertised to the public. There is little doubt that appropriate symptomatic treatment can make the patient feel better; the placebo effect also plays an important part here. For some medicines used in the treatment of colds, particularly older medicines, there is little evidence available from which to judge effectiveness.

The pharmacist's role is to select appropriate treatment based on the patient's symptoms and available evidence, and taking into account the patient's preferences. Polypharmacy abounds in the area of cold treatments and patients should not be overtreated. The discussion of medicines that follows is based on individual constituents; the pharmacist can decide whether a combination of two or more drugs is needed.

The UK Commission on Human Medicines (CHM) made recommendations in 2009 about the safer use of cough and cold medicines for children under 12 years of age. As a result, the UK Medicines and Healthcare products and Regulatory Agency (MHRA) advised that OTC cough and cold remedies should no longer be sold for children under 6 years.

Antitussives: dextromethorphan and pholcodine

Expectorants: guaifenesin and ipecacuanha

Nasal decongestants: ephedrine, oxymetazoline, phenylephrine, pseudoephedrine and xylometazoline

Antihistamines: brompheniramine, chlorphenamine, diphenhy-dramine, doxylamine, promethazine and triprolidine

Children aged between 6–12 can still use these preparations, but with an advice to limit treatment to 5 days or less. The MHRA rationale was that for children aged over 6 years, 'the risk from these ingredients is reduced because: they suffer from cough and cold less frequently and consequently require medicines less often; with increased age and size, they tolerate the medicines better; and they can say if the medicine is working'.

Decongestants
Sympathomimetics

Sympathomimetics (e.g. *pseudoephedrine*) can be effective in reducing nasal congestion. Nasal decongestants work by constricting the dilated blood vessels in the nasal mucosa. The nasal membranes are effectively shrunk, so drainage of mucus and circulation of air are improved and the feeling of nasal stuffiness is relieved. These medicines can be given orally or applied topically. Tablets and syrups are available, as are nasal sprays and drops. If nasal sprays/drops are to be recommended, the pharmacist should advise the patient not to use the product for longer than 7 days. Rebound congestion (rhinitis medicamentosa) can occur with topically applied but not oral sympathomimetics. The decongestant effects of topical products containing *oxymetazoline* or *xylometazoline* are longer lasting (up to 6 h) than those of some other preparations such as *ephedrine*. The pharmacist can give useful advice about the correct way to administer nasal drops and sprays.

Problems

Ephedrine and pseudoephedrine, when taken orally, have the theo-retical potential to keep patients awake because of their stimulating effects on the central nervous system (CNS). In general, *ephedrine* is more likely to produce this effect than does *pseudoephedrine*. A sys-tematic review found that the risk of insomnia with *pseudoephedrine* was small compared with placebo.

Sympathomimetics can cause stimulation of the heart, an increase in blood pressure and may affect diabetic control because they can increase blood glucose levels. They should be used with caution (current *British National Formulary (BNF)* warnings) in people with diabetes, those with heart disease or hypertension and those with hyperthyroidism. The hearts of the hyperthyroid patients are more vulnerable to irregularity, so stimulation of the heart is particularly undesirable.

Sympathomimetics are most likely to cause these unwanted effects when taken by mouth and are unlikely to do so when used topically. Nasal drops and sprays containing sympathomimetics can therefore be recommended for those patients in whom the oral drugs are less suitable. Saline nasal drops or the use of inhalations would be other possible choices for patients in this group.

The interaction between sympathomimetics and monoamine oxidase inhibitors (MAOIs) is potentially extremely serious; a hypertensive crisis can be induced and several deaths have occurred in such cases. This interaction can occur up to 2 weeks after a patient has stopped taking the MAOI, so the pharmacist must establish any recently discontinued medication. There is a possibility that topically applied sympathomimetics could induce such a reaction in a patient taking an MAOI. It is therefore advisable to avoid both oral and topical sympathomimetics in patients taking MAOIs.

Cautions:
  diabetes
  heart disease
  hypertension
  hyperthyroidism

Interactions: Avoid in those taking
  MAOIs (e.g. *phenelzine*)
  reversible inhibitors of monoamine oxidase A (e.g. *moclobemide*)
  beta-blockers
  tricyclic antidepressants (e.g. *amitriptyline*) – a theoretical interaction that appears not to be a problem in practice

Restrictions on sales of pseudoephedrine and ephedrine
In response to concerns about the possible extraction of *pseudoephedrine* and *ephedrine* from OTC products for use in the manufacture of methamphetamine (crystal meth), restrictions were introduced in 2007. The medicines are available only in small pack sizes, with a limit of one pack per customer, and their sale has to be made by a pharmacist.

Antihistamines (see also p. 57)
Antihistamines could theoretically reduce some of the symptoms of a cold: runny nose (rhinorrhoea) and sneezing. These effects are due

to the anticholinergic action of antihistamines. The older drugs (e.g. *chlorphenamine (chlorpheniramine), promethazine*) have more pronounced anticholinergic actions than do the non-sedating antihistamines (e.g. *loratadine, cetirizine, acrivastine*). Antihistamines are not so effective at reducing nasal congestion. Some (e.g. *diphenhydramine*) may also be included in cold remedies for their supposed antitussive action (see p. 40) or to help the patient to sleep (included in combination products intended to be taken at night). Evidence indicates that antihistamines alone are not of benefit in the common cold but that they may offer limited benefit for adults in combination with decongestants, analgesics and cough suppressants.

Interactions: The problem of using antihistamines, particularly the older types (e.g. *chlorphenamine*), is that they can cause drowsiness. Alcohol will increase this effect, as will drugs such as *benzodiazepines* or *phenothiazines* that have the ability to cause drowsiness or CNS depression. Antihistamines with known sedative effects should not be recommended for anyone who is driving, or in whom an impaired level of consciousness may be dangerous (e.g. operators of machinery at work).

Because of their anticholinergic activity, the older antihistamines may produce the same adverse effects as anticholinergic drugs (i.e. dry mouth, blurred vision, constipation and urinary retention). These effects are more likely if antihistamines are given concurrently with anticholinergics such as *hyoscine* or with drugs that have anticholinergic actions such as tricyclic antidepressants.

Antihistamines should be avoided in patients with prostatic hypertrophy and closed-angle glaucoma because of possible anticholinergic side effects. In patients with closed-angle glaucoma, they may cause increased intraocular pressure. Anticholinergic drugs can occasionally precipitate acute urinary retention in pre-disposed patients, for example, men with prostatic hypertrophy.

While the probability of such serious adverse effects is low, the pharmacist should be aware of the origin of possible adverse effects from OTC medicines.

At high doses, antihistamines can produce stimulation rather than depression of the CNS. There have been occasional reports of fits being induced at very high doses of antihistamines and it is for this reason that it has been argued that they should be avoided in epileptic patients. However, this appears to be a theoretical rather than a practical problem.

Interactions:
Alcohol
Hypnotics

Sedatives
Betahistine
Anticholinergics

Side effects:
- Drowsiness (driving, occupational hazard)
- Constipation
- Blurred vision

Cautions:
Closed-angle glaucoma
Prostatic obstruction
Epilepsy
Liver disease

Zinc

Two systematic reviews have found limited evidence that *zinc gluconate* or *acetate lozenges* may reduce continuing symptoms at 7 days compared with placebo.

Echinacea

A systematic review of trials indicated that some echinacea preparations may be better than placebo or no treatment for the prevention and treatment of colds. However, due to variations in preparations containing echinacea, there is insufficient evidence to recommend a specific product. Echinacea has been reported to cause allergic reactions and rash.

Vitamin C

A systematic review found that high-dose vitamin C (over 1 g/day) taken prophylactically reduced the duration of colds by about 8%.

Cough remedies

For discussion of products for the treatment of cough, see p. 38.

Analgesics

For details of analgesics, their uses and side effects, see p. 199.

Products for sore throats

For discussion of products for the treatment of sore throat, see p. 45.

Practical points
Inhalations

These may be useful in reducing nasal congestion and soothing the air passages, particularly if a productive cough is present. Inhalants that can be used on handkerchiefs, bedclothes and pillowcases are available. These usually contain aromatic ingredients such as eucalyptus. Such products can be useful in providing some relief, but are not as effective as steam-based inhalations in moistening the airways.

Nasal sprays or drops?

Nasal sprays are preferable for adults and children over 6 years because the small droplets in the spray mist reach a large surface area. Drops are more easily swallowed, which increases the possibility of systemic effects.

For children under 6 years, drops are preferred because in young children the nostrils are not sufficiently wide to allow the effective use of sprays. Paediatric versions of nasal drops should be used where appropriate. Nasal saline drops or sprays are a useful option to consider in nasal congestion in babies and young children.

Prevention of flu

Pharmacists should encourage those in at-risk groups to have an annual flu vaccination. In the United Kingdom, the health service now provides vaccinations to all patients over 65 years and those below that age who have chronic respiratory disease (including asthma), chronic heart disease, chronic renal failure, diabetes mellitus or immunosuppression due to disease or treatment. Community pharmacists are in a good position to use their patient medication records (PMRs) to target patients each autumn and remind them to have their vaccination.

A nasal spray containing a viscous gel is marketed with claims that it prevents progression of the first signs of a cold into a full-blown infection. It is used four times a day from the time symptoms are experienced. The theoretical basis for its action is that the gel is slightly acidic (whereas viruses are said to prefer an alkaline environment) and that its viscous nature traps the viruses. There are no published trials of effectiveness.

Increasing attention is being paid to ways of reducing transmission of the influenza virus. Routine handwashing with soap and water reduces the transmission of cold and flu viruses. Hand sanitizers have become widely used because immediate access to soap and water is difficult in many everyday settings. Transfer of the cold or flu virus usually occurs directly from person to person when an infected individual coughs or sneezes. Droplets of respiratory secretions come into contact with the mucous membranes of the mouth and nose of another person. Ethanol-based hand sanitizers are widely used in health care settings and can contribute to reducing transmission of colds and flu. The influenza virus is susceptible to alcohol in formulations of 60–95% ethanol. The rationale is that the virus in droplets can survive for 24–48 h on hard, non-porous surfaces, for 8–12 h on cloth, paper and tissue, and for

5 min on hands. Touching contaminated hands, surfaces and objects can therefore transfer the virus.

Flu pandemic

There have been three flu pandemics over the last century, occurring in 1918, 1957 and 1968. Concerns about a potential pandemic have arisen because of the emerging strains of influenza from animals or birds (zoonoses). In 1997, an avian H5N1 strain of influenza emerged, which has a high mortality rate. Although the virus is highly virulent, it does not spread easily between humans. Nearly all, if not all, cases have been spread from contact between humans and infected birds. The concern is that the virus may mutate, making transmission between humans more likely. As there is no natural immunity to this virus, a pandemic could follow, and if the virulence remained unchanged then it could be extremely deadly. It is not possible to predict how likely this scenario is. Another H1N1 influenza virus spread from pigs in 2009. Further information available from the World Health Organization (WHO) at www.who.int

The Department of Health has issued various publications detailing the evidence base for dealing with a pandemic, specifically making recommendations on vaccination, use of antivirals and antibiotics as well as the use of face masks. Anyone who is ill with influenza-type symptoms will be advised to stay at home. Further advice can be found at http://www.dh.gov.uk

Antivirals

The effectiveness of antivirals during a pandemic cannot be known until used in such a situation and can only be guessed at based on experience in seasonal influenza and in those infected with avian flu. It is believed that they are likely to reduce the chance of developing complications, reduce the chance of dying and shorten the time taken to recover from an infection. It is possible that using antivirals for the non-infected members of a household when another member has the infection could reduce the spread of the pandemic. There is uncertainty as to how much resistance to antivirals could be present in a pandemic virus.

Three antiviral products are licensed for use: *oseltamivir, zanamivir* and *amantadine.* Only the *oseltamivir* and *zanamivir* neuraminidase inhibitors are recommended by the UK Department of Health and WHO for use in a pandemic. The UK National Institute for Health and Care Excellence (NICE) does not have recommendations for a pandemic but supports the use of neuraminidase inhibitors for those who are in at-risk groups in seasonal flu outbreaks, if treatment is started within 48 h of symptom onset. *Amantadine* is generally not recommended because of its lower efficacy, side effects, and because rapid resistance can develop to its use.

Surgical face masks

The Department of Health and WHO have looked at the evidence concerning the use of surgical face masks in a flu pandemic. Their recommendations are that the general public can use them but are not encouraged to do so. There is insufficient evidence to support their use. They are, however, recommended in health-care settings, and they may be of value in infected households both for the symptomatic person and non-infected members and carers, and for symptomatic people outside the home. There is concern that the masks may not be used safely; that is, they may be worn too long and get too wet and therefore ineffective, be worn at times around the neck, not disposed of correctly, and there may be a failure to wash hands after touching the mask. There is also concern that symptomatic people wearing masks continue to meet with people outside the home when it would be best to be isolated at home.

Antibiotics

A serious complication of flu is the development of pneumonia and this can be either directly due to the flu virus or due to a secondary bacterial infection. In the case of a viral pneumonia, antibiotics are of no value although clinically it is difficult to tell the difference, and antibiotics are usually given in a hospital setting with a severe illness. Avian flu outbreaks have been mainly complicated by viral pneumonia.

Most uncomplicated infections in the community do not require antibiotics. They are now recommended for those at risk, such as people who have pre-existing COPD, compromised immunity, diabetes, heart or lung disease. In these situations, if there is no improvement within 48 h of starting antibiotics, then the person should be seen by the GP.

Typical flu symptoms include cough, retrosternal discomfort, wheeze and phlegm (symptoms of acute bronchitis), and by themselves do not require antibiotics in a person who is not at risk. However, if these symptoms worsen with a persistent or recrudescent (recurring) fever, pleuritic-type chest pain or breathlessness, then a pneumonia might be developing. In this situation, review by a GP would be essential and either treatment with antibiotics in the community or hospital admission could follow.

Colds and flu in practice

Case 1

Mrs Allen, a regular customer in her late 60s, asks what you can recommend for her husband. He has a very bad cold; the worst symptoms are his blocked nose and sore throat. Although his throat feels sore, she tells you there is only a slight reddening (she looked this morning). He has had the symptoms since last night and is not feverish. He does not have earache but has complained of a headache. When you ask her if he is taking any medicines, she says yes, quite a few for his heart. She cannot remember what they are called. You check the PMR and find that he is taking *aspirin* 75 mg daily, *ramipril* 5 mg daily, *bisoprolol* 10 mg daily and *simvastatin* 40 mg daily. Mrs Allen asks you if it is worth her husband taking extra vitamin C as she has heard this is good for colds. She wondered if this might be better than taking yet more medicines.

The pharmacist's view

The patient's symptoms indicate a cold rather than flu. He is concerned most with his congested nose and sore throat. He is taking a number of medications, which indicate that oral sympathomimetics would be best avoided. You could recommend that he take regular simple painkillers for his sore throat and a topical decongestant or an inhalation to clear his blocked nose. The symptoms may take about 1 week before they start to clear. You offer these alternatives to Mrs Allen to see what she thinks her husband might prefer. You explain that taking vitamin C might reduce the time taken for the cold to get better by about half a day. You show her some vitamin C products and tell her their cost. You also ask if Mr Allen has had a flu jab as he is in an 'at-risk' group.

The doctor's view

The advice given by the pharmacist is sensible. A simple analgesic such as *paracetamol* could help both the headache and sore throat. The development of sinusitis at such an early stage in an infection would be unlikely but it would be wise to enquire whether his colds are usually uncomplicated and to ascertain the site of his headache.

The patient's view

I came to the pharmacist because we didn't want to bother the doctor. The pharmacist asked me about which symptoms were causing Pete (my husband) the biggest problem and he gave me a choice of what to use. I wanted to know what he thought about vitamin C and he told me about how it might make the cold shorter. In the end though I decided not to bother with it because it would have been quite expensive with the other medicines as well, especially as it was unlikely to make that much difference. I thought I would give him some fresh orange juice instead.

Case 2

A man comes into the pharmacy just after Xmas asking for some cough medicine for his wife. He says that the medicine needs to be sugar-free as his wife has diabetes. On listening to him further, he says she has had a dreadful cough that keeps her awake at night. Her problem came on 5 days ago when she woke in the morning, complaining of being very achy all over and then became shivery, and developed a high temperature and cough by the evening. Since then her temperature has gone up and down and she has not been well enough to get out of bed for very long. She takes *glipizide* and *metformin* for her diabetes and he has been checking her glucometer readings, which have all been between 8 and 11 – a little higher than usual. The only other treatment she is taking is *atorvastatin*; she is not on any antihypertensives. He tells you that she will be 70 next year.

The pharmacist's view

The history indicates flu. It would be best for this woman to be seen by her GP. She has been ill for 5 days and has been mostly bedbound during this time. There are several features that suggest she might be at higher risk from flu. I would suggest that her husband call the doctor out to see her, as she does not sound well enough to go to the surgery. Sometimes people are reluctant to call the doctor as they feel they might be 'bothering' the doctor unnecessarily. The pharmacist's support is often helpful.

The doctor's view

The infection is likely to be flu. She is in the higher-risk group for developing complications (age and diabetes), so it would be reasonable to advise referral. Most cases of flu usually resolve within 7 days. The complications can include AOM, bacterial sinusitis, bacterial pneumonia and, less commonly, viral pneumonia and respiratory failure. Worldwide there are about 3–5 million severe cases of flu in seasonal outbreaks resulting in between 250 000 and 500 000 deaths per year, most of the deaths occurring over 65s (WHO, 2009, www.who.int).

In this situation, the doctor would want to check her chest for signs of a secondary infection. A persisting or worsening fever would point to a complication developing. There would be little point in prescribing an antiviral, for example, *zanamivir*, as it is only effective if started within 2 days of symptom onset. One review has found it to be effective in reducing the duration of flu symptoms by about 1 day if started soon enough. It would also be advisable to check whether or not her husband had had the flu vaccine. The incubation time for flu is 1–4 days and adults are contagious from the day before symptoms start until 5 days after the onset of symptoms.

Cough

Coughing is a protective reflex action caused when the airway is being irritated or obstructed. Its purpose is to clear the airway so that breathing can continue normally. The majority of coughs presenting in the pharmacy will be caused by a viral URTI. They will often be associated with other symptoms of a cold. The evidence to support the use of cough suppressants and expectorants is not strong but some patients report finding them helpful.

What you need to know
Age (approximate)
Baby, child, adult
Duration
Nature
Dry or productive
Associated symptoms
Cold, sore throat, fever
Sputum production
Chest pain
Shortness of breath
Wheeze
Previous history
COPD (chronic bronchitis, emphysema, chronic obstructive airways disease)
Asthma
Diabetes
Heart disease
Gastro-oesophageal reflux
Smoking habit
Present medication

Significance of questions and answers

Age

Establishing who the patient is – child or adult – will influence the choice of treatment and whether referral is necessary.

Symptoms in the Pharmacy: A Guide to the Management of Common Illness, Seventh Edition.
Alison Blenkinsopp, Paul Paxton and John Blenkinsopp.
© 2014 John Wiley & Sons, Ltd. Published 2014 by John Wiley & Sons, Ltd.

Duration

Most coughs are self-limiting and will be better within a few days with or without treatment. In general, a cough of longer than 2 weeks' duration that is not improving should be referred to the doctor for further investigation.

Patients are often concerned when a cough has lasted for, what seems to them to be, a long time. They may be worried that because the cough has not resolved, it may have a serious cause.

Nature of cough

Unproductive (dry, tickly or tight)

In an unproductive cough, no sputum is produced. These coughs are usually caused by viral infection and are self-limiting.

Productive (chesty or loose)

Sputum is normally produced. It is an oversecretion of sputum that leads to coughing. Oversecretion may be caused by irritation of the airways due to infection, allergy, etc., or when the cilia are not working properly (e.g. in smokers). Non-coloured (clear or whitish) sputum is uninfected and known as mucoid.

Coloured sputum may sometimes indicate a bacterial chest infection such as bronchitis or pneumonia and require referral. In these situations, the sputum is described as green, yellow or rust-coloured thick mucus and the patient is more unwell perhaps with a raised temperature, shivers and sweats. Sometimes blood may be present in the sputum (haemoptysis), with a colour ranging from pink to deep red. Blood may be an indication of a relatively minor problem such as a burst capillary following a bout of violent coughing during an acute infection, but may be a warning of more serious problems. Haemoptysis is an indication for referral.

Antibacterials/antibiotics are not usually indicated for previously healthy people with acute bronchitis. Most cases of acute bronchitis are caused by viral infections, so antibacterials will not help. Two systematic reviews of antibacterials for acute bronchitis found only slight benefit, possibly reducing the duration of illness by about half a day. Some people who have a tendency towards asthma develop a wheezy bronchitis with a respiratory viral infection. They may benefit from inhalation treatment used in asthma.

If a person has had repeated episodes of bronchitis over the years, they might have COPD (defined as a chronic cough, sputum, shortness of breath on exertion, wheeze, with a risk factor such as smoking when other causes of chronic cough have been excluded). So careful questioning is important to determine this.

There is general consensus that antibacterials should be considered if the person is elderly, has reduced resistance to infection, has comorbidity (such as diabetes or heart failure) or is deteriorating clinically.

In heart failure and mitral stenosis, the sputum is sometimes described as pink and frothy or can be bright red. Confirming symptoms would be breathlessness (especially in bed during the night) and swollen ankles.

Tuberculosis

Until recently thought of as a disease of the past, the number of tuberculosis (TB) cases has been rising in the United Kingdom and there is increasing concern about resistant strains. Chronic cough with haemoptysis associated with chronic fever and night sweats are classical symptoms. TB is largely a disease of poverty and more likely to present in disadvantaged communities. In the United Kingdom, most cases of respiratory TB are seen in ethnic minority groups, especially Indians and Africans. Human immunodeficiency virus (HIV) infection is a significant risk factor for the development of respiratory TB.

Croup (acute laryngotracheitis)

Croup usually occurs in infants. The cough has a harsh barking quality. It develops 1 day or so after the onset of cold-like symptoms. It is often associated with difficulty in breathing and an inspiratory stridor (noise in throat on breathing in). Referral is necessary.

Whooping cough (pertussis)

Whooping cough starts with catarrhal symptoms. The characteristic whoop is not present in the early stages of infection. The whoop is the sound produced when breathing in after a paroxysm of coughing. The bouts of coughing prevent normal breathing and the whoop represents the desperate attempt to get a breath. Referral is necessary.

Associated symptoms

Cold, sore throat and catarrh may be associated with a cough. Often there may be a temperature and generalised muscular aches present. This would be in keeping with a viral infection and be self-limiting. Chest pain, shortness of breath or wheezing are all indications for referral (see p. 62).

Postnasal drip

Postnasal drip is a common cause of coughing and may be due to sinusitis (see p. 21).

Previous history

Certain cough remedies are best avoided in diabetics and anyone with heart disease or hypertension (see p. 40).

Chronic bronchitis

Questioning may reveal a history of chronic bronchitis, which is being treated by the doctor with antibiotics. In this situation, further treatment may be possible with an appropriate cough medicine.

Asthma

A recurrent night-time cough can indicate asthma, especially in children, and should be referred. Asthma may sometimes present as a chronic cough without wheezing. A family history of eczema, hay fever and asthma is worth asking about. Patients with such a family history appear to be more prone to extended episodes of coughing following a simple URTI.

Cardiovascular

Coughing can be a symptom of heart failure (see p. 65). If there is a history of heart disease, especially with a persisting cough, then referral is advisable.

Gastro-oesophageal

Gastro-oesophageal reflux can cause coughing. Sometimes such reflux is asymptomatic apart from coughing. Some patients are aware of acid coming up into their throat at night when they are in bed.

Smoking habit

Smoking will exacerbate a cough and can cause coughing since it is irritating to the lungs. One in three long-term smokers develop a chronic cough. If coughing is recurrent and persistent, the pharmacist is in a good position to offer health education advice about the benefits of stopping smoking, suggesting nicotine replacement therapy where appropriate. However, on stopping, the cough may initially become worse as the cleaning action of the cilia is re-established during the first few days and it is worth mentioning this. Smokers may assume their cough is harmless, and it is always important to ask about any change in the nature of the cough that might suggest a serious cause (see also 'Smoking cessation' in the chapter on 'Prevention of Heart Disease').

Present medication

It is always essential to establish which medicines are currently being taken. This includes those prescribed by a doctor and any bought OTC, borrowed from a friend or neighbour or rediscovered in the family medicine chest. It is important to remember the possibility of interactions with cough medicine.

It is also useful to know which cough medicines have been tried already. The pharmacist may decide that an inappropriate preparation has been taken, for example, a cough suppressant for a productive cough. If one or more appropriate remedies have been tried for an appropriate length of time without success, then referral is advisable.

Angiotensin-converting enzyme inhibitors

Chronic coughing may occur in patients, particularly women, taking angiotensin-converting enzyme (ACE) inhibitors such as *enalapril, captopril, lisinopril* and *ramipril*. Patients may develop the cough within days of starting treatment or after a period of a few weeks or even months. The exact incidence of the reaction is not known and estimates vary from 2% to 10% of patients taking ACE inhibitors. ACE inhibitors control the breakdown of bradykinin and other kinins in the lungs, which can trigger a cough. Typically the cough is irritating, non-productive and persistent. Any ACE inhibitor may induce coughing and there seems to be little advantage to be gained in changing from one to another. The cough may resolve or may persist; in some patients, the cough is so troublesome and distressing that ACE inhibitor therapy may have to be discontinued. Any patients in whom medication is suspected as the cause of a cough should be referred to their doctor. Angiotensin-2 receptor antagonists, which have similar properties to ACE inhibitors and which do not affect bradykinin, can be used as an alternative preparation if cough is a problem.

When to refer

Cough lasting 2 weeks or more and not improving
Sputum (yellow, green, rusty or bloodstained)
Chest pain
Shortness of breath
Wheezing
Whooping cough or croup
Recurrent nocturnal cough
Suspected adverse drug reaction
Failed medication

After a series of questions, the pharmacist should be in a position to decide whether treatment or referral is the best option.

Treatment timescale

Depending on the length of time the patient has had the cough and once the pharmacist has recommended an appropriate treatment, patients should see their doctor 2 weeks after the cough started if it has not improved.

Management

Pharmacists are well aware of the debate about the clinical efficacy of the cough remedies available OTC. A systematic review concluded that 'there is no good evidence for or against the effectiveness of OTC medicines in acute cough'. However, many people who visit the pharmacy for advice do so because they want some relief from their symptoms and, while the clinical effectiveness of cough remedies is debatable, they can have a useful placebo effect.

The choice of treatment depends on the type of cough. Suppressants (e.g. *pholcodine*) are used to treat unproductive coughs, while expectorants such as *guaifenesin* (*guaiphenesin*) are used in the treatment of productive coughs. The pharmacist should check that the preparation contains an appropriate dose, since some products contain subtherapeutic amounts. Demulcents like *Simple Linctus* that soothe the throat are particularly useful in children and pregnant women as they contain no active ingredients.

The *BNF* gives the following guidance:

Expectorants are claimed to promote expulsion of bronchial secretions, but there is no evidence that any drug can specifically facilitate expectoration.
Suppressants: Where there is no identifiable cause (underlying disorder), cough suppressants may be useful; for example, if sleep is disturbed.
Demulcents: Preparations such as *Simple Linctus* have the advantage of being harmless and inexpensive. Paediatric *Simple Linctus* is particularly useful in children.

Compound preparations are on sale to the public for the treatment of cough and colds but should not be used in children under 6 years of age; the rationale for some is dubious. Care should be taken to give the correct dose and to not use more than one preparation at a time.

Productive coughs should not be treated with cough suppressants because pooling and retention of mucus in the lungs can result leading to a higher chance of infection, especially in chronic bronchitis.

There is no logic in using expectorants (which promote coughing) and suppressants (which reduce coughing) together as they have opposing effects. Therefore, products that contain both are not therapeutically sound. The UK CHM made recommendations in 2009 about safer use of cough and cold medicines for children aged under 12 (see p. 23).

Cough suppressants

Controlled trials have not confirmed any significant effect of cough suppressants over placebo on symptom reduction.

Codeine/pholcodine

Pholcodine has several advantages over *codeine* in that it produces fewer side effects (even at OTC doses *codeine* can cause constipation and, at high doses, respiratory depression) and *pholcodine* is less liable to be abused. Both *pholcodine* and *codeine* can induce drowsiness, although in practice this does not appear to be a problem. Nevertheless, it is sensible to give an appropriate warning. *Codeine* is well known as a drug of abuse and many pharmacists choose not to recommend it. Sales often have to be refused because of knowledge or likelihood of abuse. The MHRA/CHM advise that codeine-containing cough suppressants should not be used for children under 18. *Pholcodine* can be given at a dose of 5 mg to children over 6 years (5 mg of *pholcodine* is contained in 5 mL of *Pholcodine Linctus BP*). Adults may take doses of up to 15 mg three or four times daily. The drug has a long half-life and may be more appropriately given as a twice-daily dose.

Dextromethorphan

Dextromethorphan is less potent than *pholcodine* and *codeine*. It is generally non-sedating and has few side effects. Occasionally, drowsiness had been reported but, as for *pholcodine,* this does not seem to be a problem in practice. *Dextromethorphan* can be given to children of 6 years and over. *Dextromethorphan* was generally thought to have a low potential for abuse. However, there have been rare reports of mania following abuse and consumption of very large quantities, and pharmacists should be aware of this possibility if regular purchases are made.

Demulcents

Preparations such as *glycerine, lemon* and *honey* or *Simple Linctus* are popular remedies and are useful for their soothing effect. They do not contain any active ingredient and are considered to be safe in children and pregnant women. They are now the treatment recommended for children under 6.

Expectorants

Two mechanisms have been proposed for expectorants. They may act directly by stimulating bronchial mucus secretion, leading to increased liquefying of sputum, making it easier to cough up. Alternatively, they may act indirectly via irritation of the gastrointestinal tract, which has a subsequent action on the respiratory system, resulting in increased mucus secretion. This latter theory has less convincing evidence than the former to support it.

Guaifenesin (guaiphenesin)

Guaifenesin is commonly found in cough remedies. In adults, the dose required to produce expectoration is 100–200 mg, so in order to have a theoretical chance of effectiveness, any product recommended should contain a sufficiently high dose. Some OTC preparations contain sub-therapeutic doses. In the United States of America, the FDA (the licensing body) reviewed OTC medicines, and evidence from studies supporting *guaifenesin* was sufficiently strong for the FDA to be convinced of its efficacy.

Cough remedies: other constituents
Antihistamines

Examples used in OTC products include *diphenhydramine* and *promethazine*. Theoretically, these reduce the frequency of coughing and have a drying effect on secretions, but in practice they also induce drowsiness. Combinations of antihistamines with expectorants are illogical and best avoided. A combination of an antihistamine and a cough suppressant may be useful in that antihistamines can help to dry up secretions and the combination can be given as a night-time dose if the cough is disturbing sleep. This is one of the rare occasions when a side effect proves useful. The non-sedating antihistamines are less effective in symptomatic treatment of coughs and colds because of their less pronounced anticholinergic actions.

Interactions: Traditional antihistamines should not be used by patients who are taking *phenothiazines* and tricyclic antidepressants because of additive anticholinergic and sedative effects. Increased sedation will also occur with any drug that has a CNS depressant effect. Alcohol should be avoided because this will also lead to increased drowsiness. See pp. 57–58 for more details of interactions, side effects and contraindications of antihistamines.

Sympathomimetics

Pseudoephedrine is used in cough and cold remedies (see also p. 24 and p. 25 for information on restrictions on sales) for its bronchodilatory and decongestant actions. It has a stimulant effect that may theoretically lead to a sleepless night if taken close to bedtime. It may be useful if the patient has a blocked nose as well as a cough and an expectorant/decongestant combination can be useful in productive coughs. Sympathomimetics can cause raised blood pressure, stimulation of the heart and alterations in diabetic control. Oral sympathomimetics should be used with caution in patients with the following.

Diabetes
Coronary heart disease (e.g. angina)
Hypertension
Hyperthyroidism

Interactions: Avoid in those taking
monoamine oxidase inhibitors (e.g. *phenelzine*)
reversible inhibitors of monoamine oxidase A (e.g. *moclobemide*)
beta-blockers
tricyclic antidepressants (e.g. *amitriptyline*) – a theoretical interaction that appears not to be a problem in practice

Theophylline
Theophylline is sometimes included in cough remedies for its bronchodilator effect. OTC medicines containing *theophylline* should not be taken at the same time as prescribed *theophylline* since toxic blood levels and side effects may occur. The action of *theophylline* can be potentiated by some drugs, for example, *cimetidine* and *erythromycin*.

Levels of *theophylline* in the blood are reduced by smoking and drugs such as *carbamazepine, phenytoin* and *rifampicin* that induce liver enzymes, so the metabolism of *theophylline* is increased and lower serum levels result.

Side effects include gastrointestinal irritation, nausea, palpitations, insomnia and headaches. The adult dose is typically 120 mg, three or four times daily. It is not recommended in children.

Practical points
Diabetes
In short-term acute conditions, the amount of sugar in cough medicines is relatively unimportant. Diabetic control is often upset during infections and the additional sugar is now not considered to be a major problem. Nevertheless, many diabetic patients may prefer a sugar-free product, as will many other customers who wish to reduce sugar intake for themselves and their children, and many such products are now available. As part of their contribution to improving dental health, pharmacists can ensure that they stock and display a range of sugar-free medicines.

Steam inhalations
These can be useful, particularly in productive coughs. A systematic review found that there was insufficient evidence to judge whether

there might be a benefit from this treatment. The steam helps to liquefy lung secretions and patients find the warm moist air comforting. While there is no evidence that the addition of medications to water produces a better clinical effect than steam alone, some may prefer to add a preparation such as *menthol* and *eucalyptus* or a proprietary inhalant. One teaspoonful of inhalant should be added to a pint of hot (not boiling) water and the steam inhaled. Apart from the risk of scalding, boiling water volatilises the constituents too quickly. A cloth or towel can be put over the head to trap the steam.

Fluid intake

Maintaining a high fluid intake helps to hydrate the lungs, and hot drinks can have a soothing effect. General advice to patients with coughs and colds should be to increase fluid intake.

Coughs in practice

Case 1

Mrs Patel, a woman in her early 20s, asks what you can recommend for her son's cough. On questioning, you find out that her son, Dillip, aged 4 years, has had a cough on and off for a few weeks. He gets it at night and it is disturbing his sleep, although he does not seem to be troubled during the day. She took Dillip to the doctor about 3 weeks ago, and the doctor explained that antibiotics were not needed and that the cough would get better by itself. The cough is not productive and she has given Dillip some *Simple Linctus* before he goes to bed but the cough is no better. Dillip is not taking any other medicines. He has no pain on breathing or shortness of breath. He has had a cold recently.

The pharmacist's view

This is a 4-year-old child who has a night-time cough of several weeks' duration. The doctor's advice was appropriate at the time Dillip saw him. However, referral to the doctor would be advisable because the cough is only present during the night. A recurrent cough in a child at night can be a symptom of asthma, even if wheezing is not present. It is possible that the cough is occurring as a result of bronchial irritation following his recent viral URTI. Such a cough can last for up to 6 weeks and is more likely to occur in those who have asthma or a family history of atopy (a pre-disposition to sensitivity to certain common allergens such as house dust mite, animal dander and pollen). Nevertheless, the cough has been present for several weeks without improvement and medical advice is needed.

The doctor's view

Asthma is an obvious possibility. It would be interesting to know if anyone else in the family suffers from asthma, hay fever or eczema, and whether Dillip has ever had hay fever or eczema. Any of these features would make the diagnosis more likely. Mild asthma may present in this way without the usual symptoms of shortness of breath and wheezing.

An alternative diagnosis could still include a viral URTI. Most coughs are more troublesome and certainly more obvious during the night. This can falsely give the impression that the cough is only nocturnal. It should also be remembered that both diagnoses could be correct, as a viral infection often initiates an asthmatic reaction. Because the diagnosis is uncertain and inhaled oral steroids may be appropriate, referral to the doctor is advisable.

If, after further history taking and examination, the doctor feels that asthma is a possibility, then the treatment would be based on the British Thoracic Society guidelines that are summarised in the *BNF*. Naturally this would only be carried out after full discussion and agreement with the parents. Many parents are loath to have their child labelled as an asthma sufferer. The next problem is to prescribe a suitable inhalation device for a 4-year-old child. This may be an inhaler with a spacer device or a breath-actuated inhaler or a dry-powder inhaler. It would be usual to try a twice-daily dosage for 2–3 weeks and then review for future management.

The parent's view

I was hoping the pharmacist could recommend something but she seemed to think Dillip should see the doctor. She didn't really explain why though.

Case 2

A man aged about 25 years asks if you can recommend something for his cough. He sounds as if he has a bad cold and looks a bit pale. You find out that he has had the cough for a few days, with a blocked nose and a sore throat. He has no pain on breathing or shortness of breath. The cough was chesty to begin with, but he tells you it is now tickly and irritating. He has not tried any medicines and is not taking any medicines from the doctor.

The pharmacist's view

This patient has the symptoms of the common cold and none of the danger signs associated with a cough that would make referral necessary. He is not taking any medicines, so the choice of possible treatments is wide. You could recommend something to treat his congested nose as well as his cough, for example, a cough suppressant and a sympathomimetic. *Simple Linctus* and a systemic or topical decongestant would also be a possible option. If a topical decongestant were to be recommended, he should be warned to use it for no longer than 1 week to avoid the possibility of rebound congestion.

The doctor's view

The action suggested by the pharmacist is very reasonable. It may be worthwhile explaining that he is suffering from a viral infection that is self-limiting and should be better within a few days. If he is a smoker then it would be an ideal time to encourage him to stop.

Sore throat

Most people with a sore throat do not consult the doctor – only about 5% do so and many will consult their pharmacist. Most sore throats that present in the pharmacy will be caused by viral infection (90%), with only 1 in 10 being due to bacterial infection, so treatment with antibiotics is unnecessary in most cases. Clinically it is almost impossible to differentiate between the two. The majority of infections are self-limiting. Sore throats are often associated with other symptoms of a cold.

Once the pharmacist has excluded more serious conditions, an appropriate OTC medicine can be recommended.

What you need to know

Age (approximate)
  Baby, child, adult
Duration
Severity
Associated symptoms
  Cold, congested nose, cough
  Difficulty in swallowing
  Hoarseness
  Fever
Previous history
  Smoking habit
Present medication

Significance of questions and answers

Age

Establishing who the patient is will influence the choice of treatment and whether referral is necessary. Streptococcal (bacterial) throat infections are more likely in children of school age.

Symptoms in the Pharmacy: A Guide to the Management of Common Illness, Seventh Edition. Alison Blenkinsopp, Paul Paxton and John Blenkinsopp.
© 2014 John Wiley & Sons, Ltd. Published 2014 by John Wiley & Sons, Ltd.

Duration

Most sore throats are self-limiting and will be better within 7–10 days. If it has been present for longer, then the patient should be referred to the doctor for further advice.

Severity

If the sore throat is described as being extremely painful, especially in the absence of cold, cough and catarrhal symptoms, then referral should be recommended when there is no improvement within 24–48 h.

Associated symptoms

Cold, catarrh and cough may be associated with a sore throat. There may also be a fever and general aches and pains. These are in keeping with a minor self-limiting viral infection.

Both hoarseness of longer than 3 weeks' duration and difficulty in swallowing (dysphagia) are indications for referral.

Previous history

Recurrent bouts of infection (tonsillitis) would mean that referral is best.

Smoking habit

Smoking will exacerbate a sore throat, and if the patient smokes then it can be a good time to offer advice and information about quitting. Surveys indicate that two-thirds of people who smoke want to stop (see also 'Smoking cessation' in the chapter on 'Prevention of Heart Disease').

Present medication

The pharmacist should establish whether any medication has been tried already to treat the symptoms. If one or more medicines have been tried without improvement, then referral to the doctor should be considered.

Current prescriptions are important and the pharmacist should question the patient carefully about them. Steroid inhalers (e.g. *beclometasone* or *budesonide*) can cause hoarseness and candidal infections of the throat and mouth. Generally, they tend to do this at high doses. Such infections can be prevented by rinsing the mouth with water after using the inhaler. It is also worthwhile checking the patient's inhaler technique. Poor technique with metered-dose inhalers can lead to large amounts of the inhaled drug being deposited at the back of the throat. If you suspect this is the problem, discuss with the doctor whether a device that will help coordination or perhaps a different inhaler might be needed.

Any patient taking *carbimazole* and presenting with a sore throat should be referred immediately. A rare side effect of *carbimazole* is agranulocytosis (suppression of white cell production in the bone marrow). The same principle applies to any drug that can cause agranulocytosis. A sore throat in such patients can be the first sign of a life-threatening infection.

Symptoms for direct referral

Hoarseness

Hoarseness is caused when there is inflammation of the vocal cords in the larynx (laryngitis). Laryngitis is typically caused by a self-limiting viral infection. It is usually associated with a sore throat and a hoarse, diminished voice. Antibiotics are of no value and symptomatic advice (see 'Management' below), which includes resting the voice, should be given. The infection usually settles within a few days and referral is not necessary.

When this infection occurs in babies, infants or small children, it can cause croup (acute laryngotracheitis) and present difficulty in breathing and stridor (see p. 35). In this situation, referral is essential.

When hoarseness persists for more than 3 weeks, especially when it is not associated with an acute infection, referral is necessary. There are many causes of persistent hoarseness, some of which are serious. For example, laryngeal cancer can present in this way and hoarseness may be the only early symptom. A doctor will normally refer the patient to an ear, nose and throat (ENT) specialist for accurate diagnosis.

Dysphagia

Difficulty in swallowing can occur in severe throat infection. It can happen when an abscess develops in the region of the tonsils (quinsy) as a complication of tonsillitis. This will usually result in a hospital admission where an operation to drain the abscess may be necessary and high-dose parenteral antibiotics may be given.

Glandular fever (infectious mononucleosis) is one viral cause of sore throat that often produces marked discomfort and may cause dysphagia. If this is suspected, referral is necessary for an accurate diagnosis.

Most bad sore throats will cause discomfort on swallowing, but not true difficulty and do not necessarily need referral unless there are other reasons for concern. Dysphagia, when not associated with a sore throat, always needs referral (see p. 77).

Appearance of throat

It is commonly thought that the presence of white spots, exudates or pus on the tonsils is an indication for referral or a means of differentiating between viral and bacterial infection, but this is not always so. Unfortunately, the appearance can be the same in both types of infection and sometimes the throat can appear almost normal without exudates in a streptococcal (bacterial) infection.

Thrush

An exception not to be forgotten is candidal (thrush) infection that produces white plaques. However, these are rarely confined to the throat alone and are most commonly seen in babies or the very elderly. It is an unusual infection in young adults and may be associated with more serious disorders that interfere with the body's immune system, for example, leukaemia, HIV and acquired immune deficiency syndrome (AIDS), or with immunosuppressive therapy (e.g. steroids). The plaques may be seen in the throat and on the gums and tongue. When they are scraped off, the surface is raw and inflamed. Referral is advised if thrush is suspected and the throat is sore and painful. See p. 199 for more information about oral thrush.

Glandular fever

Glandular fever is a viral throat infection caused by the Epstein–Barr virus. It is well known because of its tendency to leave its victims debilitated for some months afterwards and its association with the controversial condition myalgic encephalomyelitis. The infection typically occurs in teenagers and young adults, with peak incidence between the ages of 14 and 21 years. It is known as the 'kissing disease'. A severe sore throat may follow 1 or 2 weeks of general malaise. The throat may become very inflamed with creamy exudates present. There may be difficulty in swallowing because of the painful throat. Glands (lymph nodes) in the neck and axillae (armpits) may be enlarged and tender. The diagnosis can be confirmed with a blood test, although this may not become positive until 1 week after the onset of the illness. Antibiotics are of no value; in fact if *ampicillin* is given during the infection, a measles-type rash is likely to develop in 80% of those with glandular fever. Treatment is aimed at symptomatic relief.

When to refer
Sore throat lasting 1 week or more
Recurrent bouts of infection
Hoarseness of more than 3 weeks' duration
Difficulty in swallowing (dysphagia)
Failed medication

Treatment timescale

Patients should see their doctor after 1 week if the sore throat has not improved.

Management

Most sore throats are caused by viral infections and are self-limiting in nature, with 90% of patients becoming well within 1 week of the onset of symptoms. The pharmacist can offer a selection of treatments aimed at providing some relief from discomfort and pain until the infection subsides. Oral analgesics are first-line treatment. A systematic review found that simple analgesics *(paracetamol, aspirin* and *ibuprofen)* are very effective at reducing the pain from sore throat. Lozenges and pastilles have a soothing effect. There is some evidence that *benzydamine spray* is effective in relieving sore throat pain.

Oral analgesics

Paracetamol, aspirin and *ibuprofen* have been shown in clinical trials to provide rapid and effective relief of pain in sore throat. A systematic review showed no benefit of adding other analgesic constituents. The patient can be advised to take the analgesic regularly to sustain pain relief. (For a discussion of doses, side effects, cautions and contraindications for simple analgesics, see p. 199.) *Flurbiprofen lozenges* are licensed for sore throat in adults and children aged 12 years and over. They contain 8.75 mg of *flurbiprofen,* and one lozenge is sucked or dissolved in the mouth every 3–6 h as required, to a maximum of five lozenges. *Flurbiprofen lozenges* can be used for up to 3 days at a time.

Mouthwashes and sprays

Anti-inflammatory (e.g. benzydamine)

Benzydamine is an anti-inflammatory agent that is absorbed through the skin and mucosa and has been shown to be effective in reducing pain and inflammation in conditions of the mouth and throat. Side effects have occasionally been reported and include numbness and stinging of the mouth and throat. *Benzydamine spray* can be used in children of 6 years and over, whereas the mouthwash may only be recommended for children over 12 years of age.

Local anaesthetic (e.g. benzocaine)

Benzocaine and *lidocaine* are available in throat sprays.

Lozenges and pastilles

Lozenges and pastilles can be divided into three categories.

Antiseptic (e.g. *cetylpyridinium*)
Antifungal (e.g. *dequalinium*)
Local anaesthetic (e.g. *benzocaine*)

Lozenges and pastilles are commonly used OTC treatments for sore throats, and where viral infection is the cause, the main use of antibacterial and antifungal preparations is to soothe and moisten the throat. Lozenges containing *cetylpyridinium chloride* have been shown to have antibacterial action.

Local anaesthetic lozenges will numb the tongue and throat and can help to ease soreness and pain. *Benzocaine* can cause sensitisation and such reactions have sometimes been reported.

Caution: Iodised throat lozenges should be avoided in pregnancy because they have the potential to affect the thyroid gland of the fetus.

Practical points
Diabetes

Mouthwashes and gargles are suitable and can be recommended. Sugar-free pastilles are available but the sugar content of such products is not considered important in short-term use.

Mouthwashes and gargles

Patients should be reminded that mouthwashes and gargles should not be swallowed. The potential toxicity of OTC products of this type is low and it is unlikely that problems would result from swallowing small amounts. However, there is a small risk of systemic toxicity from swallowing products containing *iodine*. Manufacturers' recommendations about whether to use the mouthwash diluted or undiluted should be checked and appropriate advice should be given to the patient.

Sore throats in practice

Case 1

A woman asks your advice about her son's very sore throat. He is 15 years old and is at home in bed. She says he has a temperature and that she can see creamy white matter at the back of his throat. He seems lethargic and has not been eating very well because his throat has been so painful. The sore throat started about 5 days ago and he has been in bed since yesterday. The glands on his neck are swollen.

The pharmacist's view

It would be best for this woman's son to be seen by the doctor. The symptoms appear to be severe and he is ill enough to be in bed.

Glandular fever is common in this age group and is a possibility. In the meantime, you might consider recommending some *paracetamol* in soluble or syrup form to make it easier to swallow. The analgesic and antipyretic effects would both be useful in this case.

The doctor's view

The pharmacist is sensible in recommending referral. The description suggests a severe tonsillitis, which will be caused by either a bacterial or viral infection. If it turns out to be viral, then glandular fever is a strong possibility. The doctor should check out the ideas, concerns and expectations of the mother and son and then explain the likely causes and treatment. Often it is not possible to rule out a bacterial (strepto-coccal) infection at this stage and it is safest to prescribe oral *penicillin*, or *erythromycin* if the patient is allergic to *penicillin*. Depending on the availability of laboratory services, the doctor may take a throat swab, which would identify a bacterial infection. If the infection has gone on for nearly 1 week, then a blood test can identify infectious mononucleosis (glandular fever). Although there is no specific treatment for glandular fever, it is helpful for the patient to know what is going on and when to expect full recovery.

Case 2

A teenage girl comes into your shop with her mother. The girl has a sore throat which started yesterday. There is slight reddening of the throat. Her mother tells you she had a slight temperature during the night. She also has a blocked nose and has been feeling general aching. She has no difficulty in swallowing and is not taking any medicines, either prescribed or OTC.

The pharmacist's view

It sounds as though this girl has a minor URTI. The symptoms described should remit within a few days. In the meantime, it would be reasonable to recommend a systemic analgesic, perhaps in combination with a decongestant.

The doctor's view

The pharmacist's assessment sounds correct. Because she has a blocked nose, a viral infection is most likely. Many patients attend their doctor with similar symptoms understandably hoping for a quick cure with antibiotics that have no place in such infections.

Case 3

A middle-aged woman comes to ask your advice about her husband's bad throat. He has had a hoarse gruff voice for about 1 month and has tried various lozenges and pastilles without success. He has been a heavy smoker (at least a pack a day) for over 20 years and works as a bus driver.

The pharmacist's view

This woman should be advised that her husband should see his doctor. The symptoms that have been described are not those of a minor throat infection. On the basis of the long duration of the problem and of the unsuccessful use of several OTC treatments, it would be best for this man to see his doctor for further investigation.

The doctor's view

A persistent alteration in voice, with hoarseness, is an indication for referral to an ENT specialist. This man should have his vocal cords examined, which requires skill and special equipment that most family doctors do not have. It is possible he may have a cancer on his vocal cords (larynx), especially as he is a smoker.

Allergic rhinitis (hay fever)

Seasonal allergic rhinitis (hay fever) affects 10–15% of people in the United Kingdom, and millions of patients rely on OTC medicines for treatment. The symptoms of allergic rhinitis occur after an inflammatory response involving the release of histamine, which is initiated by allergens being deposited on the nasal mucosa. Allergens responsible for seasonal allergic rhinitis include grass pollens, tree pollens and fungal mould spores. Perennial allergic rhinitis occurs when symptoms are present all year round and is commonly caused by the house dust mite, animal dander and feathers. Some patients may suffer from perennial rhinitis, which becomes worse in the summer months.

What you need to know
Age (approximate)
Baby, child, adult
Duration
Symptoms
Rhinorrhoea (runny nose)
Nasal congestion
Nasal itching
Watery eyes
Irritant eyes
Discharge from the eyes
Sneezing
Previous history
Associated conditions
Eczema
Asthma
Medication

Significance of questions and answers

Age

Symptoms of allergic rhinitis may start at any age, although its onset is more common in children and young adults (the condition is most

Symptoms in the Pharmacy: A Guide to the Management of Common Illness, Seventh Edition.
Alison Blenkinsopp, Paul Paxton and John Blenkinsopp.
© 2014 John Wiley & Sons, Ltd. Published 2014 by John Wiley & Sons, Ltd.

common in those in their 20s and 30s). There is frequently a family history of atopy in allergic rhinitis sufferers. Thus, children of allergic rhinitis sufferers are more likely to have the condition. The condition often improves or resolves as the child gets older. The age of the patient must be taken into account if any medication is to be recommended. Young adults who may be taking examinations should be borne in mind, because treatment that may cause drowsiness is best avoided in these patients.

Duration

Sufferers will often present with seasonal rhinitis as soon as the pollen count becomes high. Symptoms may start in April when tree pollens appear and the hay fever season may start 1 month earlier in the south than in the north of England. Hay fever peaks between the months of May and July, when grass pollen levels are highest and spells of good weather commonly cause patients to seek the pharmacist's advice. Anyone presenting with a summer cold, perhaps of several weeks' duration, may be suffering from hay fever. Fungal spores are also a cause and are present slightly later, often until September.

People can suffer from what they think are mild cold symptoms for a long period, without knowing they have perennial rhinitis.

Allergic rhinitis can be classified as:

Intermittent. Occurs less than 4 days/week or for less than 4 weeks

Persistent. Occurs more than 4 days/week and for more than 4 weeks

Mild. All of the following – normal sleep, normal daily activities, sport, leisure, normal work and school, symptoms not troublesome

Moderate. One or more of the following – abnormal sleep; impairment of daily activities, sport, leisure, problems caused at work or school, troublesome symptoms

Symptoms

Rhinorrhoea

A runny nose is a commonly experienced symptom of allergic rhinitis. The discharge is often thin, clear and watery, but can change to a thicker, coloured, purulent one. This suggests a secondary infection, although the treatment for allergic rhinitis is not altered. There is no need for antibiotic treatment.

Nasal congestion

The inflammatory response caused by the allergen produces vasodilation of the nasal blood vessels and so results in nasal congestion. Severe congestion may result in headache and occasionally earache. Secondary infection such as otitis media and sinusitis can occur (see p. 21).

Nasal itching

Nasal itching commonly occurs. Irritation is sometimes experienced on the roof of the mouth.

Eye symptoms

The eyes may be itchy and also watery; it is thought these symptoms are a result of tear duct congestion and also a direct effect of pollen grains being caught in the eye, setting off a local inflammatory response. Irritation of the nose by pollen probably contributes to eye symptoms too. People who suffer severe symptoms of allergic rhinitis may be hypersensitive to bright light (photophobic) and find that wearing dark glasses is helpful.

Sneezing

In hay fever, the allergic response usually starts with symptoms of sneezing, then rhinorrhoea, progressing to nasal congestion. Classically, symptoms of hay fever are more severe in the morning and in the evening. This is because pollen rises during the day after being released in the morning and then settles at night. Patients may also describe a worsening of the condition on windy days as pollen is scattered, and a reduction in symptoms when it rains, or after rain, as the pollen clears. Conversely, in those allergic to fungal mould spores, the symptoms worsen in damp weather.

Previous history

There is commonly a history of hay fever going back over several years. However, it can occur at any age, so the absence of any previous history does not necessarily indicate that allergic rhinitis is not the problem. The incidence of hay fever has risen during the last decade. Pollution, particularly in urban areas, is thought to be at least partly responsible for the trend.

Perennial rhinitis can usually be distinguished from seasonal rhinitis by questioning about the timing and the occurrence of symptoms. People who have had hay fever before will often consult the pharmacist when symptoms are exacerbated in the summer months.

Danger symptoms/associated conditions

When associated symptoms such as tightness of the chest, wheezing, shortness of breath or coughing are present, immediate referral is advised. These symptoms may herald the onset of an asthmatic attack.

Wheezing

Difficulty with breathing, possibly with a cough, suggests an asthmatic attack. Some sufferers experience asthma attacks only during the hay fever season (seasonal asthma). These episodes can be quite severe and require referral. Seasonal asthmatics often do not have appropriate medication at hand as their attacks occur so infrequently, which puts them at greater risk.

Earache and facial pain

As with colds and flu (see p. 21), allergic rhinitis can be complicated by secondary bacterial infection in the middle ear (otitis media) or the sinuses (sinusitis). Both these conditions cause persisting severe pain.

Purulent conjunctivitis

Irritated watery eyes are a common accompaniment to allergic rhinitis. Occasionally, this allergic conjunctivitis is complicated by a secondary infection. When this occurs, the eyes become more painful (gritty sensation) and redder, and the discharge changes from being clear and watery to coloured and sticky (purulent). A referral is needed.

Medication

The pharmacist must establish whether any prescription or OTC medicines are being taken by the patient. Potential interactions between prescribed medication and antihistamines can therefore be identified.

It would be useful to know if any medicines have been tried already to treat the symptoms, especially where there is a previous history of allergic rhinitis. In particular, the pharmacist should be aware of the potentiation of drowsiness by some antihistamines combined with other medicines. This can lead to increased danger in certain occupations and driving.

Failed medication

If symptoms are not adequately controlled with OTC preparations, an appointment with the doctor may be worthwhile. Such an appointment is useful to explore the patient's beliefs and pre-conceptions about hay fever and its management. It is also an opportunity to suggest ideas for the next season.

When to refer
Wheezing and shortness of breath
Tightness of chest
Painful ear
Painful sinuses
Purulent conjunctivitis
Failed medication

Treatment timescale

Improvement in symptoms should occur within a few days. If no improvement is noted after 5 days, the patient might be referred to the doctor for other therapy.

Management

Management is based on whether symptoms are intermittent or persistent and mild or moderate. Options include antihistamines, nasal steroids and *sodium cromoglicate* (*sodium cromoglycate*) in formulations for the nose and eyes. OTC antihistamines and steroid nasal sprays are effective in the treatment of allergic rhinitis. The choice of treatment should be rational and based on the patient's symptoms and previous history where relevant.

Many cases of hay fever can be managed with OTC treatment and it is reasonable for the pharmacist to recommend treatment. Patients with symptoms that do not respond to OTC products can be referred to the doctor at a later stage. Pharmacists also have an important role in ensuring that patients know how to use any prescribed medicines correctly (e.g. steroid nasal sprays, which must be used continuously for the patient to benefit).

Antihistamines

Many pharmacists would consider these drugs to be the first-line treatment for mild-to-moderate and intermittent symptoms of allergic rhinitis. They are effective in reducing sneezing and rhinorrhoea, less so in reducing nasal congestion. Non-sedating antihistamines available OTC include *acrivastine, cetirizine* and *loratadine*. All are effective in reducing the troublesome symptoms of hay fever and have the advantage of causing less sedation than some of the older antihistamines.

Cetirizine and *loratadine* are taken once daily, while *acrivastine* is taken three times daily. For sale OTC loratadine can be recommended for children over 2 years, cetirizine over 6 years and acrivastine over 12 years.

While drowsiness is an unlikely side effect of any of the three drugs, patients might be well advised to try the treatment for a day before driving or operating machinery. *Loratadine* may be less likely to have any sedative effect than the other two, but the incidence of drowsiness is extremely small.

Acrivastine, cetirizine and *loratadine* may be used for other allergic skin disorders such as perennial rhinitis and urticaria.

Older antihistamines such as *promethazine* and *diphenhydramine* have a greater tendency to produce sedative effects. Indeed, both drugs are available in the United Kingdom among OTC products promoted for the management of temporary sleep disorders (see p. 329). The shorter half-life of *diphenhydramine* (5–8 h compared with 8–12 h of *promethazine*) should mean less likelihood of a morning hangover/drowsiness effect.

Other older antihistamines are relatively less sedative, such as *chlorphenamine* (*chlorpheniramine*). Patients may develop tolerance to their sedation effects. Anticholinergic activity is very much lower among the newer drugs compared to the older drugs.

Interactions: The potential sedative effects of older antihistamines are increased by alcohol, hypnotics, sedatives and anxiolytics. The alcohol content of some OTC medicines should be remembered.

The plasma concentration of non-sedating antihistamines may be increased by *ritonavir;* plasma concentration of *loratadine* may be increased by *amprenavir* and *cimetidine.* There is a theoretical possibility that antihistamines can antagonise the effects of *betahistine.*

Side effects: The major side effect of the older antihistamines is their potential to cause drowsiness. Their anticholinergic activity may result in a dry mouth, blurred vision, constipation and urinary retention. These effects will be increased if the patient is already taking another drug with anticholinergic effects (e.g. tricyclic antidepressants, neuroleptics).

At very high doses, antihistamines have CNS excitatory effects rather than depressive effects. Such effects seem to be more likely to occur in children. At toxic levels, there have been reports of fits being induced. As a result, it has been suggested that antihistamines should be used with care in epileptic patients. However, this appears to be a largely theoretical risk.

Antihistamines are best avoided by patients with narrow- (closed-) angle glaucoma, since the anticholinergic effects produced can cause an increase in intraocular pressure. They should be used with caution in patients with liver disease or prostatic hypertrophy.

Decongestants

Oral or topical decongestants may be used short term to reduce nasal congestion alone or in combination with an antihistamine. They can be useful in patients starting to use a preventer such as a nasal corticosteroid (e.g. *beclometasone*) or *sodium cromoglicate* where congestion can prevent the drug from reaching the nasal mucosa. Topical decongestants can cause rebound congestion, especially with prolonged use. They should not be used for more than 1 week. Oral decongestants are occasionally included such as *pseudoephedrine.* Their use, interactions and adverse effects are considered in the section on 'Colds and flu' (see pp. 24–25).

Eye drops containing an antihistamine and sympathomimetic combination are available and may be of value in troublesome eye symptoms, particularly when symptoms are intermittent. The sympathomimetic acts as a vasoconstrictor, reducing irritation and redness. Some patients find that the vasoconstrictor causes painful stinging when first applied. Eye drops that contain a vasoconstrictor should not be used in patients who have glaucoma or who wear soft contact lenses.

Steroid nasal sprays

Beclometasone nasal spray (aqueous pump rather than aerosol version) and *fluticasone metered nasal spray* can be used for the treatment of seasonal allergic rhinitis.

A steroid nasal spray is the treatment of choice for moderate–to-severe nasal symptoms that are continuous. The steroid acts to reduce inflammation that has occurred as a result of the allergen's action. Regular use is essential for full benefit to be obtained and treatment should be continued throughout the hay fever season. If symptoms of hay fever are already present, the patient needs to know that it is likely to take several days before the full treatment effect is reached.

Dryness and irritation of the nose and throat as well as nose-bleeds have occasionally been reported; otherwise side effects are rare. *Beclometasone* and *fluticasone nasal sprays* can be used in patients over 18 years of age for up to 3 months. They should not be recommended for pregnant women or for anyone with glaucoma.

Patients are sometimes alarmed by the term 'steroid', associating it with potent oral steroids and possible side effects. Therefore, the pharmacist needs to take account of these concerns in explanations about the drug and how it works.

Sodium cromoglicate

Sodium cromoglicate is available OTC as nasal drops or sprays and as eye drops. *Cromoglicate* can be effective as a prophylactic if used correctly. It should be started at least 1 week before the hay fever season is likely to begin and then used continuously. There seem to be no significant side effects, although nasal irritation may occasionally occur.

Cromoglicate eye drops are effective for the treatment of eye symptoms that are not controlled by antihistamines. *Cromoglicate* should be used continuously to obtain full benefit. The eye drops should be used four times a day. The eye drops contain the preservative *benzalkonium chloride* and should not be used by wearers of soft contact lenses.

Topical antihistamines
Nasal treatments

Azelastine is a nasal spray used in allergic rhinitis. The *BNF* suggests that treatment should begin 2–3 weeks before the start of the hay fever season. Its place in treatment is likely to be for mild and intermittent symptoms in adults and children over 5 years. Advise the patient to keep the head upright during use to prevent the liquid trickling into the throat and causing an unpleasant taste.

Further advice

1 Car windows and air vents should be kept closed while driving. Otherwise a high pollen concentration inside the car can result.

2 Where house dust mite is identified as a problem, regular cleaning of the house to maintain dust levels at a minimum can help. Special vacuum cleaners are now on sale that are claimed to be particularly effective.

Hay fever in practice

Case 1

A young man presents in late May. He asks what you can recommend for hay fever. On questioning, he tells you that he has not had hay fever before, but some of his friends got it and he thinks he has the same thing. His eyes have been itching a little and are slightly watery, and he has been sneezing for a few days. His nose has been runny and now feels quite blocked. He will not be driving. But he is a student at the local sixth-form college and has exams coming up next week. He is not taking any medicines.

The pharmacist's view

This young man is experiencing the classic symptoms of hay fever for the first time. The nasal symptoms are causing the most discomfort; he has had rhinorrhoea and now has congestion, so it would be reasonable to recommend a corticosteroid nasal spray, provided he is aged 18 years or over. If he is under 18 years, an oral or topical antihistamine could be recommended, bearing in mind that he is sitting for exams soon and so any preparation that might cause drowsiness is best avoided. His eyes are slightly irritated, but the symptoms are not very troublesome. You know that he is not taking any other medicines, so you could recommend *acrivastine, loratadine* or *cetirizine*. If the symptoms are not better in a few days, he should see the doctor.

The doctor's view

A corticosteroid nasal spray is likely to be more effective. If he cannot use the OTC product because he is under 18 years, *acrivastine, loratadine* or *cetirizine* would be worth a try. Even though they are generally non-sedating, they can cause drowsiness in some patients. The student should be advised not to take his first dose just before the exam. If his symptoms do not settle, then referral is appropriate. He may benefit from *sodium cromoglicate eye drops* if his eye symptoms are not fully controlled by the antihistamine. It is often worthwhile trying an older antihistamine as an alternative because some people are unaffected by the sedative properties.

Case 2

A woman in her early thirties wants some advice. She tells you that she has hay fever and a blocked nose and is finding it difficult to breathe. You find out that she has had the symptoms for a few days; they have gradually got worse. She gets hay fever every summer and it is usually controlled by *chlorphenamine* tablets that she buys every year and which she is taking at the moment. As a child, she suffered quite badly from eczema and is still troubled by it occasionally. She tells you that she has been a little wheezy for the past day or so, but she does not have a cough, and has not coughed up any sputum. She is not taking any other medicines.

The pharmacist's view

This woman has a previous history of hay fever, which has, until now, been dealt adequately with *chlorphenamine* tablets. Her symptoms have worsened over a period of a few days and she is now wheezing. It seems unlikely that she has a chest infection, which could have been a possible cause of the symptoms. She should be referred to the doctor at once since her symptoms suggest more serious implications such as asthma.

The doctor's view

This woman should be referred to her doctor directly. She almost certainly has seasonal asthma. In addition to the hay fever treatment recommended by her pharmacist, it is likely that she would benefit from a steroid inhaler such as *beclometasone*. Depending on the severity of her symptoms, she would probably be prescribed a beta-agonist, such as a *salbutamol inhaler*, as well. This consultation is a complex one for a doctor to manage in the usual 10 min available in view of the time required for information-giving, explanation about the nature of the problem, the rationale for the treatments and the technique of using inhalers.

Respiratory symptoms for direct referral

Chest pain

Respiratory causes

A knifelike pain is characteristic of pleurisy. It is a localised pain which is aggravated by taking a breath or coughing. It is usually caused by a respiratory infection and may be associated with an underlying pneumonia. Less commonly, it may be caused by a pulmonary embolus (a blood clot which has lodged in a pulmonary artery after separating from a clot elsewhere in the circulation).

A pain similar to that experienced with pleurisy may arise from straining the muscles between the ribs following coughing. It may also occur with cracked or fractured ribs following injury or violent coughing. Another less common cause of pain is due to a pneumothorax where a small leak develops in the lung causing its collapse.

The upper front part of the chest may be very sore in the early stages of acute viral infections that cause inflammation of the trachea (tracheitis). Viral flu-like infections can be associated with non-specific muscular pain (myalgia).

Non-respiratory causes

Heartburn

Heartburn occurs when the acid contents of the stomach leak backwards into the oesophagus (gullet). The pain is described as a burning sensation, which spreads upwards towards the throat. Occasionally, it can be so severe as to mimic cardiac pain.

Cardiac pain

Cardiac pain typically presents as a tight, gripping, vicelike, dull pain that is felt centrally across the front of the chest. The pain may seem to move down one or both arms. Sometimes the pain spreads to the neck. When angina is present, the pain is brought on by exercise and relieved by rest. When a coronary event such as a heart attack (myocardial infarction) occurs, the pain is similar but more severe and prolonged. It may come on at rest.

Symptoms in the Pharmacy: A Guide to the Management of Common Illness, Seventh Edition. Alison Blenkinsopp, Paul Paxton and John Blenkinsopp.
© 2014 John Wiley & Sons, Ltd. Published 2014 by John Wiley & Sons, Ltd.

Anxiety

Anxiety is a commonly seen cause of chest pain in general practice. The pain probably arises as a result of hyperventilation. Diagnosis can be difficult as the hyperventilation may not be obvious.

Shortness of breath

Shortness of breath may be a symptom of a cardiac or respiratory disorder. Differential diagnosis can be difficult. It is usually a sign of a serious condition, although it can be due to anxiety.

Respiratory causes

Asthma

Occasionally, asthma may develop in later life, but it is most commonly seen in young children or young adults. The breathlessness is typically associated with a wheeze, although in mild cases the only symptom may be a recurrent nocturnal cough. Most asthmatics have normal breathing between attacks. The attacks are often precipitated by viral infections such as colds. Some are worsened in the hay fever season, others by animal fur or dust. The breathlessness is often worse at night.

Chronic bronchitis and emphysema (COPD)

Chronic bronchitis and emphysema are usually caused by cigarette smoking and give rise to permanent breathlessness, especially on exertion, with a productive cough. The breathing worsens when an infective episode develops. At such times there is also an increase in coloured sputum production.

Cardiac causes

Heart failure

Heart failure may develop gradually or present acutely as an emergency (usually in the middle of the night). The former (congestive cardiac failure) may cause breathlessness on exertion. It is often associated with ankle swelling (oedema) and is most common in the elderly. The more sudden type is called acute left ventricular failure. The victim is woken by severe breathlessness and has to sit upright. There is often a cough present with clear frothy sputum.

Other causes

Hyperventilation syndrome

Hyperventilation syndrome occurs when the rate of breathing is too high for the bodily requirements. Paradoxically, the subjective experience is that of breathlessness. The sufferer complains of difficulty in taking in a deep breath. The experience is frightening but harmless. It may be associated with other symptoms such as tingling in the hands and feet, numbness around the mouth, dizziness and various muscular aches. It may be caused by anxiety.

Wheezing

Wheezing sounds may be heard in the throat region in URTIs and are of little consequence. They are to be differentiated from wheezing emanating from the lungs. In this latter situation, there is usually some difficulty in breathing.

Wheezy bronchitis

Wheezing occurs in infants with wheezy bronchitis. It is caused by a viral infection and is completely different from chronic bronchitis seen in adults. The infection is self-limiting but requires accurate diagnosis. It may be confused with croup (laryngotracheitis) or bronchiolitis. Children who have a history of recurrent wheezy bronchitis are more likely to develop asthma.

Asthma

Wheezing is a common feature of asthma and accompanies the shortness of breath. However, in very mild asthma it is not obvious and may present with just a cough. At the other extreme, an asthma attack can be so severe that so little air moves in and out of the lungs, there is no audible wheeze.

Cardiac

Wheezing may be a symptom associated with shortness of breath in heart failure.

Sputum

Sputum may be described as thick or thin and clear or coloured. It is a substance coughed up from the lungs and is not to be confused with saliva or nasal secretions.

Bronchitis

Clear, thick sputum may be coughed up in chronic bronchitis or by regular cigarette smokers. It has a mucoid nature and may be described as white, grey or clear with black particles. Chronic bronchitics are prone to recurrent infective exacerbations during which sputum production increases and turns yellow or green.

Pneumonia

Coloured mucoid sputum may be present in other lung infections such as pneumonia. Rust-coloured sputum is a characteristic of pneumococcal (lobar) pneumonia. Usually it is associated with a high fever and sweats.

Cardiac

Clear, thin (serous) sputum may be a feature of heart failure (left ventricular failure). The sputum forms as a result of pulmonary oedema, which characteristically awakens the patient in the night with shortness of breath.

Haemoptysis

The presence of blood in sputum is always alarming. Small traces of blood can result from a broken capillary caused by coughing and is harmless. However, it can be a symptom of serious disease such as lung cancer or pulmonary TB, and should always be referred for further investigation. Occasionally, blood is coughed up after a nosebleed and is of no consequence.

Gastrointestinal Tract Problems

Mouth ulcers

Mouth ulcers are extremely common, affecting as many as one in five of the population, and are a recurrent problem in some people. They are classified as aphthous (minor or major) or herpetiform ulcers. Most cases (more than three-quarters) are minor aphthous ulcers, which are self-limiting. Ulcers may be due to a variety of causes including infection, trauma and drug allergy. However, occasionally mouth ulcers appear as a symptom of serious disease such as carcinoma. The pharmacist should be aware of the signs and characteristics that indicate more serious conditions.

What you need to know

Age
  Child, adult
Nature of the ulcers
  Size, appearance, location, number
Duration
Previous history
Other symptoms
Medication

Significance of questions and answers

Age

Patients may describe a history of recurrent ulceration, which began in childhood and has continued ever since. Minor aphthous ulcers are more common in women and occur most often between the ages of 10 and 40 years.

Nature of the ulcers

Minor aphthous ulcers usually occur in crops of one to five. The lesions may be up to 5 mm in diameter and appear as a white or yellowish centre with an inflamed red outer edge. Common sites are the tongue margin and inside the lips and cheeks. The ulcers tend to last from 5 to 14 days.

Symptoms in the Pharmacy: A Guide to the Management of Common Illness, Seventh Edition. Alison Blenkinsopp, Paul Paxton and John Blenkinsopp.
© 2014 John Wiley & Sons, Ltd. Published 2014 by John Wiley & Sons, Ltd.

Table 1 The three main types of aphthous ulcers.

Minor	Major	Herpetiform
80% of patients	10–12% of patients	8–10% of patients
2–10 mm in diameter (usually 5–6 mm)	Usually over 10 mm in diameter; may be smaller	Pinhead-sized
Round or oval	Round or oval	Round or oval, coalesce to form irregular shape as they enlarge
Usually not very painful	Prolonged and painful ulceration; may present patient with great problems – eating may become difficult	May be very painful

Other types of recurrent mouth ulcers include major aphthous and herpetiform. Major aphthous ulcers are uncommon, severe variants of the minor ones. The ulcers which may be as large as 30 mm in diameter can occur in crops of up to 10. Sites involved are the lips, cheeks, tongue, pharynx and palate. They are more common in sufferers of ulcerative colitis.

Herpetiform ulcers are more numerous, smaller and, in addition to the sites involved with aphthous ulcers, may affect the floor of the mouth and the gums. Table 1 summarises the features of the three main types of aphthous ulcers.

Systemic conditions such as Behçet's syndrome and erythema multiforme may produce mouth ulcers, but other symptoms would generally be present (see below).

Duration
Minor aphthous ulcers usually heal in less than 1 week; major aphthous ulcers take longer (10–30 days). Where herpetiform ulcers occur, fresh crops of ulcers tend to appear before the original crop has healed, which may lead patients to think that the ulceration is continuous.

Oral cancer
Any mouth ulcer that has persisted for longer than 3 weeks requires immediate referral to the dentist or doctor because an ulcer of such long duration may indicate serious pathology, such as carcinoma. Most oral cancers are squamous cell carcinomas, of which one in three affects the lip and one in four affects the tongue. The development of a cancer may be preceded by a premalignant lesion, including erythroplasia (red) and leucoplakia (white) or a speckled leucoplakia. Squamous cell carcinoma may present as a single ulcer with a raised and indurated (firm or hardened) border. Common locations include the lateral border

of the tongue, lips, floor of the mouth and gingiva. The key point to raise suspicion would be a lesion that had lasted for several weeks or longer. Oral cancer is more common in smokers than non-smokers.

Previous history
There is often a family history of mouth ulcers (estimated to be present in one in three cases). Minor aphthous ulcers often recur, with the same characteristic features of size, numbers, appearance and duration before healing. The appearance of these ulcers may follow trauma to the inside of the mouth or tongue, such as biting the inside of the cheek while chewing food. Episodes of ulceration generally recur after 1–4 months.

Ill-fitting dentures may produce ulceration and, if this is a suspected cause, the patient should be referred back to the dentist so that the dentures can be refitted. However, trauma is not always a feature of the history, and the cause of minor aphthous ulcers remains unclear despite extensive investigation.

In women, minor aphthous ulcers often precede the start of the menstrual period. The occurrence of ulcers may cease after pregnancy, suggesting hormonal involvement. Stress and emotional factors at work or home may precipitate a recurrence or a delay in healing but do not seem to be causative.

Deficiency of iron, folate, zinc or vitamin B_{12} may be a contributory factor in aphthous ulcers and may also lead to glossitis (a condition where the tongue becomes sore, red and smooth) and angular stomatitis (where the corners of the mouth become sore, cracked and red).

Food allergy is occasionally the causative factor and it is worth enquiring whether the appearance of ulcers is associated with particular foods.

Other symptoms
The severe pain associated with major aphthous or herpetiform ulcers may mean that the patient finds it difficult to eat and, as a consequence, weight loss may occur. Weight loss would therefore be an indication for referral.

In most cases of recurrent mouth ulcers, the disease eventually burns itself out over a period of several years. Occasionally, as in Behçet's syndrome, there is progression with involvement of sites other than the mouth. Most commonly, the vulva, vagina and eyes are affected, with genital ulceration and iritis (see p. 283).

Behçet's syndrome can be confused with erythema multiforme, although in the latter there is usually a distinctive rash present on the skin. Erythema multiforme is sometimes precipitated by an infection or drugs (sulphonamides being the most common).

Mouth ulcers may be associated with inflammatory bowel disorders or with coeliac disease. Therefore, if persistent or recurrent diarrhoea is present, referral is essential. Patients reporting any of these symptoms should be referred to their doctor.

Rarely, ulcers may be associated with disorders of the blood including anaemia, abnormally low white cell count or leukaemia. It would be expected that in these situations there would be other signs of illness present and the sufferer would present directly to the doctor.

Medication

The pharmacist should establish the identity of any current medication, since mouth ulcers may be produced as a side effect of drug therapy. Drugs that have been reported to cause the problem include *aspirin* and other non-steroidal anti-inflammatory drugs (NSAIDs), cytotoxic drugs, *nicorandil, beta blockers* and *sulphasalazine* (sulfasalazine). Radiotherapy may also induce mouth ulcers. It is worth asking about herbal medicines because *feverfew* (used for migraine) can cause mouth ulcers.

It would also be useful to ask the patient about any treatments tried either previously or on this occasion and the degree of relief obtained. The pharmacist can then recommend an alternative product where appropriate.

When to refer
Duration of longer than 3 weeks
Associated weight loss
Involvement of other mucous membranes
Rash
Suspected adverse drug reaction
Diarrhoea

Treatment timescale

If there is no improvement after 1 week, the patient should see the doctor.

Management

Symptomatic treatment of minor aphthous ulcers can be recommended by the pharmacist and can relieve pain and reduce healing time. Active ingredients include antiseptics, corticosteroids and local anaesthetics. There is evidence from clinical trials to support use of topical corticosteroids and *chlorhexidine mouthwash*. Gels and liquids may be more accurately applied using a cotton bud or cotton wool, provided the ulcer is readily accessible. Mouthwashes can be useful where ulcers are difficult to reach.

Chlorhexidine gluconate mouthwash

There is some evidence that *chlorhexidine mouthwash* reduces duration and severity of ulceration. The rationale for the use of antibacterial agents in the treatment of mouth ulcers is that secondary bacterial infection frequently occurs. Such infection can increase discomfort and delay healing. *Chlorhexidine* helps to prevent secondary bacterial infection but it does not prevent recurrence. It has a bitter taste and is available in peppermint as well as standard flavour. Regular use can stain teeth brown – an effect that is not usually permanent. Advising the patient to brush the teeth before using the mouthwash can reduce staining. The mouth should then be well rinsed with water as *chlorhexidine* can be inactivated by some toothpaste ingredients. The mouthwash should be used twice a day, rinsing 10 mL in the mouth for 1 min and continued for 48 h after symptoms have gone.

Topical corticosteroids

Hydrocortisone acts locally on the ulcer to reduce inflammation and pain and to shorten healing time and is available as muco-adhesive tablets for use by adults and children over 12. A tablet is held in close proximity to the ulcer until dissolved. This can be difficult when the ulcer is in an inaccessible spot. One tablet is used four times a day. The pharmacist should explain that the tablet should not be sucked, but dissolved in contact with the ulcer. Advise that the treatment is best used as early as possible. Before an ulcer appears, the affected area feels sensitive and tingling – the prodromal phase – and treatment should start then. Corticosteroids have no effect on recurrence.

Local analgesics

Benzydamine mouthwash or *spray* and *choline salicylate dental gel* are short acting but can be useful in very painful major ulcers. The mouthwash is used by rinsing 15 mL in the mouth three times a day.

Numbness, tingling and stinging can occur with *benzydamine*. Diluting the mouthwash with the same amount of water before use can reduce stinging. The mouthwash is not licensed for use in children under 12. *Benzydamine spray* is used as four sprays onto the affected area three times a day. Although *aspirin* is no longer recommended for children under 16 years of age because of possible links with Reye's syndrome, *choline salicylate dental gel* produces low levels of salicylate and can therefore be used in children.

Local anaesthetics (e.g. lidocaine (lignocaine) and benzocaine)
Local anaesthetic gels are often requested by patients. Although they are effective in producing temporary pain relief, maintenance of gels and liquids in contact with the ulcer surface is difficult. Reapplication of the preparation may be done when necessary. Tablets and pastilles can be kept in contact with the ulcer by the tongue and can be of value when just one or two ulcers are present. Any preparation containing a local anaesthetic becomes difficult to use when the lesions are located in inaccessible parts of the mouth.

Both *lidocaine* and *benzocaine* have been reported to produce sensitisation, but cross-sensitivity seems to be rare, probably because the two agents are from different chemical groupings. Thus, if a patient has experienced a reaction to one agent in the past, the alternative could be tried.

Other treatments
Polyvinylpyrrolidone (PVP) with sodium hyaluronate (SH) is available in mouthwash, spray and gel formulations. The limited evidence from clinical studies indicates that SH may reduce pain. PVP forms a protective barrier and may reduce time to healing but there is no definitive evidence.

Mouth ulcers in practice

Case 1
A man in his early 50s asks you to recommend something for painful mouth ulcers. On questioning, he tells you that he has two ulcers at the moment and has occasionally suffered from the problem over many years. Usually he gets one or two ulcers inside the cheek or lips and they last for about 1 week. He is not taking any medicines and has no other symptoms. You ask to see the lesions and note that there are two small white patches, each with an angry-looking red border. One ulcer is located on the edge of the tongue and the other inside the cheek. The patient cannot remember any trauma or injury to the mouth and has had the ulcers for a couple of days. He tells you that he has used pain-killing gels in the past and they have provided some relief.

The pharmacist's view
From what he has told you, it would be reasonable to assume that this patient suffers from recurrent minor aphthous ulcers. Treatment with *hydrocortisone muco-adhesive tablets* (one tablet dissolved in contact with the ulcers four times a day), or with a local anaesthetic or analgesic gel applied when needed, would help to relieve the discomfort until the ulcers healed. He should see his doctor if the ulcers have not healed within 3 weeks.

The doctor's view

This patient is most likely suffering from recurrent aphthous ulceration. As always, it is worthwhile enquiring about his general health, checking, in particular, that he does not have a recurrent bowel upset or weight loss. These ulcers can be helped by a topical steroid preparation.

Case 2

One of your counter assistants asks you to recommend a strong treatment for mouth ulcers for a woman who has already tried several treatments. The woman tells you that she has a troublesome ulcer that has persisted for a few weeks. She has used some pastilles containing a local anaesthetic and an antiseptic mouthwash but with no improvement.

The pharmacist's view

This woman should be advised to see her doctor for further investigation. The ulcer has been present for several weeks, with no sign of improvement, suggesting the possibility of a serious cause.

The doctor's view

Referral is correct. It is likely that the doctor will refer her to an oral surgeon for further assessment and probable biopsy as the ulcer could be malignant. Cancer of the mouth accounts for approximately 2% of all cancers of the body in Britain. It is most common after the sixth decade and is more common in men, especially pipe or cigar smokers. Cancer of the mouth is most often found on the tongue or lower lip. It may be painless initially.

Heartburn

Symptoms of heartburn are caused when there is reflux of gastric contents, particularly acid, into the oesophagus, which irritate the sensitive mucosal surface (oesophagitis). Patients will often describe the symptoms of heartburn – typically a burning discomfort/pain felt in the stomach, passing upwards behind the breastbone (retrosternally). By careful questioning, the pharmacist can distinguish conditions that are potentially more serious.

What you need to know
Age
Adult, child
Symptoms
Heartburn
Difficulty in swallowing
Flatulence
Associated factors
Pregnancy
Precipitating factors
Relieving factors
Weight
Smoking habit
Eating
Medication
Medicines tried already
Other medicines being taken

Significance of questions and answers

Age

The symptoms of reflux and oesophagitis occur more commonly in patients aged over 55 years. Heartburn is not a condition normally experienced in childhood, although symptoms can occur in young adults and particularly in pregnant women. Children with symptoms of heartburn should therefore be referred to their doctor.

Symptoms in the Pharmacy: A Guide to the Management of Common Illness, Seventh Edition.
Alison Blenkinsopp, Paul Paxton and John Blenkinsopp.
© 2014 John Wiley & Sons, Ltd. Published 2014 by John Wiley & Sons, Ltd.

Symptoms/associated factors

A burning discomfort is experienced in the upper part of the stomach in the midline (epigastrium) and the burning feeling tends to move upwards behind the breastbone (retrosternally). The pain may be felt only in the lower retrosternal area or on occasion right up to the throat, causing an acid taste in the mouth.

Deciding whether or not someone is suffering from heartburn can be helped by enquiring about precipitating or aggravating factors. Heartburn is often brought on by bending or lying down. It is more likely to occur in those who are overweight and can be aggravated by a recent increase in weight. It is also more likely to occur after a large meal. It can be aggravated and even caused by belching. Many people develop a nervous habit of swallowing to clear the throat. Each time this occurs, air is taken down into the stomach, which becomes distended. This causes discomfort which is relieved by belching but which in turn can be associated with acid reflux.

Severe pain

Sometimes the pain can come on suddenly and severely and even radiate to the back and arms. In this situation differentiation of symptoms is difficult as the pain can mimic a heart attack and urgent medical referral is essential. Sometimes patients who have been admitted to hospital apparently suffering a heart attack are found to have oesophagitis instead. For further discussion about causes of chest pain, see p. 63.

Difficulty in swallowing (dysphagia)

Difficulty in swallowing must always be regarded as a serious symptom. The difficulty may be either discomfort as food or drink is swallowed or a sensation of food or liquids sticking in the gullet. Both require referral (see 'When to refer' box below). It is possible that discomfort may be secondary to oesophagitis from acid reflux (gastro-oesophageal reflux disease (GORD)), especially when it occurs whilst swallowing hot drinks or irritant fluids (e.g. alcohol or fruit juice). A history of a sensation that food sticks as it is swallowed or that it does not seem to pass directly into the stomach (dysphagia) is an indication for immediate referral. It may be due to obstruction of the oesophagus, for example, by a tumour.

Regurgitation

Regurgitation can be associated with difficulty in swallowing. It occurs when recently eaten food sticks in the oesophagus and is regurgitated without passing into the stomach. This is due to a mechanical blockage in the oesophagus. This can be caused by a cancer or, more fortunately, by less serious conditions such as a peptic stricture. A peptic stricture is caused by long-standing acid reflux with oesophagitis. The continual inflammation of the oesophagus causes scarring. Scars contract and can therefore cause narrowing of the oesophagus. This can be treated by dilatation using a fibre-optic endoscope. However, medical examination and further investigations are necessary to determine the cause of regurgitation.

Pregnancy

It has been estimated that as many as half of all pregnant women suffer from heartburn. Pregnant women aged over 30 years are more likely to suffer from the problem. The symptoms are caused by an increase in intra-abdominal pressure and incompetence of the lower oesophageal sphincter. It is thought that hormonal influences, particularly progesterone, are important in the lowering of sphincter pressure. Heartburn often begins in mid-to-late pregnancy, but may occur at any stage. The problem may sometimes be associated with stress.

Medication

The pharmacist should establish the identity of any medication that has been tried to treat the symptoms. Any other medication being taken by the patient should also be identified; some drugs can cause the symptoms of heartburn, for example, those with anticholinergic actions, such as tricyclic antidepressants and calcium channel blockers and caffeine in compound analgesics or when taken as a stimulant.

Failure to respond to antacids and pain radiating to the arms could mean that the pain is not caused by acid reflux. Although it is still a possibility, other causes such as ischaemic heart disease (IHD) and gall bladder disease have to be considered.

When to refer
Failure to respond to antacids
Pain radiating to arms
Difficulty in swallowing
Regurgitation
Long duration
Increasing severity
Children

Treatment timescale

If symptoms have not responded to treatment after 1 week, the patient should see a doctor.

Management

The symptoms of heartburn respond well to treatments that are available over the counter (OTC), and there is also a role for the pharmacist to offer practical advice about measures to prevent recurrence of the problem. Pharmacists will use their professional judgement to decide whether to offer antacids/alginates, H_2 antagonists or a proton pump inhibitor (PPI) (*omeprazole, pantoprazole or rabeprazole*) as first-line treatment. The decision will also take into account customer preference.

Antacids

Antacids can be effective in controlling the symptoms of heartburn and reflux, more so in combination with an alginate. Choice of antacid can be made by the pharmacist using the same guidelines as in the section on indigestion (see p. 89). Preparations that are high in sodium should be avoided by anyone on a sodium-restricted diet (e.g. those with heart failure or kidney or liver problems).

Alginates

Alginates form a raft that sits on the surface of the stomach contents and prevents reflux. Some alginate-based products contain *sodium bicarbonate*, which, in addition to its antacid action, causes the release of carbon dioxide in the stomach, enabling the raft to float on top of the stomach contents. If a preparation low in sodium is required, the pharmacist can recommend one containing *potassium bicarbonate* instead. Alginate products with low sodium content are useful for the treatment of heartburn in patients on a restricted sodium diet.

H_2 antagonists (famotidine and ranitidine)

Famotidine and *ranitidine* can be used for the short-term treatment of dyspepsia, hyperacidity and heartburn in adults and children over 16 (see also p. 91). The treatment limit is intended to ensure that patients do not continuously self-medicate for long periods. Pharmacists and their staff can ask whether use has been continuous or intermittent when a repeat purchase request is made. The H_2 antagonists have both a longer duration of action (up to 8–9 h) and a longer onset of action than do antacids.

Where food is known to precipitate symptoms, the H_2 antagonist should be taken an hour before food. H_2 antagonists are also effective for prophylaxis of nocturnal heartburn. Headache, dizziness, diarrhoea and skin rashes have been reported as adverse effects but they are not common.

Manufacturers state that patients should not take OTC *famotidine* or *ranitidine* without checking with their doctor if they are taking other prescribed medicines.

Famotidine

The drug is licensed for OTC use at a maximum dose of 10 mg and a maximum daily dose of 20 mg. *Famotidine* is available as a tablet in combination with the antacids magnesium hydroxide and calcium carbonate. The idea behind this is to provide rapid symptom relief from the antacid and longer action from *famotidine*. The maximum continuous treatment period is 6 days.

Ranitidine

Ranitidine is licensed for OTC use in a dose of 75 mg with a maximum daily dose of 300 mg. It can be used for up to 2 weeks.

Proton pump inhibitors

Omeprazole, pantoprazole and rabeprazole can be used for the relief of heartburn symptoms associated with reflux in adults. PPIs are generally accepted as being amongst the most effective medicines for the relief of heartburn. It may take a day or so for them to start being fully effective. During this period a patient with ongoing symptoms may need to take a concomitant antacid. PPIs work by suppressing gastric acid secretion in the stomach. They inhibit the final stage of gastric hydrochloric acid production by blocking the hydrogen–potassium ATPase enzyme in the parietal cells of the stomach wall (also known as the proton pump).

Omeprazole and *rabeprazole* are licensed OTC as 10 mg tablets, *pantoprazole* as 20 mg tablets and their doses are shown in the table.

Strength and doses of OTC PPIs.

	Strength	Daily dose
Omeprazole	10 mg	20 mg
Pantoprazole	20 mg	20 mg
Rabeprazole	10 mg	10 mg

Patients taking a PPI should be advised not to take H_2 antagonists at the same time. The tablets should be swallowed whole with plenty of liquid prior to a meal. It is important that the tablets are not crushed or chewed. Alcohol and food do not affect the absorption of PPIs.

If no relief is obtained within 2 weeks, the patient should be referred to the doctor. PPIs should not be taken during pregnancy or whilst breastfeeding. Drowsiness has been reported but rarely. Treatment with PPIs may cause a false negative result in the 'breath test' for *helicobacter*.

Practical points

Obesity

If the patient is overweight, weight reduction should be advised (see 'Weight management' p. 350). There is some evidence that weight loss reduces symptoms of heartburn.

Food

Small meals, eaten frequently, are better than large meals, as reducing the amount of food in the stomach reduces gastric distension, which helps to prevent reflux. Gastric emptying is slowed when there is a large volume of food in the stomach; this can also aggravate symptoms. High-fat meals delay gastric emptying. The evening meal is best taken several hours before going to bed.

Posture

Bending, stooping and even slumping in an armchair can provoke symptoms and should be avoided when possible. It is better to squat rather than bend down. Since the symptoms are often worse when the patient lies down, there is evidence that raising the head of the bed can reduce both acid clearance and the number of reflux episodes. Using extra pillows is often recommended but this is not as effective as raising the head of the bed. The reason for this is that using extra pillows raises only the upper part of the body, with bending at the waist, which can result in increased pressure on the stomach contents.

Clothing

Tight, constricting clothing, especially waistbands and belts, can be an aggravating factor and should be avoided.

Other aggravating factors

Smoking, alcohol, caffeine and chocolate have a direct effect by making the oesophageal sphincter less competent by reducing its pressure and therefore contribute to symptoms. The pharmacist is in a good position to offer advice about how to stop smoking, offering a smoking cessation product where appropriate (see the chapter on 'Prevention of heart disease'). The knowledge that the discomfort of heartburn will be reduced can be a motivating factor in giving up cigarettes.

Heartburn in practice

Patient perspectives

I've been having trouble with heartburn. In fact, it is one of the reasons I wanted to lose weight. I used to get it every once in a while, but then it started to get more frequent. It used to be only during the night, but then it started happening in the middle of the day. A burning feeling in my chest and coming up into my throat. Leaving a horrible taste in the back of my throat. Because I started getting it during the day, I had to start carrying antacid tablets around in my handbag. I haven't been to a doctor. I found that getting my weight down to a certain level (out of the overweight range) got rid of my heartburn. It seems it doesn't take much extra weight before it starts again.

Case 1

Mrs Amy Beston is a woman aged about 50 years who wants some advice about a stomach problem. On questioning, you find out that sometimes she gets a burning sensation just above the breastbone and feels the burning in her throat, often with a bitter taste, as if some food has been brought back up. The discomfort is worse when in bed at night and when bending over whilst gardening. She has been having the problem for 1 or 2 weeks and has not yet tried to treat it. Mrs Beston is not taking any medicines from the doctor. To your experienced eye, this lady is at least a stone overweight. You ask Mrs Beston if the symptoms are worse at any particular time and she says they are worst shortly after going to bed at night.

The pharmacist's view

This woman has many of the classic symptoms of heartburn: pain in the retrosternal region and reflux. The problem is worse at night after going to bed, as is common in heartburn. Mrs Beston has been experiencing the symptoms for about 2 weeks and is not taking any medicines from the doctor.

It would be reasonable to advise the use of an alginate antacid product about 1 h after meals and before going to bed, an H_2 antagonist or a PPI. Practical advice could include the tactful suggestion that Mrs Beston's symptoms would be improved if she lost weight. If your pharmacy provides a weight management service, you could ask if Mrs Beston is interested in participating. Alternatively advice on healthy eating and contact with a local weight watchers group could be given. Mrs Beston could also try cutting down on tea, coffee and, if she smokes, stopping. This is a long list of potential lifestyle changes. It might be a good idea to explain the contributory factors to Mrs Beston and negotiate with her as to which one she will begin with. Success is more likely to be achieved and sustained if changes are introduced one at a time.

Menopausal women are more prone to heartburn, and weight gain at the time of menopause will exacerbate the problem.

The doctor's view

The advice given by the pharmacist is sensible. Acid reflux is the most likely explanation for her symptoms. It is not clear from the presentation whether she was seeking medication or simply asking for an opinion about the cause of her symptoms, or both. It is always helpful to explore a patient's expectations in order to produce an effective outcome to a consultation. In this instance the interchange between the pharmacist and Mrs Beston is complex as a large amount of information needs to be given, both explaining the cause of the symptoms (providing an understandable description of oesophagus, stomach, acid reflux and oesophagitis) and advising about treatment and lifestyle. It is often sensible to offer a follow-up discussion to check on progress and reinforce advice. If her heartburn was not improving, it would provide an opportunity to recommend referral to her doctor.

The doctor's next step would be very much dependent on this information. If a clear story of heartburn caused by acid reflux were obtained, then reinforcement of the pharmacist's advice concerning posture, weight, diet, smoking and alcohol would be appropriate. If medication was requested, antacids or alginates could be tried. If the symptoms were severe, an H_2 antagonist or PPI would be treatment options. In the case of persistent symptoms or diagnostic uncertainty, referral for endoscopy would be necessary. *Helicobacter pylori* eradication is not thought to play a role in the management of heartburn.

Case 2

You have been asked to recommend a 'strong' mixture for heartburn for Harry Groves, a local man in his late 50s who works in a nearby warehouse. Mr Groves tells you that he has been getting terrible heartburn for which his doctor prescribed some mixture about 1 week ago. You remember dispensing a prescription for a liquid alginate preparation. The bottle is now empty and the problem is no better. When asked if he can point to where the pain is, Mr Groves gestures across his chest and clenches his fist when describing the pain, which he says feels heavy. You ask whether the pain ever moves and Mr Groves tells you that sometimes it goes to his neck and jaw. Mr Groves is a smoker and is not taking any other medicines. When asked if the pain worsens when bending or lying down, Mr Groves says it does not, but he tells you he usually gets the pain when he is at work, especially on busy days.

The pharmacist's view

This man should see his doctor immediately. The symptoms he has described are not those that would be typical of heartburn. In addition, he has been taking an alginate preparation, which has been ineffective. Mr Groves' symptoms give cause for concern; the heartburn is associated with effort at work and its location and radiation suggest a more serious cause.

The doctor's view

Mr Groves' story is suggestive of angina. He should be advised to contact his doctor immediately. The doctor would require more details about the pain, such as duration and whether or not the pain can come on without any exertion. If the periods of pain were frequent, prolonged and unrelieved by rest, it would be usual to arrange immediate hospital admission as the picture sounds like unstable or crescendo angina.

If an urgent inpatient referral is not required, the doctor would carry out a fuller assessment that would usually include an examination, electrocardiogram (ECG), urine analysis and blood test. This in turn could lead to medication, for example, *aspirin* and *glyceryl trinitrate* (GTN), possibly a beta-blocker, a long-acting nitrate or a rate-limiting calcium channel blocker being prescribed and an urgent outpatient referral to a cardiologist. Mr Groves would be strongly advised to stop smoking.

More detailed tests are likely to be arranged in hospital. These would probably include an exercise cardiogram and an angiogram. The latter allows visualisation of the blood vessels supplying the heart muscle and assessment of whether surgery would be advisable.

Indigestion

Indigestion (dyspepsia) is commonly presented in community pharmacies and is often self-diagnosed by patients, who use the term to include anything from pain in the chest and upper abdomen to lower abdominal symptoms. Many patients use the terms indigestion and heartburn interchangeably. The pharmacist must establish whether such a self-diagnosis is correct and exclude the possibility of serious disease.

What you need to know

Symptoms
Age
  Adult, child
Duration of symptoms
Previous history
Details of pain
  Where is the pain?
  What is its nature?
  Is it associated with food?
  Is the pain constant or colicky?
  Are there any aggravating or relieving factors?
  Does the pain move to anywhere else?
Associated symptoms
  Loss of appetite
  Weight loss
  Nausea/vomiting
  Alteration in bowel habit
Diet
Any recent change of diet?
Alcohol consumption
Smoking habit
Medication
Medicines already tried
Other medicines being taken

Symptoms in the Pharmacy: A Guide to the Management of Common Illness, Seventh Edition.
Alison Blenkinsopp, Paul Paxton and John Blenkinsopp.
© 2014 John Wiley & Sons, Ltd. Published 2014 by John Wiley & Sons, Ltd.

Significance of questions and answers

Symptoms

The symptoms of typical indigestion include poorly localised upper abdominal (the area between the belly button and the breastbone) discomfort, which may be brought on by particular foods, excess food, alcohol or medication (e.g. *aspirin*).

Age

Indigestion is rare in children, who should be referred to the doctor. Abdominal pain, however, is a common symptom in children and is often associated with an infection. OTC treatment is not appropriate for abdominal pain of unknown cause and referral to the doctor would be advisable.

Be cautious when dealing with first-time indigestion in patients aged 45 years or over and refer them to the general practitioner (GP) for a diagnosis. Gastric cancer, while rare in young patients, is more likely to occur in those aged 50 years and over. Careful history taking is therefore of paramount importance here.

Duration/previous history

Indigestion that is persistent or recurrent should be referred to the doctor, after considering the information gained from questioning. Any patient with a previous history of the symptom which has not responded to treatment, or which has worsened, should be referred.

Details of pain/associated symptoms

If the pharmacist can obtain a good description of the pain, then the decision whether to advise treatment or referral is much easier. A few medical conditions that may present as indigestion but which require referral are described below.

Ulcer

Ulcers may occur in the stomach (gastric ulcer) or in the first part of the small intestine leading from the stomach (duodenal ulcer). Duodenal ulcers are more common and have different symptoms from gastric ulcers. Typically the pain of a duodenal ulcer is localised to the upper abdomen, slightly to the right of the midline. It is often possible to point to the site of pain with a single finger. The pain is dull and is most likely to occur when the stomach is empty, especially at night. It is relieved by food (although it may be aggravated by fatty foods) and antacids.

The pain of a gastric ulcer is in the same area but less well localised. It is often aggravated by food and may be associated with nausea and vomiting. Appetite is usually reduced and the symptoms are persistent and severe. Both types of ulcers are associated with *H. pylori* infection and may be exacerbated or precipitated by smoking and NSAIDs.

Gallstones

Single or multiple stones can form in the gall bladder, which is situated beneath the liver. The gall bladder stores bile. It periodically contracts to squirt bile through a narrow tube (bile duct) into the duodenum to aid the digestion of food, especially fat. Stones can become temporarily stuck in the opening to the bile duct as the gall bladder contracts. This causes severe pain (biliary colic) in the upper abdomen below the right rib margin. Sometimes this pain can be confused with that of a duodenal ulcer. Biliary colic may be precipitated by a fatty meal.

Gastro-oesophageal reflux

When a person eats, food passes down the gullet (oesophagus) into the stomach. Acid is produced by the stomach to aid digestion. The lining of the stomach is resistant to the irritant effects of acid, whereas the lining of the oesophagus is readily irritated by acid. A sphincter (valve) system operates between the stomach and the oesophagus, preventing reflux of stomach contents.

When this valve system is weak, for example, in the presence of a hiatus hernia, or where sphincter muscle tone is reduced by drugs such as beta-blockers, anticholinergics and calcium channel blockers, the acid contents of the stomach can leak backwards into the oesophagus. The symptoms arising are typically described as heartburn but many patients use the terms heartburn and indigestion interchangeably. Heartburn is a pain arising in the upper abdomen passing upwards behind the breastbone. It is often precipitated by a large meal or by bending and lying down. Heartburn can be treated by the pharmacist but sometimes requires referral (see p. 78).

Irritable bowel syndrome

Irritable bowel syndrome (IBS) is a common, non-serious, but troublesome, condition in which symptoms are caused by colon spasm (also see p. 124). There is usually an alteration in bowel habit, often with alternating constipation and diarrhoea. The diarrhoea is typically worse first thing in the morning. Pain is usually present. It is often lower abdominal (below and to the right or left of the belly button) but it may be upper abdominal and therefore confused with indigestion. Any persistent alteration in normal bowel habit is an indication for referral.

Atypical angina

Angina is usually experienced as a tight, painful constricting band across the middle of the chest. Atypical angina pain may be felt in the lower chest or upper abdomen. It is likely to be precipitated by exercise or exertion. If this occurs, referral is necessary.

More serious disorders

Persisting upper abdominal pain, especially when associated with anorexia and unexplained weight loss, may herald an underlying cancer of the stomach or pancreas. Ulcers sometimes start bleeding, which may present with blood in the vomit (haematemesis) or in the stool (melaena). In the latter, the stool becomes tarry and black. Urgent referral is necessary.

Diet

Fatty foods and alcohol can cause indigestion, aggravate ulcers and precipitate biliary colic.

Smoking habit

Smoking predisposes to, and may cause, indigestion and ulcers. Ulcers heal more slowly and relapse more often during treatment in smokers. The pharmacist is in a good position to offer advice on smoking cessation, perhaps with a recommendation to use nicotine replacement therapy.

Medication

Medicines already tried

Anyone who has tried one or more appropriate treatments without improvement or whose initial improvement in symptoms is not maintained should see the doctor.

Other medicines being taken

Gastrointestinal (GI) side effects can be caused by many drugs, so it is important for the pharmacist to ascertain any medication that the patient is taking.

NSAIDs have been implicated in the causation of ulcers and bleeding ulcers, and there are differences in toxicity related to increased doses and to the nature of individual drugs. Sometimes these drugs cause indigestion. Elderly patients are particularly prone to such problems, and pharmacists should bear this in mind. Severe or prolonged indigestion in any patient taking an NSAID is an indication for referral. Particular care is needed in elderly patients, for whom referral is always advisable. A study looked at emergency admissions to two hospitals in two areas of England for GI disease. When the results were extrapolated to the United Kingdom, the number of NSAID-associated emergency admissions in the United Kingdom per year would be about 12 000, with about 2500 deaths.

OTC medicines also require consideration: *aspirin, ibuprofen* and *iron* are among those that may produce symptoms of indigestion. Some drugs may interact with antacids (see 'Interactions with antacids' below).

<table>
<tr><td>When to refer</td></tr>
<tr><td>Age over 45 years, if symptoms develop for first time</td></tr>
<tr><td>Symptoms are persistent (longer than 5 days) or recurrent</td></tr>
<tr><td>Pain is severe</td></tr>
<tr><td>Blood in vomit or stool</td></tr>
<tr><td>Pain worsens on effort</td></tr>
<tr><td>Persistent vomiting</td></tr>
<tr><td>Treatment has failed</td></tr>
<tr><td>Adverse drug reaction is suspected</td></tr>
<tr><td>Associated weight loss</td></tr>
<tr><td>Children</td></tr>
</table>

Treatment timescale

If symptoms have not improved within 5 days, the patient should see the doctor.

Management

Once the pharmacist has excluded serious disease, treatment of dyspepsia with antacids or an H_2 antagonist may be recommended and is likely to be effective. The preparation should be selected on the basis of the individual patient's symptoms. Smoking, alcohol and fatty meals can all aggravate symptoms, so the pharmacist can advise appropriately.

Antacids

In general, liquids are more effective antacids than are solids; they are easier to take, work quicker and have a greater neutralising capacity. Their small particle size allows a large surface area to be in contact with the gastric contents. Some patients find tablets more convenient and these should be well chewed before swallowing for the best effect. It might be appropriate for the patient to have both; the liquid could be taken before and after working hours, while the tablets could be taken during the day for convenience. Antacids are best taken about 1 h after a meal because the rate of gastric emptying has then slowed and the antacid will therefore remain in the stomach for longer. Taken at this time antacids may act for up to 3 h compared with only 30 min–1 h if taken before meals.

Sodium bicarbonate

Sodium bicarbonate is the only absorbable antacid that is useful in practice. It is water soluble, acts quickly, is an effective neutraliser of acid and has a short duration of action. It is often included in OTC formulations in order to give a fast-acting effect, in combination with longer-acting agents. However, antacids containing *sodium bicarbonate* should be avoided in patients if sodium intake should be restricted (e.g. in patients with congestive heart failure). *Sodium bicarbonate* increases excretion of lithium, leading to reduced plasma levels. The contents of OTC products should therefore be carefully scrutinised, and pharmacists should be aware of the constituents of some of the traditional formulary preparations. The relative sodium contents of different antacids can be found in the *British National Formulary* (*BNF*). In addition, long-term use of *sodium bicarbonate* may lead to systemic alkalosis and renal damage. In short-term use, however, it can be a valuable and effective antacid. Its use is more appropriate in acute rather than chronic dyspepsia.

Aluminium and magnesium salts (e.g. aluminium hydroxide and magnesium trisilicate)

Aluminium-based antacids are effective; they tend to be constipating and this can be a useful effect in patients if there is slight diarrhoea. Conversely, the use of aluminium antacids is best avoided in anyone who is constipated and in elderly patients who have a tendency to be so. Magnesium salts are more potent acid neutralisers than are aluminium salts. They tend to cause osmotic diarrhoea as a result of the formation of insoluble magnesium salts and are therefore useful in patients who are slightly constipated. Combination products containing aluminium and magnesium salts cause minimum bowel disturbance and are therefore valuable preparations for recommendation by the pharmacist.

Calcium carbonate

Calcium carbonate is commonly included in OTC formulations. It acts quickly, has a prolonged action and is a potent neutraliser of acid. It can cause acid rebound and, if taken over long periods at high doses, can cause hypercalcaemia and so should not be recommended for long-term use. *Calcium carbonate* and *sodium bicarbonate* can, if taken in large quantities with a high intake of milk, result in the milk-alkali syndrome. This involves hypercalcaemia, metabolic alkalosis and renal insufficiency; its symptoms are nausea, vomiting, anorexia, headache and mental confusion.

Dimeticone (dimethicone)

Dimeticone is sometimes added to antacid formulations for its defoaming properties. Theoretically, it reduces surface tension and allows easier elimination of gas from the gut by passing flatus or eructation (belching). Evidence of benefit is uncertain.

Interactions with antacids

Because they raise the gastric pH, antacids can interfere with enteric coatings on tablets that are intended to release their contents further along the GI tract. The consequences of this may be that release of the drug is unpredictable; adverse effects may occur if the drug is in contact with the stomach. Alternatively, enteric coatings are sometimes used to protect a drug that may be inactivated by the low pH in the stomach, so concurrent administration of antacids may result in such inactivation. Taking the doses of antacids and other drugs at least 1 h apart should minimise the interaction.

Antacids may reduce the absorption of some antibiotics and antifungals (tetracyclines, *azithromycin, itraconazole, ketoconazole, ciprofloxacin, norfloxacin, rifampicin*). Absorption of angiotensin-converting enzyme (ACE) inhibitors, *phenothiazines, gabapentin* and *phenytoin*, may also be reduced (see the *BNF* for a full current list).

Sodium bicarbonate may increase the excretion of lithium and lower the plasma level, so a reduction in lithium's therapeutic effect may occur. Antacids containing *sodium bicarbonate* should not therefore be recommended for any patient on lithium therapy.

The changes in pH that occur after antacid administration can result in a decrease in iron absorption if iron is taken at the same time. The effect is caused by the formation of insoluble iron salts due to the changed pH. Taking iron and antacids at different times should prevent the problem (see the *BNF* for a detailed listing of interactions with antacids).

Famotidine and ranitidine

Famotidine and *ranitidine* can be used for the short-term treatment of dyspepsia and heartburn (see also p. 79). Treatment with *ranitidine* is limited to a maximum of 2 weeks and with *famotidine* to 6 days.

Discussing the use of H_2 antagonists with local family doctors would be valuable. Agreeing general guidelines or a protocol for their use could be a feature of the discussion.

Domperidone

Domperidone 10 mg can be used for the treatment of postprandial stomach symptoms of excessive fullness, nausea, epigastric bloating and belching, occasionally accompanied by epigastric discomfort and heartburn. It increases the rate of gastric emptying and transit time in the small intestine, and also increases the strength of contraction of the oesophageal sphincter. *Domperidone* can be used in patients aged 16 years and over. The maximum dose is 10 mg and the maximum daily dose 40 mg. When used as a prescription-only medicine (POM), *domperidone* is used to treat nausea and vomiting, but these indications are not included in the pharmacy (P) licence and patients with these symptoms would need to be referred.

In 2012, the Medicines and Healthcare Regulatory Agency (MHRA) advised that non-prescription domperidone products should only be recommended with medical supervision for patients with cardiac disease. Patients were also advised to seek medical attention immediately if experiencing symptoms such as an irregular heartbeat or fainting while taking any domperidone product.

Indigestion in practice

Case 1

Mrs Johnson, an elderly woman, complains of indigestion and an upset stomach. On questioning, you find out she has had the problem for a few days; the pain is epigastric and does not seem to be related to food. She has been feeling slightly nauseated. You ask about her diet; she has not changed her diet recently and has not been overdoing it. She tells you that she is taking four lots of tablets: for her heart, her waterworks and some new ones for her bad hip (*diclofenac* modified release 100 mg at night). She has been taking them after meals, as advised, and has not tried any medicines yet to treat her symptoms. Before the *diclofenac* she was taking *paracetamol* for the pain. She normally uses *paracetamol* as a general painkiller at home; she tells you that she cannot take *aspirin* because it upsets her stomach.

The pharmacist's view

It sounds as though this woman is suffering GI symptoms as a result of her NSAID. Such effects are more common in elderly patients. She has been taking the medicine after food, which should have minimised any GI effects, and the best course of action would be to refer her back to the doctor. It would be worth asking Mrs Johnson about the dose and frequency with which she took the paracetamol to see whether she took enough for it to be effective.

The doctor's view

Referral back to her doctor is the correct course of action. Almost certainly her symptoms have been caused by the *diclofenac*. A large clinical trial showed that risk factors for serious complications with oral NSAIDs were: age 75 years or more, history of peptic ulcer, history of GI bleeding and history of heart disease. If this woman were over 75 years and taking tablets for heart problems, she has two significant risk factors. The model predicts that for patients with none of the four risk factors, 1-year risk of a complication is 0.8%. For patients with all four risk factors, the risk is 18%.

She should be advised to stop the *diclofenac*. A blood test for *H. pylori* would be helpful and whilst awaiting the results she could be started on a PPI. If the *H. pylori* test came back positive, she would also benefit from *H. pylori* eradication therapy.

Control of her primary symptom (hip pain) will then be a problem. NSAIDs should be avoided if possible. It may be possible to change the *paracetamol* to a compound preparation containing *paracetamol* and *codeine* or *dihydrocodeine*. If an NSAID is necessary to control the pain and there is a documented history of peptic ulceration, an NSAID can be given with a PPI. Failure to control hip pain due to osteoarthritis (OA) may require referral to an orthopaedic surgeon to consider a hip replacement.

Case 2

A man aged in his early 50s comes in to ask your advice about his stomach trouble. He tells you that he has been having the problem for a couple of months but it seems to have got worse. The pain is in his stomach, quite high up; he had similar pain a few months ago, but it got better and has now come back again. The pain seems to get better after a meal; sometimes it wakes him during the night. He has been taking Rennies to treat his symptoms; they did the trick but do not seem to be working now, even though he takes a lot of them. He has also been taking some OTC *ranitidine* tablets. He is not taking any other medicines.

The pharmacist's view

This patient has a history of epigastric pain, which remitted and has now returned. At one stage, his symptoms responded to an antacid but they no longer do so, despite his increasing the dose. This long history, the worsening symptoms and the failure of medication warrant referral to the doctor.

The doctor's view

It would be sensible to recommend referral to his doctor as the information obtained so far does not permit diagnosis. It is possible that he has a stomach ulcer, acid reflux or even stomach cancer, but further information is required. An appropriate examination and investigation will be necessary.

The doctor would need to listen carefully, first by asking open questions and then by asking more direct, closed questions to find out more information; for example, how does the pain affect him? What is the nature of the pain (burning, sharp, dull, tight or constricting)? Does it radiate (to back or chest, down arms, up to neck/mouth)? Are there any associated symptoms (nausea, difficulty in swallowing, loss of appetite, weight loss or shortness of breath)? Are there any other problems (constipation or flatulence)? What are the aggravating/relieving factors? How is his general health? What is his diet like? How are things going for him generally (personally/professionally)? Does he smoke? How much alcohol does he drink? What does he think might be wrong with him? What are his expectations for treatment/management?

Nausea and vomiting

Nausea and vomiting are symptoms that have many possible causes. From the pharmacist's point of view, while there are treatments available to prevent nausea and vomiting, there is no effective OTC treatment once vomiting is established. For that reason, this section will deal briefly with some of the causes of these symptoms and then continue in the next section to consider the prevention of motion sickness, where the pharmacist can recommend effective treatments to help prevent the problem.

What you need to know
Age
Infant, child, adult, elderly
Pregnancy
Duration
Associated symptoms
Has vomiting started?
Abdominal pain
Diarrhoea
Constipation
Fever
Alcohol intake
Medication
Prescribed
OTC
Previous history
Dizziness/vertigo

Significance of questions and answers

Age

The very young and the elderly are most at risk of dehydration as a result of vomiting. Vomiting of milk in infants less than 1 year old may be due to infection or feeding problems or, rarely, an obstruction such as pyloric stenosis. In the latter, there is thickening of the

Symptoms in the Pharmacy: A Guide to the Management of Common Illness, Seventh Edition. Alison Blenkinsopp, Paul Paxton and John Blenkinsopp.
© 2014 John Wiley & Sons, Ltd. Published 2014 by John Wiley & Sons, Ltd.

muscular wall around the outlet of the stomach, which causes a blockage. It typically occurs in the first few weeks of life in a first-born male. The vomiting is frequently projectile in that the vomit is forcibly expelled a considerable distance. The condition can be cured by an operation under general anaesthetic lasting about half an hour called a pyloromyotomy. The pharmacist must distinguish, by questioning, between vomiting (the forced expulsion of gastric contents through the mouth) and regurgitation (where food is effortlessly brought up from the throat and stomach). Regurgitation sometimes occurs in babies, where it is known as possetting and is a normal occurrence. When regurgitation occurs in adults, it is associated with oesophageal disease with difficulty in swallowing and requires referral (see p. 77). Nausea is associated with vomiting but not regurgitation and this can be employed as a distinguishing feature during questioning.

Pregnancy

Nausea and vomiting are very common in pregnancy, usually beginning after the first missed period and occurring early in the morning. Pregnancy should be considered as a possible cause of nausea and vomiting in any woman of childbearing age who presents at the pharmacy complaining of nausea and vomiting. Nausea and vomiting are more common in the first pregnancy than in subsequent ones.

Duration

Generally, adults should be referred to the doctor if vomiting has been present for longer than 2 days. Children under 2 years are referred, whatever the duration, because of the risks from dehydration. Anyone presenting with chronic vomiting should be referred to the doctor since such symptoms may indicate the presence of a peptic ulcer or gastric carcinoma.

Associated symptoms

An acute infection (gastroenteritis) is often responsible for vomiting and, in these cases, diarrhoea (see p. 114) may also be present. Careful questioning about food intake during the previous 2 days may give a clue as to the cause. In young children, the rotavirus is the most common cause of gastroenteritis; this is highly infectious and so it is not unusual for more than one child in the family to be affected. In such situations, there are usually associated cold symptoms. Vomiting without other symptoms, in the very young, can be caused by serious infection such as meningitis, and is an indication for immediate referral.

The vomiting of blood may indicate serious disease and is an indication for referral, since it may be caused by haemorrhage from a peptic ulcer or gastric carcinoma. Sometimes the trauma of vomiting can cause a small bleed, due to a tear in the gut lining. Vomit with a faecal smell means that the GI tract may be obstructed and requires urgent referral.

Nausea and vomiting may be associated with a migraine. Any history of dizziness or vertigo should be noted as it may point to inner ear disease, for example, labyrinthitis or Meniere's disease as a cause of the nausea.

Alcohol intake

People who drink large quantities of alcohol may vomit, often in the morning. This may be due to occasional binge drinking or chronic ingestion of alcohol. Alcoholic patients often feel nauseous and retch in the morning. The questioning of patients about their intake of alcohol is a sensitive area and should be approached with tact. Asking about smoking habits might be a good way of introducing other social habits.

Medication

Prescribed and OTC medicines may make patients feel sick and it is therefore important to determine which medicines the patient is currently taking. *Aspirin* and NSAIDs are common causes. Some antibiotics may cause nausea and vomiting, for example, *doxycycline*. Oestrogens, steroids and narcotic analgesics may also produce these symptoms. Symptoms can sometimes be improved by taking the medication with food, but if they continue, the patient should see the doctor. *Digoxin* toxicity may show itself by producing nausea and vomiting, and such symptoms in a patient who is taking *digoxin*, especially an elderly person, should prompt immediate referral where questioning has not produced an apparent cause for the symptoms. Vomiting, with loss of fluids and possible electrolyte imbalances, may cause problems in elderly people taking *digoxin* and diuretics.

Previous history

Any history that suggests chronic nausea and vomiting would indicate referral.

Management

Patients who are vomiting should be referred to the doctor, who will be able to prescribe an anti-emetic if needed. The pharmacist can initiate rehydration therapy in the meantime.

Motion sickness and its prevention

Motion sickness is thought to be caused by a conflict of messages to the brain, where the vomiting centre receives information from the eyes, the GI tract and the vestibular system in the ear. Symptoms of motion sickness include nausea and sometimes vomiting, pallor and cold sweats. Parents commonly seek advice about how to prevent motion sickness in children, in whom the problem is most common. Any form of travel can produce symptoms, including air, sea and road. Effective prophylactic treatments are available OTC and can be selected to match the patient's needs.

What you need to know
Age
Infant, child, adult
Previous history
Mode of travel: car, bus, air, ferry, etc.
Length of journey
Medication

Significance of questions and answers

Age

Motion sickness is common in young children. Babies and very young children up to 2 years seem to only rarely suffer from the problem and therefore do not usually require treatment. The incidence of motion sickness seems to greatly reduce with age, although some adults still experience symptoms. The minimum age at which products designed to prevent motion sickness can be given varies, so for a family with several children careful product selection can provide one medicine to treat all cases.

Previous history

The pharmacist should ascertain which members of the family have previously experienced motion sickness and for whom treatment will be needed.

Symptoms in the Pharmacy: A Guide to the Management of Common Illness, Seventh Edition. Alison Blenkinsopp, Paul Paxton and John Blenkinsopp.
© 2014 John Wiley & Sons, Ltd. Published 2014 by John Wiley & Sons, Ltd.

Mode of travel/length of journey

Details of the journey to be undertaken are useful. The estimated length of time to be spent travelling will help the pharmacist in the selection of prophylactic treatment, since the length of action of available drugs varies.

Once vomiting starts there is little that can be done, so any medicine recommended by the pharmacist must be taken in good time before the journey if it is to be effective. The fact that it is important that the symptoms are prevented before they can gain a hold should be emphasised to the parents. If it is a long journey, it may be necessary to repeat the dose while travelling and the recommended dosage interval should be stressed.

The pharmacist can also offer useful general advice about reducing motion sickness according to the method of transport to be used. For example, children are less likely to feel or be sick if they can see out of the car, so appropriate seats can be used to elevate the seating position of small children. This seems to be effective in practice and is thought to be because it allows the child to see relatively still objects outside the car. This ability to focus on such objects may help to settle the brain's receipt of conflicting messages.

For any method of travel, children are less likely to experience symptoms if they are kept occupied by playing games as they are therefore concentrating on something else. However, again, it seems that looking outside at still objects remains helpful and that a simple game, for example, 'I spy', is better than reading in this respect. In fact, for many travel sickness sufferers, reading exacerbates the feeling of nausea.

Medication

In addition to checking any prescription or OTC medicines currently being taken, the pharmacist should also enquire about any treatments used in the past for motion sickness and their level of success or failure.

Management

Prophylactic treatments for motion sickness, which can be bought OTC, are effective and there is usually no need to refer patients to the doctor.

Anticholinergic activity is thought to prevent motion sickness and forms the basis of treatment by anticholinergic agents (e.g. *hyoscine*) and antihistamines, which have anticholinergic actions (e.g. *cinnarizine* and *promethazine*).

Antihistamines

Antihistamines include *cinnarizine, meclozine* and *promethazine*. Anticholinergic effects are thought to be responsible for the effectiveness of antihistamines in the prophylaxis of motion sickness. All have the potential to cause drowsiness and *promethazine* appears to be the most sedative. *Meclozine* and *promethazine theoclate* have long durations of action and are useful for long journeys since they need to be taken only once daily. *Cinnarizine* and *promethazine theoclate* are not recommended for children younger than 5 years, whereas *meclozine* can be given to those over 2 years. The manufacturers of products containing these drugs advise that they are best avoided during pregnancy.

Anticholinergic agents

The only anticholinergic used widely in the prevention of motion sickness is *hyoscine hydrobromide*, which can be given to children over 3 years. Anticholinergic drugs can cause drowsiness, blurred vision, dry mouth, constipation and urinary retention as side effects, although they are probably unlikely to do so at the doses used in OTC formulations for motion sickness. Children could be given sweets to suck to counteract any drying of the mouth.

Hyoscine has a short duration of action (from 1 h to 3 h). It is therefore suitable for shorter journeys and should be given 20 min before the start of the journey. Anticholinergic drugs and antihistamines with anticholinergic effects are best avoided in patients with prostatic hypertrophy because of the possibility of urinary retention and in glaucoma because the intraocular pressure might be increased.

Pharmacists should remember that side effects from anticholinergic agents are additive and may be increased in patients already taking drugs with anticholinergic effects, such as tricyclic antidepressants (e.g. *amitriptyline*), butyrophenones (e.g. *haloperidol*) and phenothiazines (e.g. *chlorpromazine*). It is therefore important for the pharmacist to determine the identity of any medicines currently being taken by the patient. Table 2 summarises recommended doses and length of action for the treatments discussed.

Alternative approaches to motion sickness
Ginger

Ginger has been used for many years for travel sickness. Clinical trials have produced conflicting findings in travel sickness. No mechanism of action has been identified, but it has been suggested that ginger acts on the GI tract itself rather than on the vomiting centre in the brain or on the vestibular system. No official dosage level has been suggested, but several proprietary products containing ginger are available. Ginger would be worth trying for a driver who suffered from motion sickness, since it does not cause drowsiness, and might be worth considering for use in pregnant women, for whom other anti-emetics such as anticholinergics and antihistamines are not recommended. Ginger

Table 2 Treatments for motion sickness.

Ingredient	Minimum age for use (year)	Children's dose	Adult dose	Timing of first dose in relation to journey	Recommended dose interval (h)
Cinnarizine	5	15 mg	30 mg	2 h before	8
Hyoscine hydrobromide	3	3–4 years: 75 µg	300 µg	20 min before	6
		4–7 years: 150 µg			
		7–12 years: 150–300 µg			
Meclozine	2	2–12 years: 12.5 mg	25 mg	Previous evening or 1 h before	24
Promethazine theoclate	5	5–10 years: 12.5 mg	25 mg	Previous evening or 1 h before	24
		Over 10 years: 25 mg			

has been shown to be effective in a research trial in nausea and vomiting associated with pregnancy (see the chapter on 'Women's health').

Acupressure wristbands

Elasticated wristbands that apply pressure to a defined point on the inside of the wrists are available. Evidence of effectiveness is equivocal. Such wristbands might be worth trying for drivers or pregnant women.

Constipation

Constipation is a condition that is difficult to define and is often self-diagnosed by patients. Generally, it is characterised by the passage of hard, dry stools less frequently than by the person's normal pattern. It is important for the pharmacist to find out what the patient means by constipation and to establish what (if any) change in bowel habit has occurred and over what period of time.

> ## What you need to know
>
> Details of bowel habit
>   Frequency and nature of bowel actions now
>   When was the last bowel movement?
>   What is the usual bowel habit?
>   When did the problem start?
> Is there a previous history?
> Associated symptoms
>   Abdominal pain/discomfort/bloating/distension
>   Nausea and vomiting
>   Blood in the stool
> Diet
>   Any recent change in diet?
>   Is the usual diet rich in fibre?
> Medication
>   Present medication
>   Any recent change in medication
>   Previous use of laxatives

Significance of questions and answers

Details of bowel habit

Many people believe that a daily bowel movement is necessary for good health and laxatives are often taken and abused as a result. In fact, the normal range may vary from three movements in 1 day to three in 1 week. Therefore an important health education role for the pharmacist is in reassuring patients that their frequency of bowel

Symptoms in the Pharmacy: A Guide to the Management of Common Illness, Seventh Edition. Alison Blenkinsopp, Paul Paxton and John Blenkinsopp.
© 2014 John Wiley & Sons, Ltd. Published 2014 by John Wiley & Sons, Ltd.

movement is normal. Patients who are constipated will usually complain of hard stools which are difficult to pass and less frequent than usual.

The determination of any change in bowel habit is essential, particularly any prolonged change. A sudden change, which has lasted for 2 weeks or longer, would be an indication for referral.

Associated symptoms

Constipation is often associated with abdominal discomfort, bloating and nausea. In some cases, constipation can be so severe as to obstruct the bowel. This obstruction or blockage usually becomes evident by causing colicky abdominal pain, abdominal distension and vomiting. When symptoms suggestive of obstruction are present, urgent referral is necessary as hospital admission is the usual course of action. Constipation is only one of many possible causes of obstruction. Other causes, such as bowel tumours or twisted bowels (volvulus), require urgent surgical intervention.

Blood in the stool

The presence of blood in the stool can be associated with constipation and, although alarming, is not necessarily serious, but does require medical referral for diagnosis. In such situations, blood may arise from piles (haemorrhoids) or a small crack in the skin on the edge of the anus (anal fissure). Both these conditions are thought to be caused by a diet low in fibre that tends to produce constipation. The bleeding is characteristically noted on toilet paper after defaecation. The bright red blood may be present on the surface of the motion (not mixed in with the stool) and splashed around the toilet pan. If piles are present, there is often discomfort on defaecation. The piles may drop down (prolapse) and protrude through the anus. A fissure tends to cause less bleeding but much more severe pain on defaecation. Medical referral is advisable as there are other more serious causes of bloody stools, especially where the blood is mixed in with the motion.

Bowel cancer

Large bowel cancer may also present with a persisting change in bowel habit. This condition kills about 16000 people each year in the United Kingdom. Early diagnosis and intervention can dramatically improve the prognosis. The incidence of large bowel cancer rises significantly with age. It is uncommon among people under 50 years. It is more common amongst those living in northern Europe and North America compared with southern Europe and Asia. The average age at diagnosis is 60–65 years.

Diet

Insufficient dietary fibre is a common cause of constipation. An impression of the fibre content of the diet can be gained by asking what would normally be eaten during a day, looking particularly for the presence of wholemeal cereals, bread, fresh fruit and vegetables. Changes in diet and lifestyle, for example, following a job change, loss of work, retirement or travel, may result in constipation. Inadequate intake of food and fluids, for example, in someone who has been ill, may also be responsible for constipation.

An adequate fluid intake is essential for well-being, and, for both prevention and treatment of constipation. It is thought that an inadequate fluid intake is one of the commonest causes of constipation. Research shows that by increasing fluid intake in someone who is not well hydrated the frequency of bowel actions is increased. It is particularly effective when it is increased alongside an increase in dietary fibre. The recommended daily amount of fluid is 1.8 L for men and 1.6 L for women and not all of this need to be in the form of water. Tea and coffee can be counted towards daily fluid intake.

Medication

One or more laxatives may have already been taken in an attempt to treat the symptoms. Failure of such medication may indicate that referral to the doctor is the best option. Previous history of the use of laxatives is relevant. Continuous use, especially of stimulant laxatives, can result in a vicious circle where the contents of the gut are expelled, causing a subsequent cessation of bowel actions for 1 or 2 days. This then leads to the false conclusion that constipation has recurred and more laxatives are taken and so on.

Chronic overuse of stimulant laxatives can result in loss of muscular activity in the bowel wall (an atonic colon) and thus further constipation.

Many drugs can induce constipation; some examples are listed in Table 3. The details of prescribed and OTC medications being taken should be established.

When to refer
Change in bowel habit of 2 weeks or longer
Presence of abdominal pain, vomiting, bloating
Blood in stools
Prescribed medication suspected of causing symptoms
Failure of OTC medication

Table 3 Drugs that may cause constipation.

Drug group	Drug
Analgesics and opiates	*Dihydrocodeine, codeine*
Antacids	*Aluminium salts*
Anticholinergics	*Hyoscine*
Anticonvulsants	*Phenytoin*
Antidepressants	*Tricyclics, selective serotonin reuptake inhibitors*
Antihistamines	*Chlorpheniramine, promethazine*
Antihypertensives	*Clonidine, methyldopa*
Anti-Parkinson agents	*Levodopa*
Beta-blockers	*Propranolol*
Diuretics	*Bendroflumethiazide*
Iron	
Laxative abuse	
Monoamine oxidase inhibitors	
Antipsychotics	*Chlorpromazine*

Treatment timescale

If 1 week's use of treatment does not produce relief of symptoms, the patient should see the doctor. If the pharmacist feels that it is necessary to give only dietary advice, then it would be reasonable to leave it for about 2 weeks to see if the symptoms settle.

Management

Constipation that is not caused by serious pathology will usually respond to simple measures, which can be recommended by the pharmacist: increasing the amount of dietary fibre, maintaining fluid consumption and doing regular exercise. In the short term, a laxative may be recommended to ease the immediate problem.

Stimulant laxatives (e.g. sennosides and bisacodyl)

Stimulant laxatives work by increasing peristalsis. All stimulant laxatives can produce griping/cramping pains. It is advisable to start at the lower end of the recommended dosage range, increasing the dose if needed. The intensity of the laxative effect is related to the dose taken. Stimulant laxatives work within 6–12 h when taken orally. They should be used for a maximum of 1 week. *Bisacodyl* tablets are enteric coated and should be swallowed whole because *bisacodyl* is irritant to the stomach. If it is given as a suppository, the effect usually occurs within 1 h and sometimes as soon as 15 min after insertion.

Docusate sodium appears to have both stimulant and stool-softening effects and acts within 1–days.

Bulk laxatives (e.g. ispaghula, methylcellulose and sterculia)

Bulk laxatives are those that most closely copy the normal physiological mechanisms involved in bowel evacuation and are considered by many to be the laxatives of choice. Such agents are especially useful where patients cannot or will not increase their intake of dietary fibre. Bulk laxatives work by swelling in the gut and increasing faecal mass so that peristalsis is stimulated. The laxative effect can take several days to develop.

The sodium content of bulk laxatives (as *sodium bicarbonate*) should be considered in those requiring a restricted sodium intake.

When recommending the use of a bulk laxative, the pharmacist should advise that an increase in fluid intake would be necessary. In the form of granules or powder, the preparation should be mixed with a full glass of liquid (e.g. fruit juice or water) before taking. Fruit juice can mask the bland taste of the preparation. Intestinal obstruction may result from inadequate fluid intake in patients taking bulk laxatives, particularly those whose gut is not functioning properly as a result of abuse of stimulant laxatives.

Osmotic laxatives (e.g. lactulose, macrogol)

Macrogol and lactulose work by maintaining the volume of fluid in the bowel and may take 1–2 days to work. *Lactulose is a liquid medicine.* *Macrogol* is available as sachets of powder which are dissolved in water before use. *Lactitol* is chemically related to *lactulose* and is available as sachets. The contents of the sachet are sprinkled on food or taken with liquid. One or two glasses of fluid should be taken with the daily dose. *Lactulose* and *lactitol* can cause flatulence, cramps and abdominal discomfort.

Epsom salts (*magnesium sulphate*) is a traditional remedy that, while no longer recommended, is still requested by some older customers. It acts by drawing water into the gut; the increased pressure results in increased intestinal motility. A dose usually produces a bowel movement within a few hours. Repeated use can lead to dehydration.

Glycerine suppositories have both osmotic and irritant effects and usually act within 1 h. They may cause rectal discomfort. Moistening the suppository before use will make insertion easier.

Constipation in children

Parents sometimes ask for laxatives for their children. Fixed ideas about regular bowel habits are often responsible for such requests. Numerous factors can cause constipation in children, including a change in diet and emotional causes. Simple advice about sufficient dietary fibre and fluid intake may be all that is needed. If the problem is of recent origin and there are no significant associated signs, a single *glycerine suppository* together with dietary advice may be appropriate. Referral to the doctor would be best if these measures are unsuccessful.

Constipation in pregnancy

Constipation commonly occurs during pregnancy; hormonal changes are responsible and it has been estimated that one in three pregnant women suffers from constipation. Dietary advice concerning the intake of plenty of high-fibre foods and fluids can help. Oral iron, often prescribed for pregnant women, may contribute to the problem.

Stimulant laxatives are best avoided during pregnancy; bulk-forming laxatives are preferable, although they may cause some abdominal discomfort to women when used late in pregnancy (see the chapter on 'Women's health').

Constipation in the elderly

Constipation is a common problem in elderly patients for several reasons. Elderly patients are less likely to be physically active; they often have poor natural teeth or false teeth and so may avoid high-fibre foods that are more difficult to chew; multidrug regimens are more likely in elderly patients, who may therefore suffer from drug-induced constipation; fixed ideas about what constitutes a normal bowel habit are common in older patients. If a bulk laxative is to be recommended for an elderly patient, it is of great importance that the pharmacist give advice about maintaining fluid intake to prevent the possible development of intestinal obstruction.

Laxative abuse

Two groups of patients are likely to abuse laxatives: those with chronic constipation who get into a vicious circle by using stimulant laxatives (see p. 105), which eventually results in damage to the nerve plexus in the colon, and those who take laxatives in the belief that they will control weight, for example, those who are dieting or, more seriously, women with eating disorders (anorexia nervosa or bulimia), who take very large quantities of laxatives. The pharmacist is in a position to monitor purchases of laxative products and counsel patients as appropriate. Any patient who is ingesting large amounts of laxative agents should be referred to the doctor.

Constipation in practice

Case 1

Mr Dabrowski is a middle-aged man who occasionally visits your pharmacy. Today he complains of constipation, which he has had for several weeks. He has been having a bowel movement every few days; normally they are every day or every other day. His motions are hard and painful to pass. He has not tried any medicines as he thought the problem would go of its own accord. He has never had problems with constipation in the past. He has been taking *atenolol* tablets 50 mg once a day, for over 1 year. He does not have any other symptoms, except a slight feeling of abdominal discomfort. You ask him about his diet; he tells you that since he was made redundant from his job at a local factory 3 months ago when it closed, he has tended to eat less than usual; his dietary intake sounds as if it is low in fibre. He tells you that he has been applying for jobs, with no success so far. He says he feels really down and is starting to think that he may never get another job.

The pharmacist's view

Mr Dabrowski's symptoms are almost certainly due to the change in his lifestyle and eating pattern. Now that he is not working he is likely to be less physically active and his eating pattern has probably changed. From what he has said, it sounds as if he is becoming depressed because of his lack of success in finding work. Constipation seems to be associated with depression, separately from the constipating effect of some antidepressant drugs.

It would be worth asking Mr Dabrowski if he is sleeping well (signs of clinical depression include disturbed sleep: either difficulty in getting to sleep or difficulty in waking early and not being able to get back to sleep). Weight can change either way in depression. Some patients eat for comfort, while others find their appetite is reduced. Depending on his response, you might consider whether referral to his doctor is needed.

To address the dietary problems, he could be advised to start the day with a wholegrain cereal and to eat at least four slices of wholemeal bread each day. Baked beans are a cheap, good source of fibre. Fresh vegetables are also fibre rich. It would be important to stress that fluid intake should also be increased. A high-fibre diet means patients should increase their fibre intake until they pass one large, soft stool each day; the amount of fibre needed to produce this effect will vary markedly between patients. The introduction of dietary fibre should be gradual; too rapid an increase can cause griping and wind. Mr Dabrowski also needs to make sure he is drinking the recommended daily fluid intake of 1.8 L each day. All types of drinks count.

To provide relief from the discomfort, a suppository of *glycerine* or *bisacodyl* could be recommended to produce a bowel evacuation quickly or an oral stimulant laxative taken at bedtime should produce a bowel movement the next day; in the longer term, dietary changes provide the key. He should see the doctor if the suppository does not produce an effect; if it works but the dietary changes have not been effective after 2 weeks, he should go to his doctor. Mr Johnson's medication is unlikely to be responsible for his constipation because, although beta-blockers can sometimes cause constipation, he has been taking the drug for over 1 year with no previous problems.

The doctor's view

The advice given by the pharmacist is sensible. It is likely that Mr Dabrowski's physical and mental health have been affected by the impact of a significant change in his life. The loss of his job and the uncertainty of future employment is a major and continuing source of stress. The fact that the pharmacist has taken time to check out how he has been affected will in itself be therapeutic. It also gives the pharmacist the opportunity to refer to the doctor if necessary. Many people are reluctant to take such problems to their doctor but a recommendation from the pharmacist might make the process easier. Hopefully, the advice given for constipation will at least improve one aspect of his life. If the constipation does not resolve within 2 weeks, he should see his doctor.

Case 2

Your counter assistant asks if you will have a word with a young woman who is in the shop. She was recognised by your assistant as a regular purchaser of stimulant laxatives. You explain to the woman that you will need to ask a few questions because regular use of laxatives may mean an underlying problem, which is not improving. In answer to your questions she tells you that she diets almost constantly and always suffers from constipation. Her weight appears to be within the range for her height. You show her your pharmacy's BMI (body mass index) chart and work out with her where she is on the chart, which confirms your initial feeling. However, she is reluctant to accept your advice, saying that she definitely needs to lose some more weight. You ask about her diet and she tells you that she has tried all sorts of approaches, most of which involve eating very little.

The pharmacist's view

Unfortunately this sort of story is all too common in community pharmacy, with many women who seek to achieve weight below the recommended range. The pharmacist can explain that constipation often occurs during dieting simply because insufficient bulk and fibre is being eaten to allow the gut to work normally. Perhaps the pharmacist might suggest that she join a local weight management group, or if the pharmacy provides this service, offer it. Despite the pharmacist's advice, many customers will still wish to purchase laxatives and the pharmacist will need to consider how to handle refusal of sales. Offering stimulant laxatives for sale by self-selection can only exacerbate the problems and make it more difficult to monitor sales and refuse them when necessary.

The doctor's view

This is obviously a difficult problem for the pharmacist. It is inappropriate for the young woman to continue taking laxatives and she could benefit from counselling. However, a challenge from the pharmacist could result in her simply buying the laxatives elsewhere. If, as is likely, she has an eating disorder, she may have very low self-esteem and be denying her problem. Both these factors make it more difficult for the pharmacist to intervene most effectively. An ideal outcome would be appropriate referral, which would depend on local resources but which might initially be to the doctor, or she could be advised about the Beating Eating Disorders website (www.b-eat.co.uk).

If she is seen by the doctor, an empathic approach is necessary. The most important thing is to give her full opportunity to say what she thinks about the problem, how it makes her feel and how it affects her life. Establishing a supportive relationship with resultant trust between patient and doctor is the major aim of the initial consultation. Once this has been achieved, further therapeutic opportunities can be discussed and decided on together.

Case 3

A man comes into the pharmacy and asks for some good laxative tablets. Further questioning by the pharmacist reveals that the medicine is for his dad who is aged 72 years. He does not know many details except that his dad has been complaining of increasing constipation over the last 2–3 months and has tried *senna* tablets without any benefit.

The pharmacist's view

Third-party or proxy consultations are often challenging because the person making the request may not have all of the relevant information. However, in this case the decision is quite clear. The patient needs to be referred to the doctor because of the long history of the complaint and the unsuccessful use of a stimulant laxative.

The doctor's view

Referral to the GP should be recommended in this situation. A *glycerine suppository* is a safe treatment to use in the meantime. Clearly, more information is needed to make an opinion and diagnosis. A prolonged and progressive change in bowel habit is an indication for referral to hospital for further investigations as the father could have a large bowel cancer. The GP would need to gather more information about his symptoms and would perform an examination that would include abdominal palpation and a digital rectal examination. This latter examination could confirm the presence of a rectal tumour. It is likely that an urgent referral would then be made for further investigations as an outpatient. At hospital the investigations could include sigmoidoscopy plus a barium enema X-ray and/or a colonoscopy. In colonoscopy, a flexible fibre-optic tube is passed through the anus and then up and around the whole of the large bowel to the caecum.

Diarrhoea

Community pharmacists may be asked by patients to treat existing diarrhoea or to offer advice on what course of action to take should diarrhoea occur, for example, to holidaymakers. Diarrhoea is defined as an increased frequency of bowel evacuation, with the passage of abnormally soft or watery faeces. The basis of treatment is electrolyte and fluid replacement; in addition, antidiarrhoeals are useful in adults and older children.

What you need to know

Age
  Infant, child, adult, elderly
Duration
Severity
Symptoms, associated symptoms
  Nausea/vomiting
  Fever
  Abdominal cramps
  Flatulence
Other family members affected?
Previous history
Recent travel abroad?
Causative factors
Medication
  Medicines already tried
  Other medicines being taken

Significance of questions and answers

Age
  Particular care is needed in the very young and the very old. Infants (younger than 1 year) and elderly patients are especially at risk of becoming dehydrated.

Symptoms in the Pharmacy: A Guide to the Management of Common Illness, Seventh Edition.
Alison Blenkinsopp, Paul Paxton and John Blenkinsopp.
© 2014 John Wiley & Sons, Ltd. Published 2014 by John Wiley & Sons, Ltd.

Duration

Most cases of diarrhoea will be acute and self-limiting. Because of the dangers of dehydration, it would be wise to refer infants with diarrhoea of longer than 1 day's duration to the doctor.

Severity

The degree of severity of diarrhoea is related to the nature and frequency of stools. Both these aspects are important, since misunderstandings can arise, especially in self-diagnosed complaints. Elderly patients who complain of diarrhoea may, in fact, be suffering from faecal impaction. They may pass liquid stools, but with only one or two bowel movements a day.

Symptoms

Acute diarrhoea is rapid in onset and produces watery stools that are passed frequently. Abdominal cramps, flatulence and weakness or malaise may also occur. Nausea and vomiting may be associated with diarrhoea, as may fever. The pharmacist should always ask about vomiting and fever in infants; both will increase the likelihood that severe dehydration will develop. Another important question to ask about diarrhoea in infants is whether the baby has been taking milk feeds and other drinks as normal. Reduced fluid intake predisposes to dehydration.

The pharmacist should question the patient about food intake and also about whether other family members or friends are suffering from the same symptoms, since acute diarrhoea is often infective in origin. Often there are localised minor outbreaks of gastroenteritis, and the pharmacist may be asked several times for advice and treatment by different patients during a short period of time. Types of infective diarrhoea are discussed later in this chapter.

The presence of blood or mucus in the stools is an indication for referral. Diarrhoea with severe vomiting or with a high fever would also require medical advice.

Previous history

A previous history of diarrhoea or a prolonged change in bowel habit would warrant referral for further investigation and it is important that the pharmacist distinguish between acute and chronic conditions. Chronic diarrhoea (of more than 3 weeks' duration) may be caused by bowel conditions such as Crohn's disease, IBS or ulcerative colitis and requires medical advice.

Recent travel abroad

Diarrhoea in a patient who has recently travelled abroad requires referral since it might be infective in origin. Giardiasis should be considered in travellers recently returned from South America or the Far East.

Causes of diarrhoea
Infections

Most cases of diarrhoea are short lived, the bowel habit being normal before and after. In these situations, the cause is likely to be infective (viral or bacterial).

Viral　Viruses are often responsible for gastroenteritis. In infants, the virus causing such problems often gains entry into the body via the respiratory tract (rotavirus). Associated symptoms are those of a cold and perhaps a cough. The infection starts abruptly and vomiting often precedes diarrhoea. The acute phase is usually over within 2–3 days, although diarrhoea may persist. Sometimes diarrhoea returns when milk feeds are reintroduced. This is because one of the milk-digestive enzymes is temporarily inactivated. Milk therefore passes through the bowel undigested, causing diarrhoea. The health visitor or doctor would need to give further advice in such situations.

Whilst in the majority the infection is usually not too severe and is self-limiting, it should be remembered that rotavirus infection can cause death. This is most likely in those infants already malnourished and living in poor social circumstances who have not been breastfed.

Norovirus is another common cause of gastroenteritis in people of all ages. In the United Kingdom, up to 1 million people are affected each year. The virus is spread by contact with another person, contaminated food or surfaces. After an incubation of up to 48 h, the illness begins suddenly with projectile vomiting, diarrhoea and flu-like symptoms. It usually settles fairly quickly and treatment includes the usual advice of fluid replacement.

Bacterial　These are the food-borne infections previously known as food poisoning. There are several different types of bacteria that can cause such infections: *Staphylococcus*, *Campylobacter*, *Salmonella*, *Shigella*, pathogenic *Escherichia coli*, *Bacillus cereus* and *Listeria monocytogenes*. The typical symptoms include severe diarrhoea and/or vomiting, with or without abdominal pain. Two commonly seen infections are *Campylobacter* and *Salmonella*, which are often associated with contaminated poultry, although other meats have been implicated. Contaminated eggs have also been found to be a source of *Salmonella*. Kitchen hygiene and thorough cooking are of great importance in preventing infection.

Table 4 summarises the typical features of some of the following infections:

– Bacillary dysentery is caused by *Shigella*. It can occur in outbreaks where there are people living in close proximity and may occur in travellers to Africa or Asia.

– B. *cereus* is usually associated with cooked rice, especially if it has been kept warm or has been reheated. It presents with two different clinical pictures, as shown in Table 4.

– *E. coli* infections are less common but can be severe with toxins being released into the body, which can cause kidney failure.

– *L. monocytogenes* can cause gastroenteritis or a flu-like illness. On occasion it can be more severe and cause septicaemia or meningitis, with a significant mortality rate. Pregnant women are more susceptible to it but it is still a rare infection occurring in 1 in 20 000 pregnancies. Infection during pregnancy can cause miscarriage, stillbirth or an infection of the newborn. Foods to be avoided during pregnancy include unpasteurised cheese, soft ripe cheeses, blue-veined cheeses, pates, cold cuts of meat and smoked fish. Care needs to be taken with the storage and handling of chilled ready-to-eat food in the home. Pregnant women with diarrhoea or fever should be referred immediately to their midwife or GP.

Antibiotics are generally unnecessary as most food-borne infections resolve spontaneously. The most important treatment is adequate fluid replacement. Antibiotics are used for *Shigella* infections and the more severe *Salmonella* or *Campylobacter* ones. *Ciprofloxacin* may be used in such circumstances.

– *Protozoan* infections are uncommon in Western Europe but may occur in travellers from further afield. Examples include *Entamoeba histolytica* (amoebic dysentery) and *Giardia lamblia* (giardiasis). Diagnosis is made by sending stool samples to the laboratory.

Chronic diarrhoea

Recurrent or persistent diarrhoea may be due to an irritable bowel or, more seriously, a bowel tumour, an inflammation of the bowel (e.g. ulcerative colitis or Crohn's disease), an inability to digest or absorb

Table 4 Features of some infections causing diarrhoea.

Infection	Incubation	Duration	Symptoms
Staphylococcus	2–6 h	6–24 h	Severe, short lived; especially vomiting
Salmonella	12–24 h	1–7 days	Mainly diarrhoea
Campylobacter	2–7 days	2–7 days	Diarrhoea with abdominal colic
B. *cereus*	1–5 h	6–24 h	Vomiting
B. *cereus* (two types of infection)	8–16 h	12–24 h	Diarrhoea
L. monocytogenes	3–70 days		Flu-like, diarrhoea

food (malabsorption, e.g. coeliac disease) or diverticular disease of the colon.

Irritable bowel syndrome (see p. 124) This non-serious, but troublesome condition is one of the more common causes of recurrent bowel dysfunction in adolescents and young adults. The patient usually describes the frequent passage of small volumes of stool rather than true diarrhoea. The stools are typically variable in nature, often loose and semi-formed. They may be described as being like rabbit droppings or pencil shaped. The frequency of bowel action is also variable as the diarrhoea may alternate with constipation. Often the bowels are open several times in the morning before the patient leaves for work. The condition is more likely to occur at times of stress, it may be associated with anxiety and, occasionally, it may be triggered by a bowel infection. Inadequate or insoluble dietary fibre may also be of significance. It is possible that certain foods can irritate the bowel, but this may be difficult to prove.

There is no blood present within the motion in an irritable bowel. Bloody diarrhoea may be a result of an inflammation or tumour of the bowel, and always requires urgent referral. The latter is more likely with increasing age (from middle age onwards) and is likely to be associated with a prolonged change in bowel habit; in this case, diarrhoea might sometimes alternate with constipation.

Medication
Medicines already tried
The pharmacist should establish the identity of any medication that has already been taken to treat the symptoms in order to assess its appropriateness.

Other medicines being taken
Details of any other medication being taken (both OTC and prescribed) are also needed, as the diarrhoea may be drug induced (Table 5). OTC

Table 5 Some drugs that may cause diarrhoea.

Antacids: *Magnesium salts*
Antibiotics
Antihypertensives: *methyldopa*; beta-blockers (rare)
Digoxin (toxic levels)
Diuretics (*furosemide*)
Iron preparations
Laxatives
Misoprostol
Non-steroidal anti-inflammatory drugs
Selective serotonin reuptake inhibitors

medicines should be considered; commonly used medicines such as magnesium-containing antacids and iron preparations are examples of medicines that may induce diarrhoea. Laxative abuse should be considered as a possible cause.

When to refer

Diarrhoea of greater than
1 day's duration in children younger than 1 year
2 days' duration in children under 3 years and elderly patients
3 days' duration in older children and adults
   Association with severe vomiting and fever
   Recent travel abroad
   Suspected drug-induced reaction to prescribed medicine
   History of change in bowel habit
   Presence of blood or mucus in the stools
   Pregnancy

Treatment timescale

One day in children; otherwise two days.

Management

Oral rehydration therapy

The risk of dehydration from diarrhoea is greatest in babies, and rehydration therapy is considered to be the standard treatment for acute diarrhoea in babies and young children. Oral rehydration sachets may be used with antidiarrhoeals in older children and adults.

Rehydration may still be initiated even if referral to the doctor is advised. Sachets of powder for reconstitution are available; these contain sodium as chloride and bicarbonate, along with glucose and potassium. The absorption of sodium is facilitated in the presence of glucose. A variety of flavours are available.

It is essential that appropriate advice be given by the pharmacist about how the powder should be reconstituted. Patients should be reminded that only water should be used to make the solution (never fruit or fizzy drinks) and that boiled and cooled water should be used for children younger than 1 year. Boiling water should not be used, as it would cause the liberation of carbon dioxide. The solution can be kept for 24 h if stored in a refrigerator. Fizzy, sugary drinks should never be used to make rehydration fluids, as they will produce a hyperosmolar solution that may exacerbate the problem. The sodium content of such drinks, as well as the glucose content, may be high.

Table 6 Amount of rehydration solution to be offered to patients.

Age	Quantity of solution (per watery stool)
Under 1 year	50 mL (quarter of a glass)
1–5 years	100 mL (half a glass)
6–12 years	200 mL (one glass)
Adult	400 mL (two glasses)

Home-made salt and sugar solutions should not be recommended, since the accuracy of electrolyte content cannot be guaranteed, and this accuracy is essential, especially in infants, young children and elderly patients. Special measuring spoons are available; their correct use would produce a more acceptable solution, but their use should be reserved for the treatment of adults, where electrolyte concentration is less crucial.

Quantities

Parents sometimes ask how much rehydration fluid should be given to children. The following simple rules can be used for guidance; the amount of solution offered to the patient is based on the number of watery stools that are passed. Table 6 provides the volumes required per watery stool.

Other therapy

Loperamide

Loperamide is an effective antidiarrhoeal treatment for use in older children and adults. When recommending *loperamide* the pharmacist should remind patients to drink plenty of extra fluids. Oral rehydration sachets may be recommended. *Loperamide* may not be recommended for use in children under 12 years.

Diphenoxylate/atropine (Co-phenotrope)

Co-phenotrope can be used as an adjunct to rehydration to treat diarrhoea in those aged 16 years and over.

Kaolin

Kaolin has been used as a traditional remedy for diarrhoea for many years. Its use was justified on the theoretical grounds that it would absorb water in the GI tract and would absorb toxins and bacteria onto its surface, thus removing them from the gut. The latter has not been shown to be true and the usefulness of the former is questionable. The use of *kaolin*-based preparations has largely been superseded by oral rehydration therapy, although patients continue to ask for various products containing *kaolin*.

Morphine

Morphine, in various forms, has been included in antidiarrhoeal remedies for many years. The theoretical basis for its inclusion is that *morphine*, together with other narcotic drugs such as *codeine*, is known to slow the action of the GI tract; indeed, constipation is a well-recognised side effect of such drugs. However, at the doses included in most OTC preparations, it is unlikely that such an effect would be produced. *Kaolin* and *morphine* mixture remains a popular choice for some patients, despite the lack of evidence of its effectiveness.

Probiotics

A systematic review concluded that, when used with rehydration, probiotics appear to reduce stool frequency and shorten the duration of infectious diarrhoea. Many of the studies were in otherwise healthy people and the researchers also concluded that more research is needed before recommendations could be made to guide the use of probiotics.

Practical points

1 Patients with diarrhoea should be advised to drink plenty of clear, non-milky fluids, such as water and diluted squash.

2 National Health Service (NHS) Clinical Knowledge Summaries (CKS) say that the patient can be advised to continue their usual diet but that fatty foods and foods with a high sugar content might be best avoided as they may not be well tolerated.

3 Breast- or bottle-feeding should be continued in infants. The severity and duration of diarrhoea are not affected by whether milk feeds are continued. A well-nourished child should be the aim, particularly where the infant is poorly nourished to begin with and where the withholding of milk feeds may be more detrimental than in a well-nourished infant, where temporary withdrawal is unimportant. Some doctors continue nevertheless to advise the discontinuation of milk, especially bottle, during the acute phase of infection.

Diarrhoea in practice

Case 1

Mrs Robinson asks what you can recommend for diarrhoea. Her son David, aged 11 years, has diarrhoea and she is worried that her other two children, Natalie, aged 4 years, and Tom, aged just over 1 year, may also get it. David's diarrhoea started yesterday; he went to the toilet about five times and was sick once, but has not been sick since. He has griping pains, but is generally well and quite lively. Yesterday he had pie and chips from the local takeaway during his lunch break at school. No one else in the family ate the same food. Mrs Robinson has not given him any medicine.

The pharmacist's view

It sounds as if David has a bout of acute diarrhoea, possibly caused by the food he ate yesterday during lunchtime. He has vomited once, but now the diarrhoea is the problem. The child is otherwise well. He is 11 years old, so the best plan would be to start oral rehydration with some proprietary sachets, with advice to his mother about how they should be reconstituted. If either or both the other children get diarrhoea, they can also be given some rehydration solution. David should see the doctor the day after tomorrow if his condition has not improved.

The doctor's view

David's diarrhoea could well be due to food poisoning. Oral rehydration is the correct treatment. He should also be told not to eat anything for the next 24 h or so until the diarrhoea has settled. If he wants to drink other fluids in addition to the electrolyte mixture, he should be told to avoid milk.

His symptoms should settle down over the next few hours. If they persist or he complains of worsening abdominal pain, particularly in the lower right side of the abdomen, his mother should contact the doctor. An atypical acute appendicitis may present with symptoms of a bowel infection.

Case 2

Mrs Choudry is collecting her regular repeat prescription for antihypertensive treatment. You ask how she and the family are, and she tells you that several members of the family have been suffering with diarrhoea on and off. You know that the family recently returned from a trip to India where they had been visiting relatives to attend a family wedding. In answer to your questions, Mrs Choudry tells you that the problem with the diarrhoea started after they returned.

The pharmacist's view

Referral to the GP is needed here as the diarrhoea may be related to the recent travel.

The doctor's view

Referral is a sensible course of action. Clearly, more information is required, for example, the date of onset of symptoms and the date of return to the United Kingdom. It does not sound as if any of the family are acutely ill but it would be necessary to ensure that no one is dehydrated. If the diarrhoea is persisting, it would be helpful to send stool samples to the local public health laboratory for analysis. It is possible that they may be suffering from giardiasis, which can be treated with *metronidazole*. Sometimes stool samples come back showing no signs of infection, in which case the diarrhoea is considered as being due to postinfection irritability of the bowel. This usually resolves spontaneously with no specific treatment.

Case 3

Mrs Jean Berry wants to stock up on some medicines before her family sets off on their first holiday abroad; they will be going to Spain next week. Mrs Berry tells you that she has heard of people whose holidays have been ruined by holiday diarrhoea and she wants you to recommend a good treatment. On questioning, you find out that Mr and Mrs Berry and their two boys aged 10 and 14 years will be going on the holiday.

The pharmacist's view

Holiday diarrhoea can often easily be dealt with. Mrs Berry could be advised to buy some *loperamide* capsules, which would be suitable treatment for her, Mr Berry and their 14-year-old son. In addition, she should purchase some oral rehydration sachets for the younger son. The sachets could also be used by other family members.

The pharmacist could also give some valuable advice about the avoidance of potential problems by the Berry family on their first foreign holiday. Fresh fruit should be peeled before eating and hot food should not be eaten other than in restaurants. Roadside snack stalls are best avoided. The question of the quality of drinking water often crops up. Good advice to travellers would be to check with the tour company representative as to the advisability of drinking local water. If in doubt, bottled mineral water can be drunk; such water (still rather than sparkling) could also be used to reconstitute rehydration sachets. Ice in drinks may be best avoided, depending on the water supply.

Holiday diarrhoea is usually self-limiting, but if it is still present after several days, medical advice should be sought. If the diarrhoea persists or is recurrent after returning home, the doctor should be seen. Finally, patients would be well advised to be wary of buying OTC medicines abroad. In some countries, a large range of drugs including oral steroids and antibiotics can be purchased OTC. Each year, patients return to Britain with serious adverse effects following the use of oral *chloramphenicol*, for example, which has been prescribed or purchased.

The doctor's view

The pharmacist has covered all the important points. The most likely cause of diarrhoea would be contaminated food or water. The best treatment of acute diarrhoea is to stop eating and to drink bottled mineral water (with or without electrolyte reconstitution powders). It would be sensible to take an antidiarrhoeal such as *loperamide*.

Case 4

Mr Radcliffe is an elderly man who lives alone. Today, his home help asks what you can recommend for diarrhoea, from which Mr Radcliffe has been suffering for 3 days. He has been passing watery stools quite frequently and feels rather tired and weak. He has sent the home help because he dare not leave the house and go out of reach of the toilet. You check your patient medication records (PMRs), which confirm your memory that he takes several different medicines: *digoxin*, *furosemide* and *paracetamol*. Last week you dispensed a prescription for a course of *amoxicillin*. The home help tells you that he has been eating his usual diet and there does not seem to be a link between food and his symptoms.

The pharmacist's view

Mr Radcliffe's diarrhoea may be due to the *amoxicillin*, which he started to take a few days ago. It would be best to call the patient's doctor to discuss the appropriate course of action because Mr Radcliffe's other drug therapy means that fluid loss and dehydration may cause electrolyte imbalance and put him at further risk. The doctor may decide to stop the *amoxicillin*.

The doctor's view

It is likely that the *amoxicillin* has caused the diarrhoea. The most important consideration in management is to ensure adequate fluid and electrolyte replacement. This is particularly so as the elderly (and babies) are not as resilient to the effects of dehydration. In Mr Radcliffe's case, things are further complicated by his other medication: *furosemide* and *digoxin*. He is not on any potassium supplement or a potassium-sparing diuretic. Although there may be good reason for this, diuretics such as *furosemide* can lower the plasma potassium level and make *digoxin* dangerously toxic. Unfortunately, potassium can also be lost in diarrhoea, further aggravating this problem. It is therefore reasonable to ask for the doctor to visit and assess.

There is also a possibility that the diarrhoea could be due to a bacterium (*Clostridium difficile*) in the colon. It is thought that antibiotics (Mr Radcliffe was given *amoxicillin*) upset the normal bowel flora allowing *C. difficile* to flourish. This condition can be caused by most antibiotics, but has been reported most often with *clindamycin*, *ampicillin*, *amoxicillin* and the cephalosporins. The condition is more likely to occur in those over the age of 65 years. It is now most commonly seen in hospitals where it is thought that the infection is spread by health workers.

The diarrhoea of a C. *difficile* infection can range from mild self-limiting symptoms to severe protracted or recurrent episodes and can sometimes be fatal. There is often a low-grade fever, and abdominal pain/cramps may occur. The symptoms usually begin within 1 week of starting antibiotic treatment but may start up to 6 weeks after a course of antibiotics. It is sometimes necessary to treat severe cases with *metronidazole* or *vancomycin*.

Irritable bowel syndrome

Irritable bowel syndrome is defined as a chronic, functional bowel disorder in which abdominal pain is associated with intermittent diarrhoea, sometimes alternating with constipation, and a feeling of abdominal distension. IBS is estimated to affect 20% of adults in the industrialised world, most of whom (up to three quarters) do not consult a doctor. More women with IBS consult a health professional than do men and the incidence of the condition appears to be higher in women. The cause is unknown. IBS can sometimes develop after a bout of gastroenteritis. It often seems to be triggered by stress, and many IBS sufferers have symptoms of anxiety and depression. Some sufferers have food intolerances which trigger their symptoms.

What you need to know

Age
  Child, adult
Symptoms
  GastrointestinalAbdominal pain
  Abdominal distension/bloating
  Disturbed bowel habit; diarrhoea and/or constipation
  Nausea
Other symptoms
  Urinary symptoms, especially frequency
  Dyspareunia (pain during intercourse)

Significance of questions and answers

Age
Because of the difficulties in diagnosis of abdominal pain in children, it is best to refer.

IBS usually develops in young adult life. If an older adult is presenting for the first time with no previous history of bowel problems, a referral should be made.

Symptoms in the Pharmacy: A Guide to the Management of Common Illness, Seventh Edition.
Alison Blenkinsopp, Paul Paxton and John Blenkinsopp.
© 2014 John Wiley & Sons, Ltd. Published 2014 by John Wiley & Sons, Ltd.

Symptoms

IBS has three key symptoms: abdominal pain (which may ease following a bowel movement), abdominal distension/bloating and disturbance of bowel habit.

Abdominal pain

The pain can occur anywhere in the abdomen. It is often central or left sided and can be severe. When pain occurs in the upper abdomen, it can be confused with peptic ulcer or gall bladder pain. The site of pain can vary from person to person and even for an individual. Sometimes the pain comes on after eating and can be relieved by defaecation.

Bloating

A sensation of bloating is commonly reported. Sometimes it is so severe that clothes have to be loosened.

Bowel habit

Diarrhoea and constipation may occur; sometimes they alternate. A morning rush is common, where the patient feels an urgent desire to defaecate several times after getting up in the morning and following breakfast, after which the bowels may settle. There may be a feeling of incomplete emptying after a bowel movement. The motion is often described as loose and semi-formed rather than watery. Sometimes it is like pellets or rabbit droppings, or pencil shaped. There may be mucus present but never blood.

Other symptoms

Nausea sometimes occurs; vomiting is less common.

Patients may also complain of apparently unrelated symptoms such as backache, feeling lethargic and tired. Urinary symptoms may be associated with IBS, for example, frequency, urgency and nocturia (the need to pass urine during the night). Some women report dyspareunia.

Duration

Patients may present when the first symptoms occur or may describe a pattern of symptoms, which has been going on for months or even years. If an older person is presenting for the first time, referral is most appropriate.

Previous history

You need to know whether the patient has consulted his/her doctor about the symptoms and, if so, what they were told. A history of travel abroad and gastroenteritis sometimes appears to trigger an irritable bowel. Referral is necessary to exclude an unresolved infection. Any history of previous bowel surgery would suggest a need for referral.

Aggravating factors

Stress appears to play an important role and can precipitate and exacerbate symptoms.

Caffeine often worsens symptoms and its stimulant effect on the bowel and irritant effect on the stomach are well known in any case.

The sweeteners sorbitol and fructose have also been reported to aggravate IBS. Other foods that have been implicated are milk and dairy products, chocolate, onions, garlic, chives and leeks.

Medication

The patient may already have tried prescribed or OTC medicines to treat the condition. You need to know what has been tried and whether it produced any improvement. It is also important to know what other medicines the patient is taking. In many patients, IBS is associated with anxiety and depression, but it is not known whether this is cause or effect.

When to refer
Children
Older person with no previous history of IBS
Pregnant women
Blood in stools
Unexplained weight loss
Caution in patients aged over 45 years with changed bowel habit
Signs of bowel obstruction
Unresponsive to appropriate treatment

Treatment timescale

Symptoms should start to improve within 1 week.

Management

Antispasmodics

Antispasmodics are the mainstay of OTC treatment of IBS, and research trials show some improvement in abdominal pain with smooth muscle relaxants. *Alverine citrate, peppermint, mebeverine* and *hyoscine* are used. They work by a direct effect on the smooth muscle of the gut, causing relaxation and thus reducing abdominal pain. The patient should see an improvement within a few days of starting treatment and should be asked to return to you in 1 week, so you can monitor progress. It is worth trying a different antispasmodic if the first has not worked. Side effects from antispasmodics are rare.

All antispasmodics are contraindicated in paralytic ileus, a serious condition that fortunately occurs only rarely (e.g. after abdominal operations and in peritonitis). Here the gut is not functioning and is obstructed. The symptoms would be severe pain, no bowel movements and possibly vomiting of partly digested food. Immediate referral is needed.

Alverine citrate

Alverine citrate is given in a dose of 60–120 mg (one or two capsules) up to three times a day. Remind the patient to take the capsules with water and not to chew them. Side effects are rare, but nausea, dizziness, pruritus, rash and headache have occasionally been reported. The drug should not be recommended for pregnant or breastfeeding women or for children. *Alverine citrate* is also available in a combination product with *sterculia* (see 'Bulking agents' below).

Peppermint oil

Peppermint oil has been used for many years as an aid to digestion and has an antispasmodic effect. Capsules containing 0.2 mL of the oil are taken in a dose of one or two capsules three times a day, 15–30 min before meals. They are enteric coated, with the intention that the *peppermint oil* is delivered beyond the stomach and upper small bowel. Patients should be reminded not to chew the capsules as not only will this render the treatment ineffective, it will also cause irritation of the mouth and oesophagus.

This treatment should not be recommended for children. Occasionally, *peppermint oil* causes heartburn and so is best avoided in patients who already suffer from this problem. Allergic reactions can occur and are rare; rash, headache and muscle tremor have been reported in such cases. One trial involving 110 people showed improvement in symptoms of abdominal pain, distension and stool frequency.

Mebeverine hydrochloride

Mebeverine hydrochloride is used at a dose of 135 mg three times a day. The dose should be taken 20 min before meals. The drug should not be recommended for pregnant or breastfeeding women, for children under 10 or for patients with porphyria.

Hyoscine

Hyoscine butylbromide 10 mg tablets can be used in adults and children aged over 6. On starting treatment, adults should take one tablet three times a day, increasing if necessary to two tablets four times a day. The anticholinergic effects of hyoscine may intensify those of other anticholinergics by increasing anticholinergic load.

Bulking agents

Traditionally, patients with IBS were told to eat a diet high in fibre, and raw wheat bran was often recommended as a way of increasing the fibre intake. Bran is no longer recommended in IBS (see 'Practical points: Diet'). Bulking agents such as ispaghula containing soluble fibre can help some patients. It may take a few weeks of experimentation to find the dose that suits the individual patient. Remind the patient to increase fluid intake to take account of the additional fibre. Bulking agents are also available in combination with antispasmodics. The evidence for benefit is not strong, as studies have involved small numbers of patients. Possible positive benefit has been shown for ispaghula husk.

Antidiarrhoeals

Patients who complain of diarrhoea may be describing a frequent urge to pass stools, but the stools may be loose and formed rather than watery. Use of OTC antidiarrhoeals such as *loperamide* is appropriate only on an occasional, short-term basis. In two studies involving a total of 100 patients, *loperamide* improved diarrhoea, including frequency of bowel movements, but not abdominal pain or distension.

Practical points
Diet

Patients with IBS should follow the recommendations for a healthy (low-fat, low-sugar, high-fibre) diet.

Foods that contain soluble fibre include:

- oats
- barley
- rye
- fruit, such as bananas and apples
- root vegetables, such as carrots and potatoes
- golden linseeds

Foods that contain insoluble fibre include:

- wholegrain bread
- bran
- cereals
- nuts and seeds (except golden linseeds)

Patients who have IBS with diarrhoea may find it helpful to eat less insoluble fibre and to avoid the skin, pith and pips from fruit and vegetables. Patients who have IBS with constipation can try increasing the amount of soluble fibre and the amount of water drunk.

Bran (which contains insoluble fibre) used to be widely recommended but it tends to ferment in the bowel and can lead to feelings of bloating and discomfort, and can make symptoms worse.

Some patients find that excluding foods which they know exacerbate their symptoms is helpful (see 'Aggravating factors' above). The sweeteners sorbitol and fructose can make symptoms worse and they are found in many foods the patient needs to check labels at the supermarket. Cutting out caffeine, milk and dairy products and chocolate may be worth trying. Although some patients benefit from the withdrawal of milk and dairy products, there is no evidence of lactase deficiency in IBS. Remind patients that caffeine is included in many soft drinks and so they should check labels.

Complementary therapies

Some patients find relaxation techniques helpful. Videos and audio tapes are available to teach complementary therapies.

Studies have shown that hypnotherapy is of benefit in IBS. If patients want to try this, they should consult a registered hypnotherapist. Others may benefit from traditional acupuncture, reflexology, aromatherapy or homoeopathy.

Irritable bowel syndrome in practice

Case 1

Joanna Mathers is a 29-year-old woman who asks to speak to the pharmacist. She has seen an advertisement for an antispasmodic for IBS and wonders whether she should try it. On questioning, she tells you that she has been getting stomach pains and bowel symptoms for several months, two or three times a month. She thinks her symptoms seem to be associated with business lunches and dinners at important meetings and include abdominal pain, a feeling of abdominal fullness, diarrhoea, nausea and sometimes vomiting. In answer to your specific question about morning symptoms, Joanna says that sometimes she feels the need to go to the toilet first thing in the morning and may have to go several times. Sometimes she has been late for work because she felt she could not leave the house due to the diarrhoea. Joanna tells you that she works as a marketing executive and that her job is pressurised and stressful when there are big deadlines or client meetings. Joanna drinks six or seven cups of coffee a day and says her diet is 'whatever I can get at work and something from the freezer when I get home'. She is not taking any other medicines and has not been to the doctor about her problems as she did not want to bother him.

The pharmacist's view

The picture that has emerged indicates IBS. She has the key symptoms and there is a link to stress at work. It would be worth trying an antispasmodic (*alverine*, *peppermint oil*, *mebeverine* or *hyoscine*) for 1 week and asking Joanna to come back at the end of that time. She also needs a careful explanation of aggravating factors for IBS and might want to try a gradual reduction in her intake of coffee over the next few days. If there is no improvement, a different antispasmodic could be tried for a further week, with referral then if needed.

The doctor's view

Joanna gives a clear history of IBS. Her symptoms are likely to settle with the pharmacist's advice and treatment. There is up to a 60% placebo response rate in IBS sufferers, so it would be surprising if she did not improve when next reviewed. If there were no improvement, then a referral would be sensible. A referral would give her doctor an opportunity to deal with her concerns about what was wrong, confirm the diagnosis and give her an appropriate explanation of IBS. She could also be given some time to consider how she might tackle her work pressures. Plenty of information is available on the web, which she could be advised to look at, for example, NHS Choices.

Case 2

Jane Dawson asks to see the pharmacist. She is in her early 20s and says she has been getting some upper abdominal pain after food. She wants to try a stomach medicine. On further questioning, she says that she has had an irritable bowel before but this is different, although she does admit that her bowels have been troublesome recently and she has noticed some urinary frequency. Jane says that she has been constipated and felt bloated. She says that she went to her doctor last year and was told she had IBS. The doctor said it was all due to stress, which had upset her. Over the last year, she has started a new job and moved into new accommodation. She eats a healthy diet and exercises regularly.

The pharmacist's view

The history here is not straightforward and although Jane's symptoms are indicative of IBS, which she says she has had before, the symptoms are different on this occasion. The best course of action is to refer her to the doctor for further investigation.

The doctor's view

Jane probably has IBS but there is insufficient information so far to make that diagnosis. It is not uncommon to have upper abdominal pain with IBS, but other possibilities need to be considered. It sounds as though Jane thinks it is coming from her stomach. She may fear that she has an ulcer. She also mentions urinary frequency, which may well be associated with IBS but could be a urinary infection. A referral to her doctor is sensible to make a complete assessment of her symptoms. It is likely that the assessment would just involve listening to her description of her problem, gathering more information and a brief examination of her abdomen. A urine sample would show whether or not she had a urinary infection. If there was still doubt about the diagnosis, a referral to a gastroenterologist at the local hospital could be made. Between 20% and 50% of referrals to gastroenterologists turn out to be due to IBS. The main purpose of referral is for a diagnosis.

If the doctor thinks Jane has IBS, an explanation of the syndrome would be helpful in addition to dealing with her concerns about a stomach ulcer. Whether or not psychological factors cause IBS, there is no doubt that the stresses of life can aggravate symptoms. It therefore makes sense to help sufferers to make this connection, so they can consider different ways of dealing with stress.

Often the above approach is an effective treatment in itself. However, if Jane did want some medication, a bulk bowel regulator to help her constipation plus some antispasmodic tablets would be of value.

Haemorrhoids

Haemorrhoids (commonly known as piles) can produce symptoms of itching, burning, pain, swelling and discomfort in the perianal area and anal canal and rectal bleeding. Haemorrhoids are swollen veins, rather like varicose veins, which protrude into the anal canal (internal piles). They may swell so much that they hang down outside the anus (external piles). Haemorrhoids are often caused or exacerbated by inadequate dietary fibre or fluid intake. The pharmacist must, by careful questioning, differentiate between this minor condition and others that may be potentially more serious.

What you need to know

Duration and previous history
Symptoms
    Itching, burning
    Soreness
    Swelling
    Pain
    Blood in stools
    Constipation
    Bowel habit
    Pregnancy
Other symptoms
    Abdominal pain/vomiting
    Weight loss
    Medication

Significance of questions and answers

Duration and previous history

As an arbitrary guide, the pharmacist might consider treating haemorrhoids of up to 3 weeks' duration. It would be useful to establish whether the patient has a previous history of haemorrhoids and if the doctor has been seen about the problem. A recent examination by

Symptoms in the Pharmacy: A Guide to the Management of Common Illness, Seventh Edition.
Alison Blenkinsopp, Paul Paxton and John Blenkinsopp.
© 2014 John Wiley & Sons, Ltd. Published 2014 by John Wiley & Sons, Ltd.

the doctor that has excluded serious symptoms would indicate that treatment of symptoms by the pharmacist would be appropriate.

Symptoms

The term haemorrhoids includes internal and external piles, which can be further classified as (1) those which are confined to the anal canal and cannot be seen, (2) those which prolapse through the anal sphincter on defaecation and then reduce by themselves or are pushed back through the sphincter after defaecation by the patient and (3) those which remain persistently prolapsed and outside the anal canal. These three types are sometimes referred to as first, second and third degree, respectively. Predisposing factors for haemorrhoids include diet, sedentary occupation and pregnancy and there is thought to be a genetic element.

Pain

Pain is not always present; if it is, it may take the form of a dull ache and may be worse when the patient is having a bowel movement. A severe, sharp pain on defaecation may indicate the presence of an anal fissure, which can have an associated sentinel pile (a small skin tag at the posterior margin of the anus) and requires referral. A fissure is a minute tear in the skin of the anal canal. It is usually caused by constipation and can often be managed conservatively by correcting this and using a local anaesthetic-containing cream or gel. In severe cases a minor operation is sometimes necessary.

Irritation

The most troublesome symptom for many patients is itching and irritation of the perianal area rather than pain. Persistent or recurrent irritation, which does not improve, is sometimes associated with rectal cancer and should be referred.

Bleeding

Blood may be deposited onto the stool from internal haemorrhoids as the stool passes through the anal canal. This fresh blood will appear bright red. It is typically described as being splashed around the toilet pan and may be seen on the surface of the stool or on the toilet paper. If blood is mixed with the stool, it must have come from higher up the GI tract and will be dark in colour (altered blood). If rectal bleeding is present, the pharmacist would be well advised to suggest that the patient see the doctor so that an examination can be performed to exclude more serious pathology such as tumour or polyps. Colorectal cancer can cause rectal bleeding. The disease is unusual in patients under 50 and the pharmacist should be alert for the middle-aged patient with rectal bleeding. This is particularly so if there has been a significant and sustained alteration in bowel habit.

Constipation

Constipation is a common causatory or exacerbatory factor in haemorrhoids. Insufficient dietary fibre and inadequate fluid intake may be involved, and the pharmacist should also consider the possibility of drug-induced constipation.

Straining at stool will occur if the patient is constipated; this increases the pressure in the haemorrhoidal blood vessels in the anal canal and haemorrhoids may result. If piles are painful, the patient may try to avoid defaecation and ignoring the call to open the bowels will make the constipation worse.

Bowel habit

A persisting change in bowel habit is an indication for referral, as it may be caused by a bowel cancer. Seepage of faecal material through the anal sphincter (one form of faecal incontinence) can produce irritation and itching of the perianal area and may be caused by the presence of a tumour.

Pregnancy

Pregnant women have a higher incidence of haemorrhoids than non-pregnant women. This is thought to be due to pressure on the haemorrhoidal vessels due to the gravid uterus. Constipation in pregnancy is also a common problem because raised progesterone levels mean that the gut muscles tend to be more relaxed. Such constipation can exacerbate symptoms of haemorrhoids. Appropriate dietary advice can be offered by the pharmacist (see the chapter on 'Women's health').

Other symptoms

Symptoms of haemorrhoids remain local to the anus. They do not cause abdominal pain, distension or vomiting. Any of these more widespread symptoms suggest other problems and require referral.

Tenesmus (the desire to defaecate when there is no stool present in the rectum) sometimes occurs when there is a tumour in the rectum. The patient may describe a feeling of often wanting to pass a motion but no faeces being present. This symptom requires urgent referral.

Medication

Patients may already have tried one or more proprietary preparations to treat their symptoms. Some of these products are advertised widely, since the problem of haemorrhoids is perceived as potentially embarrassing and such advertisements may sometimes discourage patients from describing their symptoms. It is therefore important for the pharmacist to identify the exact nature of the symptoms being experienced and details of any products used already. If the patient is constipated, the use of any laxatives should be established.

Present medication

Haemorrhoids may be exacerbated by drug-induced constipation and the patient should be carefully questioned about current medication, including prescription and OTC medicines. A list of drugs that may cause constipation can be found on p. 105. Rectal bleeding in a patient taking *warfarin* or another anticoagulant is an indication for referral.

When to refer

Duration of longer than 3 weeks
Presence of blood in the stools
Change in bowel habit (persisting alteration from normal bowel habit)
Suspected drug-induced constipation
Associated abdominal pain/vomiting

Treatment timescale

If symptoms have not improved after 1 week, patients should see their doctor.

Management

Symptomatic treatment of haemorrhoids can provide relief from discomfort but, if present, the underlying cause of constipation must also be addressed. The pharmacist is in a good position to offer dietary advice, in addition to treatment, to prevent the recurrence of symptoms in the future.

Local anaesthetics (e.g. benzocaine and lidocaine (lignocaine))

Local anaesthetics can help to reduce the pain and itching associated with haemorrhoids. There is a possibility that local anaesthetics may cause sensitisation and their use is best limited to a maximum of 2 weeks.

Skin protectors

Many antihaemorrhoidal products are bland, soothing preparations containing skin protectors (e.g. *zinc oxide* and *kaolin*). These products have emollient and protective properties. Protection of the perianal skin is important, because the presence of faecal matter can cause symptoms such as irritation and itching. Protecting agents form a barrier on the skin surface, helping to prevent irritation and loss of moisture from the skin.

Topical steroids

Ointment and suppositories containing *hydrocortisone* with skin protectors are available. The steroid reduces inflammation and swelling to give relief from itching and pain. The treatment should be used each morning and at night and after a bowel movement. The use of such products is restricted to those over 18. Treatment should not be used continuously for longer than 7 days.

Astringents

Astringents such as zinc oxide, hamamelis (witch hazel) and *bismuth salts* are included in products on the theoretical basis that they will cause precipitation of proteins when applied to mucous membranes or skin which is broken or damaged. A protective layer is then thought to be formed, helping to relieve irritation and inflammation. Some astringents also have a protective and mild antiseptic action (e.g. *bismuth*).

Antiseptics

These are among the ingredients of many antihaemorrhoidal products, including medicated toilet tissues. They do not have a specific action in the treatment of haemorrhoids. *Resorcinol* has antiseptic, antipruritic and exfoliative properties. The exfoliative action is thought to be useful by removing the top layer of skin cells and aiding penetration of medicaments into the skin. *Resorcinol* can be absorbed systemically via broken skin if there is prolonged use and its antithyroid action can lead to the development of myxoedema (hypothyroidism).

Counterirritants

Counterirritants such as *menthol* are sometimes included in antihaemorrhoidal products on the basis that their stimulation of nerve endings gives a sensation of cooling and tingling, which distracts from the sensation of pain. *Menthol* and *phenol* also have antipruritic actions.

Shark liver oil/live yeast

These agents are said to promote healing and tissue repair, but there is no scientific evidence to support such claims.

Laxatives

The short-term use of a laxative to relieve constipation might be considered. A stimulant laxative (e.g. *senna*) could be supplied for 1 or 2 days to help deal with the immediate problem while dietary fibre and fluids are being increased. For patients who cannot or choose not to adapt their diet, bulk laxatives may be used long term.

Practical points

Self-diagnosis

Patients may say that they have piles, or think they have piles, but careful questioning by the pharmacist is needed to check whether this self-diagnosis is correct. If there is any doubt, referral is the best course of action.

Hygiene

The itching of haemorrhoids can often be improved by good anal hygiene, since the presence of small amounts of faecal matter can cause itching. The perianal area should be washed with warm water as frequently as is practicable, ideally after each bowel movement. Soap will tend to dry the skin and could make itching worse, but a mild soap could be tried if the patient wishes to do so. Moist toilet tissues are available and these can be very useful where washing is not practical, for example, at work during the daytime, and some patients prefer them. These tissues are better used with a patting rather than a rubbing motion, which might aggravate symptoms. Many people with haemorrhoids find that a warm bath soothes their discomfort.

An increased intake of dietary fibre will increase bowel output, so patients should be advised to take care in wiping the perianal area and to use soft toilet paper to avoid soreness after wiping.

How to use OTC products

Ointments and creams can be used for internal and external haemorrhoids and should be applied in the morning, at night and after each bowel movement. An applicator is included in packs of ointments and creams and patients should be advised to take care in its use, to avoid any further damage to the perianal skin.

Suppositories can be recommended for internal haemorrhoids. After removing the foil or plastic packaging (patients have been known to try and insert them with the packaging left on), a suppository should be inserted in the morning, at night and after bowel movements. Insertion is easier if the patient is crouching or lying down.

Haemorrhoids in practice

Case 1

Tom Harris, a customer whom you know quite well, asks if you can recommend something for his usual problem. You ask him to tell you more about it: Mr Harris suffers from piles occasionally; you have dispensed prescriptions for Anusol HC and similar products in the past and have previously advised him about dietary fibre and fluid intake. He has been away on holiday for 2 weeks and says he has not been eating the same foods he does when at home. His symptoms are itching and irritation of the perianal area but no pain and he has a small swelling, which hangs down from the anus after he has passed a motion, but which he is able to push back again. He is a little constipated, but he is not taking any medicines.

The pharmacist's view

Mr Harris has a previous history of haemorrhoids, which have been diagnosed and treated by his doctor. It is likely that his holiday and temporary change in diet have caused a recurrence of the problem, so he now has a second-degree pile, and it would be reasonable to suggest symptomatic treatment for a few days. You could recommend the use of an ointment preparation containing *hydrocortisone* and skin protectors for up to 1 week and remind Mr Harris that the area should be kept clean and dry. You might consider recommending a laxative to ease the constipation until Mr Harris's diet gets back to normal (you advise that he return to his usual high-fibre diet) and makes sure his daily fluid intake is sufficient; a small supply of a stimulant laxative (perhaps a stimulant/stool softener such as *docusate sodium*) would be reasonable. He should see his doctor after 1 week if the problem has not cleared up.

The doctor's view

The treatment suggested by the pharmacist should settle Mr Harris's symptoms within 1 week. The treatment is, of course, symptomatic and not curative. If he continues to suffer from frequent relapse, referral should be considered. His doctor could advise whether or not to refer him for injection or removal of the piles.

Case 2

Mr Briggs is a local shopkeeper in his late 50s who wants you to recommend something for his piles. He tells you that he has had them for quite a while – a couple of months. He has tried several different ointments and suppositories, all to no avail. The main problem now is bleeding, which has become worse. In fact he tells you, somewhat embarrassed, that he has been buying sanitary towels because this is the only way he can prevent his clothes from becoming stained. He is not constipated and has no pain.

The pharmacist's view

Mr Briggs should be referred to his doctor at once. His symptoms have a history of 2 months and there must be quite profuse rectal bleeding, which may well be due to a more serious disease. He has already tried some OTC treatments, with no success. His age and the description of his symptoms mean that further investigation is needed.

The doctor's view

Mr Briggs should be advised to see his doctor. This is not a typical presentation of piles. He will need a more detailed assessment by his doctor who will need to look for a cancer of the colon or rectum. Piles can bleed at times other than when defaecating, but this is uncommon. The doctor would gather more information by questioning and from an examination. The examination would usually include a digital rectal assessment to determine whether or not a rectal tumour is present. It is quite likely that this man would require outpatient hospital referral for further investigations, which would involve sigmoidoscopy and barium enema.

Case 3

Caroline Andrews is a young woman in her mid-20s, who works as a graphic designer in a local art studio. She asks your advice about an embarrassing problem: she is finding it very painful to pass motions. On questioning, she tells you that she has had the problem for a few days and has been constipated for about 2 weeks. She eats a diet that sounds relatively low in fibre and has been eating less than usual because she has been very busy at work. Caroline says she seldom takes any exercise. She takes the contraceptive pill but is not taking any medicines and has no other symptoms such as rectal bleeding.

The pharmacist's view

Caroline would probably be best advised to see her doctor, since the symptoms and pain which she has described might be due to an anal fissure, though they may be caused by a haemorrhoid.

The doctor's view

An anal fissure would be the most likely cause of Caroline's problem. An examination by her doctor should quickly confirm this. Correction of the constipation and future preventative dietary advice could well solve the problem. The discomfort could be helped by a local anaesthetic-containing cream or gel. If this is applied prior to a bowel action, the discomfort would be less. In severe cases that are not settling, referral to a specialist surgeon is necessary in order to release one of the muscles in spasm for rapid relief of pain. Topical nitrate (e.g. *GTN 0.2–0.3% ointment*) is now also used by hospital specialists to treat anal fissure (unlicensed indication).

Skin Conditions

Eczema/dermatitis

Eczema is a term used synonymously with dermatitis. The latter is more commonly used when an external precipitating factor is present (contact dermatitis). The rashes produced have similar features but the distribution on the body varies and can be diagnostic. Atopic eczema affects up to 20% of children, in many of whom it disappears or greatly improves with age such that 2–10% of adults are affected. Atopy is a term that has been used to describe a group of diseases, for example, eczema, asthma and hay fever, which run in families.

The rash of eczema typically presents as dry flaky skin that may be inflamed and have small red spots (Plate 1). The skin may be cracked and weepy and sometimes becomes thickened. The rash is irritating and can be extremely itchy. Many cases of mild-to-moderate eczema can be managed by the patient with support from the pharmacist.

What you need to know
Age
Distribution of rash
Occupation/contact
Previous history
History of hay fever/asthma
Aggravating factors
Medication

Significance of questions and answers

Age/distribution

The distribution of the rash tends to vary with age. In infants, it is usually present around the nappy area, neck, back of scalp, face, limb creases and backs of the wrists (Plate 2).

In white children, the rash is most marked in the flexures: behind the knees, on the inside of the elbow joints, around the wrists, as well as the hands, ankles, neck and around the eyes. In black and Asian children, the rash is often on the extensor surface of the joints and may have a more follicular appearance.

Symptoms in the Pharmacy: A Guide to the Management of Common Illness, Seventh Edition.
Alison Blenkinsopp, Paul Paxton and John Blenkinsopp.
© 2014 John Wiley & Sons, Ltd. Published 2014 by John Wiley & Sons, Ltd.

In adults, the neck, the backs of the hands, the groin, around the anus, the ankles and the feet are the most common sites. The rash of intertrigo is caused by a fungal infection and is found in skinfolds or occluded areas such as under the breasts in women and in the groin or armpits.

Occupation/contact

Contact dermatitis may be caused by substances that irritate the skin or spark off an allergic reaction. Irritant contact dermatitis is most commonly caused by prolonged exposure to water (wet work). Typical occupations include cleaning, hairdressing, food processing, fishing and metal engineering. Substances that can irritate the skin include alkaline cleansing agents, degreasing agents, solvents and oils. Such substances either cause direct and rapid damage to the skin or, in the case of weaker irritants, exert their irritant effect after continued exposure. Nappy rash (napkin dermatitis) is an example of irritant dermatitis and can be complicated by infection, for example, thrush.

In other cases, the contact dermatitis is caused by an allergic response to substances which include chromates (present in cement and rust-preventive paint), nickel (present in costume jewellery and as plating on scissors), rubber and resins (two-part glues and the resin colophony in adhesive plasters), dyes, certain plants (e.g. primula), oxidising and reducing agents (as used by hairdressers when perming hair) and medications (including *topical corticosteroids, lanolin, neomycin* and *cetyl stearyl alcohol*). Eye make-up can also cause allergic contact dermatitis.

Clues as to whether or not a contact problem is present can be gleaned from knowledge of site of rash, details of job and hobbies, onset of rash and agents handled and improvement of rash when away from work or on holiday.

Previous history

Patients may ask the pharmacist to recommend treatment for eczema, which has been diagnosed by the doctor. In cases of mild-to-moderate eczema, it would be reasonable for the pharmacist to recommend the use of emollients and to advise on skin care. *Topical hydrocortisone, clobetasone* and *alclometasone* preparations can be recommended for the treatment of mild-to-moderate eczema. However, where severe or infected exacerbations of eczema have occurred, the patient is best referred to the doctor.

Pharmacists are sometimes asked for over-the-counter (OTC) *topical hydrocortisone, clobetasone* or *alclometasone* by patients on the recommendation of their doctor or nurse. It can be difficult to explain why such a sale cannot legally be made if the product is for use on the face or anogenital area or for severe eczema. Pharmacists can minimise such problems by ensuring that local family doctors (especially those in training) are aware of the restrictions that apply to the sale of hydrocortisone and clobetasone OTC. Pharmacists use their professional judgement regarding individual cases.

History of hay fever/asthma

Many eczema sufferers have associated hay fever and/or asthma. There is often a family history (in about 80% of cases) of eczema, hay fever or asthma. Eczema occurring in such situations is called atopic eczema. The pharmacist can enquire about the family history of these conditions.

Aggravating factors

Atopic eczema may be worsened during the hay fever season and by house dust or animal danders. Factors that dry the skin such as soaps or detergents and cold wind can aggravate the condition. Certain clothing such as woollen material can irritate the skin. In a small minority of sufferers (less than 5%), cow's milk, eggs and food colouring (tartrazine) have been implicated. Emotional factors, stress and worry can sometimes exacerbate eczema. Antiseptic solutions applied directly to the skin or added to the bathwater can irritate the skin.

Medication

Contact dermatitis may be caused or made worse by sensitisation to topical medicaments. The pharmacist should ask which treatments have already been used. Topically applied local anaesthetics, antihistamines, antibiotics and antiseptics can all provoke allergic dermatitis. Some preservatives may cause sensitisation. Information about different preparations and their formulations can be obtained from the local pharmacist or from the manufacturer of the product. The *British National Formulary (BNF)* is also a good source of information on this subject, with a list of additives for each topical product and excipients that may be associated with sensitisation.

If the patient has used a preparation which the pharmacist considers appropriate for the condition correctly but there has been no improvement or the condition has worsened, the patient should see the doctor.

When to refer

Evidence of infection (weeping, crusting, spreading)
Severe condition: badly fissured/cracked skin, bleeding
Failed medication
No identifiable cause (unless previously diagnosed as eczema)
Duration of longer than 2 weeks

Treatment timescale

Most cases of mild-to-moderate atopic eczema, irritant and allergic dermatitis should respond to skin care and treatment with OTC products. If no improvement has been noted after 1 week, referral to the doctor is advisable.

Management

Skin rashes tend, quite understandably, to cause much anxiety. There is also a social stigma associated with skin disease. Many patients will therefore have been seen by their doctor. Pharmacists are most likely to be involved when the diagnosis has already been made or when the condition first presents but is very mild.

However, with increasing recognition that patients can manage mild-to-moderate eczema, and as much of the management involves advice and the use of emollients, the pharmacist is in a good position to help, with short-term use of OTC topical steroids where needed. Where the pharmacist is able to identify a cause of irritant or allergic dermatitis, an OTC topical steroid may be recommended.

Emollients

Emollients are the key to managing eczema and are medically inert creams and ointments which can be used to soothe the skin, reduce irritation, prevent the skin from drying, act as a protective layer and be used as a soap substitute. They may be applied directly to the skin or added to the bathwater.

There are many different types of emollient preparations that vary in their degree of greasiness. The greasy preparations such as white soft paraffin are often the most effective, especially with very dry skin, but have the disadvantage of being messy and unpleasant to use. Patient preference is very important and plays a major part in compliance with emollient treatments. Patients will understandably not use a preparation they find unacceptable. Patients may need to try several different emollients before they find one that suits them, and they may need to have several different products (e.g. for use as a moisturiser, for use in the bath and for use as a soap substitute when washing or showering). Emollient preparations should be used as often as needed to keep the skin hydrated and moist. Several and frequent applications each day may be required to achieve this.

Standard soaps have a drying effect on the skin and can make eczema worse. Aqueous cream can be used as a soap substitute. It should be applied to dry skin and rinsed off with water. Proprietary skin washes are also available. Adding emulsifying ointment or a proprietary bath oil to the bath is helpful. Emulsifying ointment should first be mixed with water (one or two tablespoonfuls of ointment in a bowl of hot water) before being added to the bath to ensure distribution in the bathwater. Some patients with eczema believe, incorrectly, that bathing will make their eczema worse. This is not the case, provided appropriate emollient products are used and standard soaps and perfumed bath products are avoided, and in fact, bathing to remove skin debris and crusts is beneficial.

Advice

This could include the identification of possible aggravating or precipitating factors. If the history is suggestive of an occupationally associated contact dermatitis, then referral is advisable. The doctor may in turn feel that referral to a dermatologist is appropriate. It is sometimes necessary for a specialist to perform patch testing to identify the cause of contact dermatitis.

Further advice could be given regarding the use of ordinary soaps that tend to dry the skin and their alternatives (soap substitutes). If steroid creams have been prescribed and emollients are to be used, the pharmacist is in a good position to check that the patient understands the way in which they should be used.

Topical corticosteroids

Hydrocortisone cream and ointment, *alclometasone* 0.05% and *clobetasone* 0.05% can be sold OTC for a limited range of indications. Their steroid potency is classed as mild (*hydrocortisone*) and moderate (*alclometasone and clobetasone*). *Topical hydrocortisone* OTC is licensed for the treatment of irritant and allergic dermatitis, insect bites and mild-to-moderate eczema. OTC *hydrocortisone* is contraindicated where the skin is infected (e.g. athlete's foot or cold sores, in acne and on the face and anogenital areas). Children aged over 10 years and adults can be treated, and any course must not be longer than 1 week. Only proprietary OTC brands of *topical hydrocortisone* can be used; dispensing packs may not be sold.

Topical alclometasone 0.05% and *clobetasone* 0.05% can be used for the short-term treatment and control of patches of eczema and dermatitis in people aged 12 years and over. The indications include atopic eczema and primary irritant or allergic dermatitis and exclude seborrhoeic dermatitis.

OTC topical corticosteroids should not be used on the groin, breastfold, genitals or between the toes because these are common sites of fungal infections, or on the face as they can cause perioral dermatitis and acneiform pustules.

All should be used sparingly and explaining patients the use of fingertip units is helpful. A fingertip unit is the amount of cream you can squeeze on to your fingertip from the tip to the first crease. Half a fingertip unit will cover a patch of skin the same size as the palm of the hand.

Antipruritics

Antipruritic preparations are sometimes useful, although evidence of effectiveness is lacking. The itch of eczema is not histamine related, so the use of antihistamines other than that of sedation at night is not indicated. *Calamine* or *crotamiton* can be used in cream or lotion. A combination product containing *crotamiton* with *hydrocortisone* is available. Indications for use are the same as those for *topical hydrocortisone* for contact dermatitis (irritant or allergic), insect bites or stings and mild-to-moderate eczema. The same restrictions apply on use (see 'Topical corticosteroids' above).

Support for patients

The National Eczema Society provides information and support through its website www.eczema.org, a telephone helpline and written information.

Eczema and dermatitis in practice

Patient perspectives

I have lived with eczema all my life. I am now 33. My father had eczema and asthma. And the youngest of my three children also suffers with eczema. I know the heartache of this disease well. I have learned to control my eczema through my lifetime, but it takes quite a lot of trial and error to find the things that work and to avoid the things that set it off. Parents of kids with eczema need to listen to them and be patient with them because they are probably miserable, like I was as a child.

By the time I was about 18 or 19 my eczema had practically gone. My skin is still very sensitive and quite dry but is mostly OK. I go through phases where it breaks out behind my knees, on my forearms, on the back of my neck and on my lower back. When this happens, extra moisturiser and OTC *hydrocortisone cream* bring it under control again.

Managing atopic dermatitis is like taking care of the family car. When the car breaks down, you take it to the mechanic and get it fixed. That's like managing a flare-up of eczema with topical steroids … but the maintenance is still needed. Your car may be mended, but you still have to put oil in it regularly or the engine will seize up. And, like your car, you can do everything right – change the oil when you're supposed to – and it can still break down on you.

Case 1

Samixa Shah asks your advice about her 4-year-old daughter Aisha whose eczema has worsened recently. She tells you that she has been using Chinese herbs, which have proved very helpful until the last week or so. The eczema has flared up especially on her arms and legs. She would like to use a safe cream but not a steroid cream as she has heard about its side effects. Aisha is not with her mother.

The pharmacist's view

Chinese herbal treatments have become popular for eczema. Their exact contents and the amounts of their constituent active ingredients are difficult to identify. Ironically, analysis of some of these herbal treatments showed them to contain active ingredients with steroidal effects. Aisha should be seen by the family doctor as the eczema has flared up and without seeing the child it is difficult to assess its severity. However, the mother's comments and the history indicate that medical assessment would be helpful.

The doctor's view

The flare-up of her eczema could be due to an infection. The dry flaky skin can be an ideal site for infections to thrive. If that happens, the eczema is further worsened. It would be advisable for Aisha to be referred to her general practitioner (GP). The GP might take a skin swab to confirm an infection and start oral antibiotics with a steroid cream, which could be combined with a topical antibiotic. In this case, it would be necessary to check out Mrs Shah's concerns about steroid creams. With appropriate information she may well be persuaded to try one. Advise her that Chinese herbs may not be subject to quality control and regulation, and have been associated with liver toxicity.

Case 2

Ray Timpson is a local man in his mid-30s and a regular customer. Today, he wants to buy some *clobetasone* cream for his eczema, which has worsened. He has had eczema for many years and usually obtains his cream on a repeat prescription from his doctor. As a child, Mr Timpson was asthmatic, and both asthma and hay fever are present in some members of his family. He has just seen an advert for *clobetasone* and says he would prefer to buy his supplies from you in the future to save both himself and the doctor some time. The eczema affects his ankles, shins and hands; the skin on his hands is cracked and weeping.

The pharmacist's view

Mr Timpson needs to see his doctor because the eczema on his hands is infected. Topical steroids, including *clobetasone*, should not be used on infected skin.

The doctor's view

The description given suggests widespread atopic eczema with an area of infection on his hands. Although he has had this problem for many years, it would make sense for him to be referred to the GP, especially in view of the likely infection. It would be helpful for the GP to gain an understanding of Mr Timson's ideas, concerns and expectations about his eczema and its management. It would be useful to identify any aggravating factors, for example, pets, soaps, washing powders, working environment and stress. It would be helpful to enquire which emollients have been used and how helpful they have been. It could be useful to take a swab to confirm the infection, which is most likely due to *Staphylococcus aureus*. In this situation, a 10-day course of *flucloxacillin,* or *erythromycin* if the patient is *penicillin* sensitive, is indicated. If he is subject to repeated infection, he could try an antiseptic bath oil and emollient. It might be appropriate for him to use a prescribed potent topical steroid, for example, *betamethasone* 0.1% for a short period to control symptoms, rather than persist with a weaker one in the long term. Once his symptoms are under control, he could continue with an OTC corticosteroid as required plus his usual emollient.

Case 3

Romiz Miah, a young adult, asks your advice about his hands, which are sore and dry. The skin is flaky but not broken and there is no sign of secondary infection such as weeping or pus. He says the problem is spreading and now affecting his arms as well. He has occasionally had the problem before, but not as severely. On further questioning, you discover that he has recently started working in his family's restaurant and has been doing a lot of washing up and cleaning.

The pharmacist's view

The most likely cause is an irritant dermatitis caused by increased recent exposure to water and detergents. There are no signs of infection and it would be reasonable to recommend treatment with *topical hydrocortisone, alclometasone* or *clobetasone*. The skin is dry, so an ointment formulation would be helpful. Wearing rubber gloves to protect the skin would help. Regular and frequent use of an emollient will also be helpful.

The doctor's view

If his skin does not settle with the pharmacist's advice over the next week or two, it would be appropriate to suggest seeing his GP. In the consultation with the GP, it would be helpful to find out what his understanding of the problem is, how he thinks it is caused and what concerns he may have. He might, for example, think that it is caused solely by an infection and be contagious. Similarly, his expectations of what can be done to help need to be explored. He might, for instance, be expecting a complete cure; some people expect oral medication rather than topical creams. Exploration of his ideas, concerns and expectations will lead to a more satisfactory outcome. He will be more likely to adhere to the advice and treatment.

In this case, he might benefit from a stronger steroid cream (0.1% *betamethasone*) and a change of emollient. The most important aspect for the future would be prevention by protection from frequent contact with detergents.

Case 4

You are asked to speak to a patient on the phone about some cream she purchased at your pharmacy earlier today. The patient says she bought some *clobetasone* eczema and dermatitis cream for a rash caused by a new deodorant. However, when she got back home and read the patient information leaflet (PIL), she discovered that it should not be used by breastfeeding mothers without medical advice. She had her first baby 4 months ago and is breastfeeding.

The pharmacist's view

I didn't realise that the PIL said this about breastfeeding, so this phone call put me on the spot. I thought about the possible risk and decided it was very small. The treatment was going to be used only for a few days and the amount of steroid that might be absorbed through the skin would be absolutely tiny. However, I didn't want to undermine her confidence. I was also a bit worried about where I stood if I gave advice that was different from the PIL. But in the end I decided to use my own judgement. I told her that I would explain why the warning is in the leaflet, would give her my opinion and then see what she wanted to do. I said that if she would prefer it, she could use a simple soothing cream on the rash. I also said that if it was inconvenient for her to come back to the pharmacy, I could arrange for the other cream to be delivered by our prescription delivery van.

The patient's view

I was really worried when I got home and read the leaflet. You don't expect that putting something on a rash might mean you can't breast-feed. I thought maybe something in the cream could be dangerous to my baby. The pharmacist spent time talking it through with me and in the end I decided to go for the soothing cream instead, to be on the safe side.

The doctor's view

It is unlikely that the *corticosteroid* would cause any problems for the baby, especially as the treatment is going to be very short term. The advice given about corticosteroids and breastfeeding in the *BNF* states that 'maternal doses of up to 40-mg *prednisolone* daily by mouth are unlikely to cause any systemic effects in infants'. As so little of this topical moderate-potency steroid is likely to be absorbed, the chances of any problems are unlikely. It is possible that the warning is included in the PIL because there is no research evidence available in this situation.

Acne

The incidence of acne in teenagers is extremely high and it has been estimated that over half of all adolescents will experience some degree of acne. Most acne sufferers resort, at least initially, to self-treatment. Mild acne often responds well to correctly used OTC treatments. Acne has profound effects on patients, and pharmacists should remember that even mild acne is seen as stigmatising for teenagers and moderate-to-severe acne can be a major problem and a source of depression for some. A sympathetic response to requests for help, together with an invitation to return and report progress, can be as important as the treatment selected.

What you need to know
Age
Severity
Mild, moderate, severe
Affected areas
Duration
Medication

Significance of questions and answers

Age

Acne commonly occurs during the teenage years and its onset is most common at puberty, although it may start to appear a year or so earlier. Acne can persist for anything from a few months to several years; with onset at puberty, acne may continue until the late teens or even early 20s. The hormonal changes that occur during puberty, especially the production of androgens, are thought to be involved in the causation of acne. Increased keratin and sebum production during adolescence are thought to be important contributory factors; the increased amount of keratin leads to blockages of the follicles and the formation of microcomedones. A microcomedone can develop into a non-inflammatory lesion (comedone), which may be open (black-head) or closed (whitehead), or into an inflammatory lesion (papule,

Symptoms in the Pharmacy: A Guide to the Management of Common Illness, Seventh Edition. Alison Blenkinsopp, Paul Paxton and John Blenkinsopp.

pustule or nodule). Excess sebum encourages the growth of bacteria, particularly *Propionibacterium acnes*, which are involved in the development of inflammatory lesions. Acne can thus be non-inflammatory or inflammatory in nature.

Very young

Acne is extremely rare in young children and babies and any such cases should be referred to the doctor for investigation since an androgen-secreting (hormone-producing) tumour may be responsible.

Older

For patients in whom acne begins later than the teenage years, other causes should be considered, including drug therapy (discussed below) and occupational factors. Oils and greases used at work can precipitate acne and it would be worth asking whether the patient comes into contact with such agents. Acne worsens just before or during menstruation in some women; this is thought to be due to changes in progesterone levels.

Severity

OTC treatment may be recommended for mild acne. Comedones may be open or closed; the sebum in closed comedones cannot reach the surface of the skin. The plug of keratin, which is at the entrance to the follicle in a comedone, is initially white (a whitehead), later becoming darker coloured because of the accumulation of melanin (a blackhead). However, sebum is still produced, so swelling occurs and the comedone eventually ruptures, discharging its contents under the skin's surface. The released sebum causes an inflammatory response; if the response is not severe, small red papules appear. In more severe acne, angry-looking red pustules are seen and referral to the doctor for alternative forms of treatment such as topical or systemic antibiotics is needed.

Affected areas

In acne, affected areas may include the face, neck, centre of the chest, upper back and shoulders, that is, all areas with large numbers of sebaceous glands. Rosacea is a skin condition that is sometimes confused with acne (Plate 3). Occurring in young and middle-aged adults, rosacea has characteristic features of reddening, papules and pustules. Only the face is affected.

Duration

The information gained here should be considered in conjunction with facts about medication (prescribed or OTC) tried already and other medicines being taken. Acne of long duration where several OTC preparations have been correctly used without success indicates referral to the doctor.

Medication

The pharmacist should establish the identity of any treatment tried already and its method of use. Inappropriate use of medication, for example, infrequent application, could affect the chances of success.

Information about current therapy is important, since acne can sometimes be drug induced. *Lithium, phenytoin* and the progestogens, levonorgestrel and norethisterone (e.g. in the combined oral contraceptive pill), may be culprits. If acne is suspected as a result of drug therapy, patients should be advised to discuss this with their doctor.

When to refer
Severe acne
Failed medication
Suspected drug-induced acne

Treatment timescale

A patient with mild acne which has not responded to treatment within 8 weeks should be referred to the doctor.

Management

Dozens of products are marketed for the treatment of acne. The pharmacist can make a logical selection based on knowledge of likely efficacy. The general aims of therapy are to remove follicular plugs so that sebum is able to flow freely and to reduce the number of bacteria on the skin. Treatment should therefore reduce comedone formation. The most useful formulations are lotions, creams and gels. Gels with an alcoholic base dry quickly but can be irritating. Those with an aqueous base dry slower but are less likely to irritate the skin. A non-comedogenic moisturiser can help if the skin becomes dry as a result of treatment.

Benzoyl peroxide

Benzoyl peroxide has both antibacterial and anticomedogenic actions and is the first-line OTC treatment for inflammatory and non-inflammatory acne. Anti-inflammatory action occurs at all strengths. Anticomedogenic action is low and has the greatest effect at higher strengths. It has a keratolytic action, which increases the turnover of skin cells, helping the skin to peel. Regular application can result in improvement of mild acne. At first, *benzoyl peroxide* is very likely to produce reddening and soreness of the skin, and patients should be warned of this (see 'Practical points' below). Treatment should start with a 2.5% or 5% product, moving gradually to the 10% strength if needed. Gels can be helpful for people with oily skin and creams for those with dry skin. Washing the skin with a mild soap or cleansing product rinsed off with water before applying *benzoyl peroxide* can help by reducing the amount of sebum on the skin.

Benzoyl peroxide prevents new lesions forming rather than shrinking existing ones. Therefore, it needs to be applied to the whole of the affected area, not just to individual comedones, and is best applied to skin following washing. During the first few days of use, the skin is likely to redden and may feel slightly sore. Stinging, drying and peeling are likely. Warning should be given that such an irritant effect is likely to occur; otherwise treatment may be abandoned inappropriately.

One approach to minimise reddening and skin soreness is to begin with the lowest strength preparation and to apply the cream, lotion or gel sparingly and infrequently during the first week of treatment. Application once daily or on alternate days could be tried for a week and then frequency of use increased to twice daily. After 2 or 3 weeks, a higher strength preparation may be introduced. If irritant effects do not improve after 1 week or are severe, use of the product should be discontinued.

Sensitisation

Occasionally, sensitisation to *benzoyl peroxide* may occur. The skin becomes reddened, inflamed and sore, and treatment should be discontinued.

Bleaching

Warning should be given that *benzoyl peroxide* can bleach clothing and bedding. If it is applied at night, white sheets and pillowcases are best used and patients can be advised to wear an old T-shirt or shirt to minimise damage to good clothes. Contact between *benzoyl peroxide* and the eyes, mouth and other mucous membranes should be avoided.

Other keratolytics

Other keratolytics include *potassium hydroxyquinoline sulphate* and *salicylic acid*. They are second-line treatments.

Nicotinamide

Topical nicotinamide has a mild anti-inflammatory action and is applied twice daily. There is limited evidence of effectiveness. Side effects may include skin dryness and/or irritation. Several weeks' treatment may be needed to see the full effects.

Antibacterials

Skin washes and soaps containing antiseptic agents such as chlorhexidine are available. Such products may be useful in acne by degreasing the skin and reducing the skin flora. There is limited evidence of effectiveness.

Practical points

Information on acne for teenagers

The website www.teenagehealthfreak.com is a useful source of practical information for teenagers with health concerns including acne. As well as explaining what acne is and what can be used to treat it, site users can read other teenagers' queries about acne.

Diet

There is no evidence to link diet with acne, despite a common belief that chocolate and fatty foods cause acne or make it worse.

Sunlight

It is commonly believed that there are beneficial effects of sunlight on acne, thought to be due to its peeling effect, which helps to unblock follicles, and its drying or degreasing effect. A systematic review found that 'convincing direct evidence for a positive effect of sunlight exposure on acne is lacking'.

Antibiotics

The resistance of *P. acnes* to antibiotics is increasing. The pharmacist is in a good position to ensure that acne treatments are used correctly. Oral antibiotic therapy usually consists of tetracyclines (*minocycline* is more commonly used as there is less resistance, better absorption and it needs a dose only once daily) and patients should be reminded not to eat or drink dairy products up to 1 h before or after taking the antibiotic. The same rule applies to antacid or iron preparations. Evidence suggests that failure of antibiotic therapy in acne in the past may have been due to subclinical levels of antibiotic because of chelation by metal ions in dairy products or antacids. *Erythromycin* is also used in acne. Bacterial resistance to *erythromycin* is now high, so it may not be effective.

Topical antibiotics are used as an alternative to oral antibiotics but are not as effective. They are useful in inflammatory acne. Topical *erythromycin* combined with *benzoyl peroxide* or *zinc* may induce less bacterial resistance than oral therapy alone.

Continuous treatment

Acne is notoriously slow to respond to treatment and a period of up to 6 months may be required for maximum benefit. It is generally agreed that keratolytics such as *benzoyl peroxide* require a minimum of 6–8 weeks' treatment for benefit to be shown. Patients should therefore be encouraged to persevere with treatment, whether with OTC or prescription products, and told not to feel discouraged if results are not immediate. Research has shown that many teenagers have unrealistic expectations of the time needed for improvement to be seen, perhaps created by the advertising for some treatments. The patient also needs to understand that acne is a chronic condition and continuous treatment is needed to keep the problem under control.

Skin hygiene

Acne is not caused by poor hygiene or failure to wash the skin sufficiently often. Regular washing of the skin with soap and warm water or with an antibacterial soap or skin wash can be helpful as it degreases the skin and reduces the number of bacteria present. However the evidence for face cleansing in the management of acne is mostly from poor-quality studies.

Since personal hygiene is a sensitive area, an initial enquiry about the kind of soap or wash currently being used might be a tactful way to introduce the subject. Dermabrasion with facial scrubs removes the outer layer of dead skin and must be done gently. There is no evidence of effectiveness of this approach in acne.

OTC topical corticosteroids and acne

The use of *topical hydrocortisone, alclometasone or clobetasone* is contraindicated in acne because steroids can potentiate the effects of androgenic hormones on the sebaceous glands, hence making acne worse.

Make-up

Heavy, greasy make-up can only exacerbate acne. If make-up is to be worn, water-based rather than oily foundations are best, and they should be removed thoroughly at the end of the day.

Athlete's foot

The incidence of athlete's foot (tinea paedis) is not, as its name might suggest, limited to those of an athletic disposition. The fungus that causes the disease thrives in warm, moist conditions. The spaces between the toes can provide a good growth environment and the infection therefore has a high incidence. The problem is more common in men than in women and responds well to OTC treatment.

What you need to know
Duration
Appearance
Severity
Broken skin
Soreness
Secondary infection
Location
Previous history
Medication

Significance of questions and answers

Duration
Considered together with its severity, a long-standing condition may make the pharmacist decide to refer the patient. However, most cases of athlete's foot are minor in nature and can be treated effectively with OTC products.

Appearance
Athlete's foot usually presents as itchy, flaky skin in the web spaces between the toes. The flakes or scales of skin become white and macerated and begin to peel off. Underneath the scales, the skin is usually reddened and may be itchy and sore. The skin may be dry and scaly or moist and weeping. (see Plate 4).

Symptoms in the Pharmacy: A Guide to the Management of Common Illness, Seventh Edition. Alison Blenkinsopp, Paul Paxton and John Blenkinsopp.
© 2014 John Wiley & Sons, Ltd. Published 2014 by John Wiley & Sons, Ltd.

Severity

Athlete's foot is usually a mild fungal infection, but occasionally the skin between the toes becomes more macerated and broken and deeper and painful fissures may develop. The skin may then become inflamed and sore. Once the skin is broken, there is the potential for secondary bacterial infection to develop. If there are indications of bacterial involvement, such as weeping, pus or yellow crusts, then referral to the doctor is needed.

Location

Classically, the toes are involved, the web space between the fourth and fifth toes being the most commonly affected. More severe infections may spread to the sole of the foot and even to the upper surface in some cases. This type of spread can alter the appearance of the condition and severe cases are probably best referred to the doctor for further investigation. When other areas of the foot are involved, the appearance can be confused with that of allergic dermatitis. However, in eczema or dermatitis, the spaces between the toes are usually spared, in contrast to athlete's foot.

If the toenails appear to be involved, referral to the doctor may be necessary depending on how many toenails are affected and severity. Systemic antifungal treatment may be required to deal with infection of the nail bed where OTC treatment is not appropriate.

Previous history

Many people occasionally suffer from athlete's foot. The pharmacist should ask about previous bouts and about the action taken in response. Any diabetic patient who presents with athlete's foot is best referred to the doctor. Diabetics may have impaired circulation or innervation of the feet and are more prone to secondary infections in addition to poorer healing of open wounds.

Medication

One or more topical treatments may have been tried before the patient seeks advice from the pharmacist. The identity of any treatment and the method of use should be established. Treatment failure may occur simply because it was not continued for sufficiently long enough. However, if an appropriate antifungal product has been used correctly without remission of symptoms, the patient is best referred to the doctor, especially if the problem is of long duration (several weeks).

Treatment timescale

If athlete's foot has not responded to treatment within 2 weeks, patients should see their doctor.

Management

Many preparations are available for the treatment of athlete's foot. Formulations include creams, powders, solutions, sprays and paints. A systematic review of clinical evidence compared topical allylamines (e.g. *terbinafine*), azoles (e.g. *clotrimazole, miconazole, ketoconazole and bifonazole*), *undecenoic acid* and *tolnaftate*. All are more effective than placebo. Topical allylamines have been tested against topical azoles; cure rates were the same. However, *terbinafine* was more effective in preventing recurrence. *Terbinafine* and *ketoconazole* have a 1 week treatment period, which some patients may prefer.

Pharmacists should instruct patients on how to use the treatment correctly and on other measures that can help to prevent recurrence (see 'Practical points' below). Regular application of the recommended product to clean, dry feet is essential, and treatment must be continued after symptoms have gone to ensure eradication of the fungus. Individual products state the length of treatment and generally advise use for 1–2 weeks after the disappearance of all signs of infection.

Azoles (e.g. clotrimazole, miconazole)

Topical azoles can be used to treat many topical fungal infections, including athlete's foot. They have a wide spectrum of action and have been shown to have both antifungal and antibacterial activity. (The latter is useful as secondary infection can occur.) The treatment should be applied two or three times daily. Formulations include creams, powders and sprays. *Miconazole, clotrimazole, bifonazole* and *ketoconazole* have occasionally been reported to cause mild irritation of the skin. *Ketoconazole* has a 1 week treatment period.

Terbinafine

Terbinafine is available as cream, solution, spray and gel formulations. Their licensed indications and treatment schedules are shown in the table below. There is evidence that *terbinafine* is better than the azoles in preventing recurrence, so it will be useful where frequent bouts of athlete's foot are a problem. *Terbinafine* can cause redness, itching and stinging of the skin; contact with the eyes should be avoided. *Terbinafine* products are not recommended for use in children.

	Cream (16 and over)	Spray (16 and over)	Solution (18 and over)	Gel (16 and over)
Athlete's foot	Apply once or twice daily for 1 week	Apply once daily for 1 week	Apply once between the toes and to the soles and sides of the feet. Leave in contact for 24 h.	Apply once daily for 1 week
Dhobi itch ('jock itch')	Apply once or twice daily for 1–2 weeks	Apply once daily for 1 week	–	Apply once daily for 1 week
Ringworm	–	Apply once daily for 1 week	–	Apply once daily for 1 week

Griseofulvin

Griseofulvin 1% spray can be used OTC for the treatment of athlete's foot. The spray is used once a day and the maximum treatment period is 4 weeks.

Tolnaftate

Tolnaftate is available in powder, cream, aerosol and solution formulations and is effective against athlete's foot. It has antifungal, but not antibacterial, action. It should be applied twice daily and treatment should be continued for up to 6 weeks. *Tolnaftate* may sting slightly when applied to infected skin.

Undecenoates (e.g. zinc undecenoate, undecenoic acid and methyl and propyl undecylenate)

Undecenoic acid is an antifungal agent, sometimes formulated with zinc salt to give additional astringent properties. Treatment should be continued for 4 weeks.

Hydrocortisone cream or ointment

Hydrocortisone may be sold OTC for allergic and irritant dermatitis, insect bites or stings and mild-to-moderate eczema. *Topical hydrocortisone* cannot be recommended in athlete's foot because, although it would reduce inflammation, used alone it would not deal with the fungal infection, which might then worsen. Combination products containing *hydrocortisone* together with an antifungal agent are, however, available OTC for use in athlete's foot and intertrigo (described as 'sweat rash' on product packaging and information). Treatment is limited to 7 days.

Practical points
Footwear
Sweating of the feet can produce the kind of hot, moist environment in which the fungus is able to grow. Shoes that are too tight and that are made of synthetic materials make it impossible for moisture to evaporate. If possible, the patient should wear leather shoes, which will allow the skin to breathe. In summer, open-toed sandals can be helpful, and shoes should be left off where possible. The wearing of cotton socks can facilitate the evaporation of moisture, whereas nylon socks will prevent this.

Foot hygiene
The feet should be washed and carefully and thoroughly dried, especially between the toes, before the antifungal preparation is applied.

Transmission of athlete's foot
Athlete's foot is easily transmitted and is thought to be acquired by walking barefoot, for example, on changing room floors in workplaces, schools and sports clubs. There is no need to avoid sports but wearing some form of footwear, such as rubber sandals, is advisable.

Prevention of reinfection
Care should be taken to ensure that shoes and socks are kept free of fungus. Socks should be changed and washed regularly. Shoes can be dusted with a fungicidal powder to eradicate the fungus. The use of a fungicidal dusting powder on the feet and in the shoes can be a useful prophylactic measure and can also help to absorb moisture and prevent maceration. Patients should be reminded to treat all shoes, since fungal spores may be present.

Ringworm
Ringworm of the body (tinea corporis) is a fungal infection, which occurs as a circular lesion that gradually spreads after beginning as a small, red papule. Often there is only one lesion and the characteristic appearance is of a central, cleared area with a red advancing edge (Plate 5). Topical azoles such as *miconazole* are effective treatments for ringworm.

Ringworm of the groin (tinea cruris) presents as an itchy red area in the genital region and often spreads to the inside of the thighs. The problem is more common in men than in women and is commonly known as jock itch in the United States. Treatment consists of topical antifungals; the use of powder formulations can be particularly valuable because they absorb perspiration.

Ringworm of the scalp (tinea capitis) is most common in preadolescent children, although it can occur in adolescents and adults. There may be associated hair loss and affected hairs come out easily (see Plate 6). Treatment is with oral antifungals and referral is required (see also 'Hair loss').

Fungal nail infections (onychomycosis)

Onychomycosis is a fungal infection in which mild cases involve the nail plate and sometimes the nail bed that lies underneath (see Plate 7). A nail lacquer containing 5% *amorolfine* can be used for the treatment of mild infection involving one or two nails in people aged over 18 years. Plate 8 shows an onychomycotic nail. The lacquer should be applied to the affected finger or toenails once weekly. Treatment length is 6 months for fingernails and 9–12 months for toenails. Refer where there is a predisposing condition such as diabetes, peripheral circulatory problems and immunosuppression. *Amorolfine* should not be used by pregnant or breastfeeding women. Reported adverse effects include nail discolouration and broken or brittle nails. (These can also be effects of the infection itself.) A burning sensation of the skin is rarely experienced, as is contact dermatitis from *amorolfine*.

Fungal infections in practice

Case 1

John Chen, the local plumber, is in his early twenties and captains the local football team on Sunday mornings. Today he wants to buy something for his athlete's foot, which he says he just can't get rid of. His girlfriend bought him some cream a few days ago but it doesn't seem to be having any effect. The skin between the third and fourth toes and between the second and third toes is affected. John tells you the skin is itchy and that it looks flaky. He tells you that he has had athlete's foot before and that it keeps coming back again. He wears trainers most of the time (he has them on now) and has used the cream his girlfriend bought on most days.

The pharmacist's view

From the answers he has given, it sounds as though John has athlete's foot. Once you have ascertained the identity of the cream he has been using, it might be appropriate to suggest the use of one of the azoles or *terbinafine*. Advice is also needed about foot hygiene and footwear and about regular use of treatment. If the problem has not cleared up after 2 weeks, John should see his doctor.

The doctor's view

He probably does have athlete's foot (tinea paedis), although it is unusual for the skin not to be affected between the fourth and fifth toes. Athlete's foot usually starts with the skin being affected in this area. If his symptoms don't settle with the pharmacist's suggested treatment and management then he should see his GP. The GP could confirm the diagnosis. It would be helpful to know whether he has a history of other skin problems such as eczema or dermatitis, and it would be important to examine his foot. If the diagnosis was in doubt, a swab could be taken to identify whether or not it was a fungal infection.

Case 2

Linda Green asks if you can recommend anything for athlete's foot. She tells you that it affects her toes and the soles and top of her feet, and is extremely itchy. When asked about the skin between her toes, she tells you she does not think the rash is between the toes. She says the skin is dry and red and has been like this for several days. Ms Green has not tried any medication to treat it.

The pharmacist's view

The symptoms that Linda Green has described do not sound like those of athlete's foot. The skin between the toes is not affected, so dermatitis is a possibility. Rather than recommend a product without being able to identify the cause of the problem, it would be better to refer Ms Green to her doctor.

The doctor's view

The description that the pharmacist has obtained does not sound like athlete's foot, which usually involves the cleft between the fourth and fifth toes. Referral to the doctor for diagnosis would be sensible. It is possible she may have pompholyx and/or eczema. It would be helpful to know if she suffers, or has suffered, from any skin problems elsewhere on the body, for example, psoriasis or eczema. Pompholyx is also known as vesicular or dyshidrotic eczema and typically affects the hands and feet. An early feature of pompholyx is the development of tiny blisters deep in the skin of the fingers palms or toes. This can progress to scaling, cracking or crusting. About half of sufferers have a history of allergy or eczema. It appears more common in conditions that lead to increased sweating, such as a hot, humid climate and stress. The condition tends to come and go and is often not a problem for long periods of time. Treatment is similar to that for ordinary eczema and may include emollients, topical steroids and, if the pompholyx has become infected, topical or systemic antibiotics.

Psoriasis can also affect the soles of the feet and cause thickened dry skin associated with deep painful cracks. The differential diagnosis is made easier if there are signs of psoriasis present elsewhere, such as thickened, reddened skin around the knee caps and elbows.

Cold sores

Cold sores (herpes labialis) are caused by one of the most common viruses affecting humans worldwide. The virus responsible is the herpes simplex virus (HSV), of which there are two major types: HSV1 and HSV2. HSV1 typically causes infection around or in the mouth, whereas HSV2 is responsible for genital herpes infection. Occasionally, however, this situation is reversed with HSV2 affecting the face and HSV1 the genital area.

What you need to know
Age
Duration
Symptoms and appearance
Tingling
Pain
Location (current and previous)
Precipitating factors
Sunlight
Infection
Stress
Previous history
Medication

Significance of questions and answers

Age

Although initial infection, which is usually subclinical and goes unnoticed, occurs in childhood, cold sores are most commonly seen in adolescents and young adults. Following the primary attack, the virus is not completely eradicated and virus particles lie dormant in nerve roots until they are reactivated at a later stage. Although herpes infection is almost universal in childhood, not all those affected later experience cold sores, and the reason for this is not fully understood. Recurrent cold sores occur in up to 25% of all adults and the frequency declines

Symptoms in the Pharmacy: A Guide to the Management of Common Illness, Seventh Edition. Alison Blenkinsopp, Paul Paxton and John Blenkinsopp.
© 2014 John Wiley & Sons, Ltd. Published 2014 by John Wiley & Sons, Ltd.

with age, although cold sores occur in patients of all ages. The incidence of cold sores is slightly higher in women than in men.

In active primary herpes infection of childhood, the typical picture is of a febrile child with a painful ulcerated mouth and enlarged lymph nodes. The herpetic lesions last for 3–6 days and can involve the outer skin surface as well as the inside of the mouth. Such patients should be referred to the doctor.

Duration

The duration of the symptoms is important as treatment with *aciclovir* (*acyclovir*) is of most value if started early in the course of the infection (during the prodromal phase). Usually the infection is resolved within 1–2 weeks. Any lesions that have persisted longer need medical referral.

Symptoms and appearance

The symptoms of discomfort, tingling or irritation (prodromal phase), may occur in the skin for 6–24 h before the appearance of the cold sore. The cold sore starts with the development of minute blisters on top of inflamed, red, raised skin. The blisters may be filled with white matter. They quickly break down to produce a raw area with exudation and crusting by about the fourth day after their appearance. By around 1 week later, most lesions will have healed.

Cold sores are extremely painful and this is one of the critical diagnostic factors. Oral cancer can sometimes present a similar appearance to a cold sore. However, cancerous lesions are often painless and their long duration differentiates them from cold sores. Another cause of a painless ulcer is that of a primary oral chancre of syphilis. Chancres normally occur in the genital area but can be found on the lips. The incidence of syphilis has increased since 1997 in major cities in Europe, North America and Australia. In the United Kingdom outbreaks have occurred in Bristol, London, Manchester, Nottingham and Newcastle upon Tyne.

When a cold sore occurs for the first time, it can be confused with a small patch of impetigo. Impetigo is usually more widespread, does not start with blisters and has a honey-coloured crust. Impetigo tends to spread out to form further patches and does not necessarily start close to the lips. It is less common than cold sores and tends to affect children. Since impetigo requires either topical or oral antibiotic treatment, the condition cannot be treated by the pharmacist. If there is any doubt about the cause of the symptoms, the patient should be referred.

Location

Cold sores occur most often on the lips or face. Lesions inside the mouth or affecting the eye need medical referral.

Precipitating factors

It is known that cold sores can be precipitated by sunlight, wind, fever (during infections such as colds and flu) and menstruation, being rundown and local trauma to the skin. Physical and emotional stress can also be triggers. Whilst it is often not possible to avoid these factors completely, the information is usually helpful for the sufferer.

Previous history

The fact that the cold sore is recurrent is helpful diagnostically. If a sore keeps on returning in the same place in a similar way, then it is likely to be a cold sore. Most sufferers experience one to three attacks each year. Cold sores occur throughout the year, with a slightly increased incidence during the winter months. Information about the frequency and severity of the cold sore is helpful when recommending referral to the doctor, although the condition can usually be treated by the pharmacist.

In patients with atopic eczema, herpes infections can be severe and widespread. Such patients must be referred to their doctor.

Medication

It is helpful to enquire what creams and lotions have been used so far, what was used in previous episodes and what, if anything, helped last time.

Immunocompromised patients, for example, those undergoing cytotoxic chemotherapy, are at risk of serious infection and should always be referred to their doctor.

When to refer

Babies and young children
Failure of an established sore to resolve
Severe or worsening sore
History of frequent cold sores
Sore lasting longer than 2 weeks
Painless sore
Patients with atopic eczema
Eye affected
Uncertain diagnosis
Immunocompromised patient

Management

Aciclovir and penciclovir

Aciclovir cream and *penciclovir creams* are antivirals that reduce time to healing by one half to 1 day and reduce pain experienced from the lesion. Treatment should be started as soon as symptoms are felt and before the lesion appears. Once the lesion has appeared, evidence of effectiveness is less convincing. The treatments are therefore a helpful recommendation for patients who suffer repeated attacks and know when a cold sore is going to appear. Such patients can be told that they should use treatment as soon as they feel the characteristic tingling or itching which precedes the appearance of a cold sore.

Aciclovir cream can be used by adults and children and should be applied 4 hourly during waking hours (approximately five times a day) to the affected area for 5 days. If healing is not complete, treatment can be continued for up to 5 more days, after which medical advice should be sought if the cold sore has not resolved. *Penciclovir cream* can be used by those aged 12 years and over and is applied 2 hourly during waking hours (approximately eight times a day) for 4 days. Some patients experience a transient stinging or burning sensation after applying the creams. The affected skin may become dry and flaky.

Bland creams

Keeping the cold sore moist will prevent drying and cracking, which might predispose to secondary bacterial infection. For the patient who suffers only an occasional cold sore, a simple cream, perhaps containing an antiseptic agent, can help to reduce discomfort.

Hydrocolloid gel patch

This patch is applied as soon as symptoms start and replaced as needed. The thin hydrocolloid gel patch is used for its wound healing properties. There is limited evidence of efficacy in cold sores.

Complementary therapies

Balm mint extract and tea tree oil applied topically may have an effect on pain, dryness and itching. There is insufficient evidence to assess whether they have an effect on healing, time to crusting, severity of an attack or rate of recurrence. Low-energy, non-thermal narrow-waveband light within the infrared spectrum may have an effect on cold sores, although there is insufficient evidence currently.

Practical points
Preventing cross infection

Patients should be aware that HSV1 is contagious and transmitted by direct contact. Tell patients to wash their hands after applying treatment to the cold sore. Women should be careful in applying eye make-up when they have a cold sore to prevent infection affecting the eye. It is sensible not to share cutlery, towels, toothbrushes or face flannels until the cold sore has cleared up. Oral sex with someone who has a cold sore means a risk of genital herpes and should be avoided until the cold sore has gone.

Use of sunscreens

Sunscreen creams (SPF 15 or above) applied to and around the lips when patients are subject to increased sun exposure (e.g. during skiing and beach holidays) can be a useful preventive measure.

Stress

Sources of stress in life could be looked at to see if changes are possible. It might be worthwhile to recommend a discussion with the doctor about this.

Eczema herpeticum (Kaposi's varicelliform eruption)

Patients with atopic eczema are very susceptible to herpetic infection and show an abnormal response to the virus with widespread lesions and sometimes involvement of the central nervous system. These patients should avoid contact with anyone who has an active cold sore.

Impetigo

In some parts of the UK pharmacists now assess and treat impetigo using a Patient Group Direction (PGD). Localised crusted impetigo is usually treated with topical fusidic acid. Washing the hands with soap and water after applying treatment and not sharing face cloths and towels can help to prevent spread.

Warts and verrucae

Warts and verrucae are caused by a viral infection of the skin and have a high incidence in schoolchildren. Once immunity to the infecting virus is sufficiently high, the lesions will disappear, but many patients and parents prefer active treatment for cosmetic reasons. Effective preparations are available OTC, but correct use is essential if damage to surrounding skin is to be minimised.

What you need to know
Age
Adult, child
Appearance and number of lesions
Location
Duration and history
Medication

Significance of questions and answers

Age

Warts can occur in children and adults; they are more common in children and the peak incidence is found between the ages of 12 and 16 years. The peak incidence is thought to be due to higher exposure to the virus in schools and sports facilities. Warts and verrucae both are caused by the human papilloma virus, differing in their location.

Appearance

Warts appear as raised lesions with a roughened surface that are usually flesh coloured. Plantar warts occur on the weight-bearing areas of the sole and heel (verrucae). They have a different appearance from warts elsewhere on the body because the pressure from the body's weight pushes the lesion inwards, eventually producing pain when weight is applied during walking. Warts have a network of capillaries and, if pared, thrombosed, blackened capillaries or bleeding points will be seen. The presence of these capillaries provides a useful distinguishing feature between callouses and verrucae on the feet: if a corn

Symptoms in the Pharmacy: A Guide to the Management of Common Illness, Seventh Edition. Alison Blenkinsopp, Paul Paxton and John Blenkinsopp.
© 2014 John Wiley & Sons, Ltd. Published 2014 by John Wiley & Sons, Ltd.

or callous is pared, no such dark points will be seen; instead layers of white keratin will be present. The thrombosed capillaries are sometimes thought, incorrectly, to be the root of the verruca by the patient. The pharmacist can correct this misconception when explaining the purpose and method of treatment (discussed below).

Multiple warts

Warts may occur singly or as several lesions. Molluscum contagiosum is a condition in which the lesions may resemble warts and where another type of viral infection is the cause. Closer examination shows that the lesions contain a central plug of material (consisting of viral particles), which can be removed by squeezing. The location of molluscum contagiosum tends to differ from that of warts – the eyelids, face, armpits and trunk may be involved. Such cases are best referred to the doctor, since self-treatment would be inappropriate.

Location

The palms or backs of the hands are common sites for warts, as is the area around the fingernails. People who bite or pick their nails are more susceptible to warts around them. Warts sometimes occur on the face and referral to the doctor is the best option in such cases. Since treatment with OTC products is destructive in nature, self-treatment of facial warts can lead to scarring and should never be attempted.

Parts of the skin that are subject to regular trauma or friction are more likely to be affected, since damage to the skin facilitates entry of the virus. Plantar warts (verrucae) are found on the sole of the foot and may be present singly or as several lesions.

Anogenital

Anogenital warts are caused by a different type of human papilloma virus and require medical referral for examination, diagnosis and treatment. They are sexually transmitted and patients can self-refer to their local genitourinary clinic.

Duration and history

It is known that most warts will disappear spontaneously within a period of 6 months to 2 years. The younger the patient, the more quickly the lesions are likely to remit.

Any change in the appearance of a wart should be treated with suspicion and referral to the doctor is advised. Skin cancers are sometimes mistakenly thought to be warts by patients, and the pharmacist can establish how long the lesion has been present and any changes that have occurred. Signs related to skin cancer are described in 'Practical points' below.

Medication

Diabetic patients should not use OTC products to treat warts or verrucae since impaired circulation can lead to delayed healing, ulceration or even gangrene. Peripheral neuropathy may mean that even extensive damage to the skin may not provoke a sensation of pain.

Warts can be a major problem if the immune system is suppressed by either disease (e.g. HIV infection and lymphoma) or drugs (e.g. ciclosporin (cyclosporin) to prevent rejection of a transplant).

The pharmacist should ask whether any treatment has been attempted already and if so, its identity and the method of use. Commonly, treatments are not used for a sufficiently long period of time because patients' expectations are often of a fast cure.

When to refer

Changed appearance of lesions: size and colour
Bleeding
Itching
Genital warts
Facial warts
Immunocompromised patients

Treatment timescale

Treatment with OTC preparations should produce a successful outcome within 3 months; if not, referral is necessary.

Management

Treatment of warts and verrucae aims to reduce the size of the lesion by gradual destruction of the skin. Continuous application of the selected preparation for several weeks or months may be needed and it is important to explain this to the patient if compliance with treatment is to be achieved. Surrounding healthy skin should be protected during treatment (see 'Practical points' below).

Salicylic acid

Salicylic acid may be considered to be the treatment of choice for warts; it acts by softening and destroying the skin, thus mechanically removing infected tissue. Preparations are available in a variety of strengths, sometimes in collodion-type bases that help to retain the *salicylic acid* in contact with the wart. *Lactic acid* is included in some preparations with the aim of enhancing availability of the *salicylic acid*. It is a keratolytic and has an antimicrobial effect. Ointments, gels and plasters containing *salicylic acid* provide a selection of methods of

---

application. Preparations should be kept well away from the eyes and applied with an orange stick or other applicator, not with the fingers.

Cryotherapy

Dimethyl ether propane can be used to freeze warts and is available in an application system for home use for adults and children over 4. There is little evidence from which to judge its effectiveness in home use rather than when applied by a doctor. The treatment should not be used by people with diabetes or by pregnant women. The wart should fall off about 10 days after application.

Duct tape

Application of a piece of duct tape to the wart has been widely used in the United States and little used in the United Kingdom. The tape is left in place for up to 6 days at a time after which the wart is soaked in warm water for 5 min and then gently abraded with an emery board. Treatment takes up to 8 weeks. A randomised controlled trial (RCT) comparing duct tape with OTC cryotherapy found similar effectiveness.

Formaldehyde

Formaldehyde is used for the treatment of verrucae; it is considered to be less suitable for warts on the hands because of its irritant effect on the skin. The thicker skin layer on the sole of the feet protects against this irritant action. A gel formulation is available for the treatment of verrucae and is applied twice a day. Both *formaldehyde* and *glutaraldehyde* have an unpredictable action and are not first-line treatments for warts, though they may be useful in resistant cases.

Glutaraldehyde

Glutaraldehyde is used in a 5% or 10% gel or solution to treat warts; it is not used for anogenital warts and is generally used for verrucae. Its effect on viruses is variable. Patients should be warned that *glutaraldehyde* will stain the skin brown, although this will fade after treatment has stopped.

Practical points
Application of treatments

Treatments containing *salicylic acid* should be applied daily. The treatment is helped by prior soaking of the affected hand or foot in warm water for 5–10 min to soften and hydrate the skin, increasing the action of the *salicylic acid*. Removal of dead skin from the surface of the wart by gentle rubbing with a pumice stone or emery board ensures that the next application reaches the surface of the lesion. Occlusion of the wart using an adhesive plaster helps to keep the skin macerated, maximising the effectiveness of *salicylic acid*.

Protection of the surrounding skin is important and can be achieved by applying a layer of petroleum jelly to prevent the treatment from making contact with healthy skin. Application of the liquid or gel using an orange stick will help to confine the substance to the lesion itself.

Warts and skin cancer

Premalignant and malignant lesions can sometimes be thought to be warts by the patient. There are different types of skin cancer. They can be divided into two categories: non-pigmented (i.e. skin-coloured) and pigmented (i.e. brown).

Non-pigmented In this group, which is more likely to occur in the elderly, the signs might include a persisting small ulcer or sore that slowly enlarges but never seems to heal. Sometimes a crust forms but when it falls off, the lesion is still present. In the case of a basal cell carcinoma (rodent ulcer), the lesion typically has a circular, raised and rolled edge.

Pigmented Pigmented lesions or moles can turn malignant. These can occur in patients of a much younger age than the first group. Changes in nature or appearance of pigmented skin lesions that warrant referral for further investigation include:

Increase in size
Irregular outline (surface and edge)
Colour change, especially to black
Itching or bleeding
Satellite lesions (near main lesion)

Plates 9 and 10 show a melanoma and a superficial spreading melanoma.

Length of treatment required

Several weeks' continuous treatment is usually needed up to 3 months for both warts and verrucae. Patients need to know that a long period of treatment will be required and that they should not expect instant or rapid success. An invitation to come back to see the pharmacist and report progress can help the pharmacist monitor the treatment. If treatment has not been successful after 3 months, referral for removal using liquid nitrogen may be required.

Verrucae and swimming pools

Viruses are able to penetrate moist skin more easily than dry skin, and it has been suggested that the high level of use of swimming pools has contributed to the high incidence of verrucae. Theoretically, walking barefoot on abrasive surfaces by the pool or changing area can lead to infected material from the verruca being rubbed into the flooring. There has been controversy about whether wearing rubber socks can protect against the spread of verrucae. Also, the wearing of this conspicuous article might in itself create stigma for the child involved.

Scabies

Infestation by the scabies mite, *Sarcoptes scabiei,* causes a character-istically intense itching, which is worse during the night. The itch of scabies can be severe and scratching can lead to changes in the appear-ance of the skin. It is therefore necessary to take a careful history. Scabies goes through peaks and troughs of prevalence, with a peak occurring every 15–20 years, and pharmacists need to be aware when a peak is occurring.

What you need to know
Age
Infant, child, adult
Symptoms
Itching, rash
Presence of burrows
History
Signs of infection
Medication

Significance of questions and answers

Age

Scabies infestation can occur at any age from infancy onwards. The pharmacist may feel it best to refer infants and young children to the doctor if scabies is suspected.

Symptoms

The scabies mite burrows down into the skin and lives under the surface. The presence of the mites sets up an allergic reaction, thought to be due to the insect's coat and exudates, resulting in intense itching. A characteristic feature of scabies is that itching is worse at night and can lead to loss of sleep.

Burrows can sometimes be seen as small thread-like grey lines. The lines are raised, wavy and about 5–10 mm long. Commonly infested sites include the web space of the fingers and toes, wrists, armpits,

Symptoms in the Pharmacy: A Guide to the Management of Common Illness, Seventh Edition. Alison Blenkinsopp, Paul Paxton and John Blenkinsopp.
© 2014 John Wiley & Sons, Ltd. Published 2014 by John Wiley & Sons, Ltd.

buttocks and genital area. Patients may have a rash that does not always correspond to the areas of infestation. The rash may be patchy and diffuse or dense and erythematous. It is more commonly found around the midriff, underarms, buttocks, inside the thighs and around the ankles.

In adults, scabies rarely affects the scalp and face, but in children aged 2 years or under and in the elderly, involvement of the head is more common, especially the postauricular fold.

Burrows may be indistinct or may have been disguised by scratching which has broken and excoriated the skin. Scabies can mimic other skin conditions and may not present with the classic features. The itch tends to be generalised rather than in specific areas. In immunocompromised or debilitated patients (e.g. the elderly), scabies presents differently. The affected skin can become thickened and crusted. Mites survive under the crust and any sections that become dislodged are infectious to others because of the living mites they contain.

History

The itch of scabies can take several (6–8) weeks to develop in someone who has not been infested previously. The scabies mite is transmitted by close personal contact, so patients can be asked whether anyone else they know is affected by the same symptoms, for example, other family members, boyfriends and girlfriends.

Signs of infection

Scratching can lead to excoriation, so secondary infections such as impetigo can occur. The presence of a weeping yellow discharge or yellow crusts would be indications for referral to the doctor for treatment.

Medication

It is important for the pharmacist to establish whether any treatment has been tried already and, if so, its identity. The patient should be asked about how any treatment has been used, since incorrect use can result in treatment failure. The itch of scabies may continue for several days or even weeks after successful treatment, so the fact that itching has not subsided does not necessarily mean that treatment has been unsuccessful.

When to refer
Babies and children
Infected skin
Treatment failure
Unclear diagnosis

Management

There is relatively little evidence from RCTs of scabies treatment. *Permethrin cream* is an effective scabicide (acaricide) and *malathion* can be used where *permethrin* is not suitable. Two treatments are recommended, 7 days apart. Aqueous lotions are used in preference to alcoholic versions because the latter sting and irritate excoriated skin. Medical supervision is required for the treatment of scabies in children under 2 years.

The treatment is applied to the entire body including the neck, face, scalp and ears in adults. Particular attention should be paid to the webs of fingers, toes and soles of the feet, and under the ends of the fingernails and toenails.

Permethrin

The cream formulation is used in the treatment of scabies. For a single application in an adult, 30–60 g of cream (one to two 30-g tubes) is needed. The cream is applied to the whole body and left on for 8–12 h before being washed off. If the hands are washed with soap and water within 8 h of application, cream should be reapplied to the hands. Medical supervision is required for its use in children under 2 years and in elderly patients (aged 70 years and over). *Permethrin* can itself cause itching and reddening of the skin.

Malathion

Malathion is effective for the treatment of scabies and pediculosis (head lice). For one application in an adult, 100 mL of lotion should be sufficient. The aqueous lotion should be used in scabies. The lotion is applied to the whole body. The lotion can be poured into a bowl and then applied on cool, dry skin using a clean, broad paintbrush or cotton wool. The lotion should be left on for 24 h, without bathing, after which it is washed off. If the hands are washed with soap and water during the 24 h, *malathion* should be reapplied to the hands. Skin irritation may sometimes occur. Medical supervision is needed for children under 6 months.

Practical points

1 The itch will continue and may become worse in the first few days after treatment. The reason for this is thought to be the release of allergen from dead mites. Patients need to be told that the itch will not stop straightaway after treatment. *Crotamiton cream* or lotion could be used to relieve the symptoms, provided the skin is not badly excoriated. An oral antihistamine may be considered if the itch is severe.

2 The treatment should be applied to cool, dry skin. Good advice would be to apply the treatment immediately before bedtime (leaving time for the cream to be absorbed or the lotion to dry). Because the hands are likely to be affected by scabies, it is important not to wash the hands after application of the treatment and to reapply the preparation if the hands are washed within the treatment period.

3 All members of the family or household should be treated, preferably, on the same day. Because the itch of scabies may take several weeks to develop, people may be infested but symptomless. It is thought that patients may not develop symptoms for up to 8 weeks after infestation. The incubation period of the scabies mite is 3 weeks, so reinfestation may occur from other family or household members.

4 The scabies mite can live only for around 1 day after leaving its host and transmission is almost always caused by close personal contact. It is possible that reinfestation could occur from bedclothes or clothing and this can be prevented by washing them at a minimum temperature of 50°C after treatment.

5 Other possible infestations include those caused by pet fleas and bedbugs. Pet fleas are common and patients may present with small, reddened swellings, often on the lower legs and around the ankles where the pet has come into contact with the skin. Questioning may reveal that a pet cat or dog has recently been acquired or that a pet has not been treated with insecticide for some time. Regular checks for fleas and use of insecticides will prevent the problem occurring in the future. A range of proprietary products is available to treat either the pet or bedding and carpets. A second treatment should be applied 2 weeks after the first to eradicate any fleas that have hatched since the first application. Pet flea bites can be treated with topical *hydrocortisone* in anyone over 10 years. Alternatively, an antipruritic such as *crotamiton* (with or without *hydrocortisone) or calamine cream* can be recommended.

Dandruff

Dandruff is a chronic relapsing condition of the scalp, which responds to treatment but returns when treatment is stopped. The condition usually appears during puberty and reaches a peak in early adulthood. Dandruff has been estimated to affect one in two people aged between 20 and 30 years and up to four in ten of those aged between 30 and 40 years. Dandruff is considered to be a mild form of seborrhoeic dermatitis, associated with the yeast *Malassezia furfur*. Diagnosis is straightforward and effective treatments are available OTC.

What you need to know

Appearance
Presence of scales
Colour and texture of scales
Location: scalp, eyebrows, paranasal clefts and others
Severity
Previous history
    Psoriasis
    Seborrhoeic dermatitis
Aggravating factors
Medication

Significance of questions and answers

Appearance

Dandruff is characterised by greyish-white flakes or scales on the scalp and an itchy scalp as a result of excessive scaling. In dandruff the epidermal cell turnover is at twice the rate of those without the condition. A differential diagnosis for severe dandruff could be psoriasis. In the latter conditions, both the appearance and the location would be different. In more severe cases of seborrhoeic dermatitis the scales are yellowish and greasy looking and there is usually some inflammation with reddening and crusting of the affected skin (Plate 11). In psoriasis the scales are silvery-white and associated with red, patchy plaques and inflammation (Plate 12).

Symptoms in the Pharmacy: A Guide to the Management of Common Illness, Seventh Edition. Alison Blenkinsopp, Paul Paxton and John Blenkinsopp.
© 2014 John Wiley & Sons, Ltd. Published 2014 by John Wiley & Sons, Ltd.

Location

In dandruff the scalp is the only area affected. More widespread seborrhoeic dermatitis affects the areas where there is greatest sebaceous gland activity, so it can affect eyebrows, eyelashes, moustache, paranasal clefts, behind the ears, nape of neck, forehead and chest.

In infants seborrhoeic dermatitis is common and occurs as cradle cap, appearing in the first 12 weeks of life.

Psoriasis can affect the scalp but other areas are involved. The knees and elbows are commonly involved but the face is rarely affected. This latter point distinguishes psoriasis from seborrhoeic dermatitis, where the face is often affected.

Severity

Dandruff is generally a mild condition. However, the itching scalp may lead to scratching, which may break the skin, causing soreness and the possibility of infection. If the scalp is very sore or there are signs of infection (crusting or weeping), referral should be indicated.

Previous history

Since dandruff is a chronic relapsing condition there will usually be a previous history of fluctuating symptoms. There is a seasonal variation in symptoms, which generally improve in summer in response to UVB light. *M. furfur* is unaffected by UVA light.

Aggravating factors

Hair dyes and perms can irritate the scalp. Inadequate rinsing after shampooing the hair can leave traces of shampoo causing irritation and itching.

Psoriasis can be exacerbated by drugs (e.g. *chloroquine*).

Medication

Various treatments may already have been tried. It is important to identify what has been tried and how it was used. Dandruff treatments need to be applied to the scalp and be left for at least 5 min for best effect. However, if an appropriate treatment has been correctly used with no improvement, referral should be considered.

When to refer

Suspected psoriasis
Signs of infection
Unresponsive to appropriate treatment

Treatment timescale

Dandruff should start to improve within 12 weeks of beginning treatment.

Management

The aim of the treatment is to reduce the level of M. *furfur* on the scalp; therefore, agents with antifungal action are effective. *Ketoconazole, selenium sulphide, zinc pyrithione* and coal tar are effective. The results from studies suggest that *ketoconazole* is the most and coal tar is the least effective. All treatments need to be left on the scalp for 3–5 min for full effect.

Ketoconazole

Ketoconazole 2% shampoo is used twice a week for 2–4 weeks, after which usage should reduce to weekly or fortnightly as needed to prevent recurrence. It is considered first line in moderate-to-severe dandruff.

The shampoo can also be used in seborrhoeic dermatitis. Whilst shampooing the lather can be applied to the other affected areas and left before rinsing.

Ketoconazole is not absorbed through the scalp and side effects are extremely rare. There have been occasional reports of allergic reactions.

Zinc pyrithione

Zinc pyrithione is effective against dandruff and has a cytostatic effect. It should be used twice weekly for the first 2 weeks and then once weekly as required.

Selenium sulphide 2.5%

Selenium sulphide has been shown to be effective and works by reducing the cell turnover rate (cytostatic effect). Twice-weekly use for the first 2 weeks is followed by weekly use for the next 2 weeks; then it can be used as needed. The hair and scalp should be thoroughly rinsed after using *selenium sulphide* shampoo; otherwise, discoloration of blond, grey or dyed hair can result. Frequent use can make the scalp greasy and therefore exacerbate seborrhoeic dermatitis. Products containing *selenium sulphide* should not be used within 48 h of colouring or perming the hair. Contact dermatitis has occasionally been reported. *Selenium sulphide* should not be applied to inflamed or broken skin.

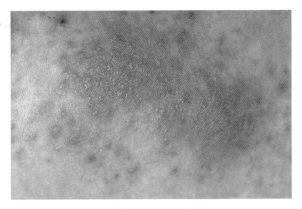

Plate 1 Typical eczema dermatitis rash.

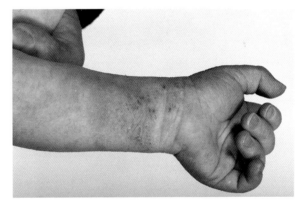

Plate 2 Atopic eczema.

Symptoms in the Pharmacy: A Guide to the Management of Common Illness, Seventh Edition.
Alison Blenkinsopp, Paul Paxton and John Blenkinsopp.
© 2014 John Wiley & Sons, Ltd. Published 2014 by John Wiley & Sons, Ltd.

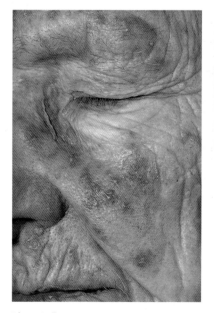

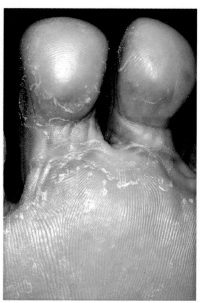

Plate 3 Rosacea.

Plate 4 Athlete's foot.

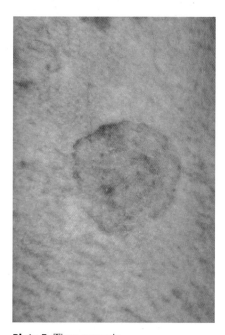

Plate 5 Tinea corporis.

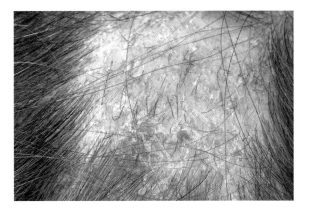

Plate 6 Tinea capitis.

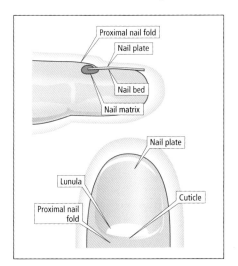

Plate 7 The nail.

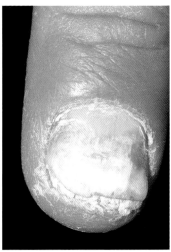

Plate 8 Tinea of a fingernail.

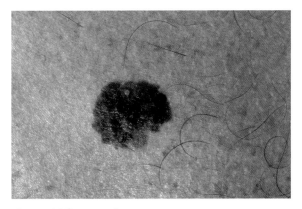

Plate 9 Malignant melanoma.

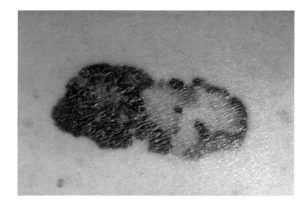

Plate 10 Superficial spreading melanoma.

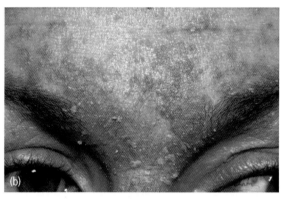

Plate 11 Seborrhoeic dermatitis.

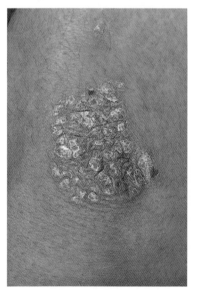

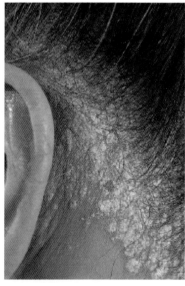

Plate 12 Psoriasis vulgaris. **Plate 13** Scalp psoriasis.

Coal tar

Findings from research studies indicate that coal tar is the least effective of the antidandruff agents. Modern formulations are pleasanter than the traditional ones but some people still find the smell of coal tar unacceptable. Coal tar can cause skin sensitisation and is a photosensitiser.

Practical points

Continuing treatment

Patients need to understand that the treatment will not cure their dandruff permanently and that it will be sensible to use the treatment on a less frequent basis to prevent their dandruff from coming back.

Treating the scalp

It is the scalp that needs to be treated rather than the hair. The treatment should be applied to the scalp and massaged gently. All products need to be left on the scalp for 5 min before rinsing for the full effect to be gained.

Standard shampoos

There is debate amongst experts as to whether dandruff is caused by infrequent hairwashing. However, it is generally agreed that frequent washing (at least three times a week) is an important part of managing dandruff. Between applications of their treatment the patients can continue to use their normal shampoo. Some may wish to wash their hair with their normal shampoo before using the dandruff treatment shampoo.

Hair products

Gel, mousse and hairspray can still be used and will not adversely affect treatment for dandruff.

Psoriasis

People with psoriasis usually present to the doctor rather than the pharmacist. At the time of first presentation, the doctor is the most appropriate first line of help and pharmacists should always refer cases of suspected, but undiagnosed, psoriasis. The diagnosis is not always easy and needs confirming. In the situation of a confirmed diagnosis in a relatively chronic situation, the pharmacist can offer continuation of the treatment where the products are available OTC.

This is a condition where continued management and monitoring by the pharmacist is reasonable, with referral back to the doctor when there is an exacerbation or for periodic review. Jointly agreed guidelines between pharmacist and doctors are valuable here.

Psoriasis occurs worldwide with variation in incidence between different ethnic groups. The incidence for white Europeans is about 2%. Although there is a genetic influence, environmental factors are thought to be important.

What you need to know
Appearance
Psychological factors
Diagnosis
Medication

Significance of questions and answers

Appearance
In its most common form there are raised, large, red, scaly patches/plaques over the extensor surfaces of the elbow and knee (Plate 12). The patches are symmetrical and sometimes there is a patch present over the lower back area. The scalp is often involved (see Plate 13). Psoriasis can affect the soles of the feet.

Psychological factors
In some people these patches are very long standing and show little change. With others, the skin changes worsen and spread to other

Symptoms in the Pharmacy: A Guide to the Management of Common Illness, Seventh Edition. Alison Blenkinsopp, Paul Paxton and John Blenkinsopp.
© 2014 John Wiley & Sons, Ltd. Published 2014 by John Wiley & Sons, Ltd.

parts of the body sometimes in response to a stressful event. This is particularly distressing for the person involved who then has to cope with the stress of having a relapse of psoriasis as well as the precipitating event.

The psychological impact of having a chronic skin disorder such as psoriasis must not be underestimated. There is still a significant stigma connected with skin disease. There can be a mistaken belief that the rash is contagious. There is a cultural pressure to have a perfect body as defined by the fashion industry and media. Psoriasis can understandably cause loss of self-esteem, embarrassment and depression. However each person will react differently, with some being psychologically affected by relatively minor patches whist others are untroubled by a more widespread rash. In the United Kingdom further information and support can be accessed at https://www.psoriasis-association.org.uk/.

Diagnosis

The diagnosis of psoriasis can be confusing. In the typical situation described above, it is straightforward. In addition to affecting the extensor surfaces, psoriasis can typically involve the scalp (also see p. 182). Often the fingernails show signs of pitting, which is a useful diagnostic guide. However, psoriasis can present with differing patterns that can be confused with other skin disorders. In guttate psoriasis a widespread rash of small, scaly patches develops abruptly, affecting large areas of the body. This most typically occurs in children or young adults and may be triggered by a streptococcal sore throat. In general practice the most common differential diagnosis to guttate psoriasis is pityriasis rosea. This latter condition is self-limiting and usually settles down within 8 weeks.

Psoriasis can also involve the flexor surfaces, the groin area, palms, soles and nails. The most common alternative diagnostic possibilities in these situations include eczema or fungal infections. For some people who have psoriasis there is an associated arthritis, which most commonly affects the hands and feet.

Medication

It is worthwhile enquiring about routine medications taken as *lithium*, beta-blockers, non-steroidal anti-inflammatory drugs and antimalarials can exacerbate psoriasis.

Management

Management is dependent on many factors, for example, nature and severity of psoriasis, understanding the aims of the treatment, ability to apply creams and whether the person is pregnant. (Some treatments are teratogenic.) As always, it is particularly important for the doctor to deal with the person's ideas, concerns and expectations to appreciate how that person's life is affected by the condition to give a relevant, understandable explanation and to mutually agree whether to treat or not, and if so, how.

Topical treatments

The doctor is likely to offer a topical treatment, usually an emollient alone or in conjunction with active therapy. Emollients are important in psoriasis and may be underused. The pharmacist can ask the patient when and how they are being used.

Calcipotriol or tacalcitol

Vitamin D derivatives are available as *calcipotriol* or *tacalcitol*. This does not smell or stain and has been widely used in the treatment of mild-to-moderate psoriasis. A systematic review has shown it to be as beneficial in efficacy as *dithranol*. If overused, there is a risk of causing hypercalcaemia. It is available as a scalp application as well as an ointment.

Topical steroids

Topical steroids should generally be restricted to use in the flexures or on the scalp. Although effective in suppressing skin plaques on the body, large amounts are required over time as the condition is a chronic one, resulting in severe steroid side effects (striae, skin atrophy and adrenocortical suppression). Also, stopping steroid preparations can result in a severe flare-up of the psoriasis.

There is a combination cream with *betamethasone* and *calciptriol*, which is effective but licensed for use only on up to 30% of body surface for up to 4 weeks.

Dithranol

Dithranol has been a traditional, effective and safe treatment for psoriasis and is available as proprietary creams (0.1–2.0%) which can be used for one short-contact (30 min) period each day and removed using an emollient. Some people are very sensitive to *dithranol* as it can cause a quite severe skin irritation. It is usual to start with the lowest concentration and build up slowly to the strongest that can be tolerated. Users should wash their hands after application. It should not be applied to the face, flexures or genitalia. There are some people who are unable to tolerate it at all.

Second-line treatment

Referral by a doctor to a dermatologist may be necessary when there is diagnostic uncertainty, when the doctor's treatment fails or in severe cases. Second-line treatment may include phototherapy (PUVA)

---

or systemic therapy with *methotrexate, etretinate* or *ciclosporin (cyclosporin)*. Unfortunately, all of these have potentially serious side effects. *Methotrexate* has been shown to be effective in non-randomised trials but relapse usually occurs within 6 months of discontinuation. Long-term *methotrexate* treatment carries the risk of liver damage. Those not responding to PUVA or systemic therapy may be prescribed biologics (*etanercept, adalimumab or ustekinumab*), which block part of the immune system involved in causing inflammation.

Painful Conditions

Headache

The most common types of headache that the community pharmacist is likely to encounter are tension headache, migraine and sinusitis. Careful questioning can distinguish causes that are potentially more serious, so referral to the doctor can be advised.

What you need to know

Age
  Adult, child
Duration
Nature and site of pain
Frequency and timing
Previous history
  Fits, faints, blackouts
Associated symptoms
  Nausea, vomiting, photophobia
Precipitating factors
  Foods, alcohol, stress, hormonal
Recent trauma or injury
Falls
Recent eye test
Medication

Significance of questions and answers

Age

The pharmacist would be well advised to refer any child with a headache to the doctor, especially if there is an associated history of injury or trauma to the head, for example, from a fall. Children with severe pain across the back of the head and neck rigidity should be referred immediately. Elderly patients sometimes suffer a headache a few days after a fall involving a bang to the head. Such cases may be the result of a slow bleed into the brain, causing a subdural haematoma, and require immediate referral.

Symptoms in the Pharmacy: A Guide to the Management of Common Illness, Seventh Edition.
Alison Blenkinsopp, Paul Paxton and John Blenkinsopp.
© 2014 John Wiley & Sons, Ltd. Published 2014 by John Wiley & Sons, Ltd.

It is unusual for patients to present with their first migraine episode over the age of 40 years and such patients should be referred. In the United States, the peak incidence of migraine without aura in males is between ages 10 and 11 years and in females between ages 14 and 17 years. The incidence of migraine with aura peaks in males at age 5 years and females between ages 12 and 13 years (Best Practice BMJ group).

Duration
Any headache that does not respond to over-the-counter (OTC) analgesics within a day requires referral.

Nature and site of pain
Tension headaches are the most common form. The pain is often described as being around the base of the skull and the upper part of the neck. Sometimes the pain extends up and over the top of the head to above the eyes. It is not associated with any neck stiffness. The sub-occipital muscles can feel tender to touch. The pain may be described like a band around the head. The pain is usually of a dull nature rather than the pounding or throbbing sensation associated with migraines. However, the nature of the pain alone is not sufficient evidence on which to decide whether the headache is likely to be from a minor or more serious cause.

A steady, dull pain that is deep seated, severe and aggravated by lying down requires referral, since it may be due to raised intracranial pressure from a brain tumour, infection or other cause. This is rare and usually there would be other associated symptoms such as altered consciousness, unsteadiness, poor coordination and, in the case of an infection, a raised temperature.

Classic migraine is unilateral, affecting one side of the head, especially over the forehead.

Rarely, a sudden severe pain that develops at the back of the head may signify a subarachnoid haemorrhage (SAH). The incidence rate for SAH in the general population is 6 cases per 100 000 person-years. It occurs when a small blood vessel at the base of the brain leaks blood into the cerebrospinal fluid surrounding the brain. It may be associated with raised blood pressure. Emergency medical referral is essential. Sometimes sudden headaches at the back of the head are related to exercise (exertional headaches). These are not dangerous but may need differentiation from haemorrhagic ones by computed tomography and magnetic resonance angiography.

Frequency and timing of symptoms
Pharmacists should regard a headache that is worse in the morning and improves during the day as particularly serious, since this may

be a sign of raised intracranial pressure. Cluster headaches typically happen daily for 2–3 months and each episode of pain can last up to 3 h. A person who has headaches of increasing frequency or severity should be referred.

Previous history

It is always reassuring to know that the headache experienced is the usual type for that person. In other words, it has similar characteristics in nature and site but not necessarily in severity to headaches experienced over previous years. This fact makes it much less likely to be from a serious cause, whereas new or different headaches (especially in people over 45 years) may be a warning sign of a more serious condition. Migraine patients typically suffer from recurrent episodes of headaches. In some cases, the headaches occur in clusters. The pain may be present daily for 2–3 weeks and then be absent for months or years.

Associated symptoms

Children and adults with unsteadiness and clumsiness associated with a headache should be referred immediately.

Migraine

Migraine affects over 15% of the UK population and two-thirds of sufferers are women. There are two common types of migraine: migraine without aura (common migraine), which occurs in 75% cases, and migraine with aura (classic migraine).

Classic migraine. Classic migraine is often associated with alterations in vision before an attack starts, the so-called prodromal phase. Patients may describe seeing flashing lights or zigzag lines. During the prodromal phase, patients may experience tingling or numbness on one side of the body, in the lips, fingers, face or hands. Migraines are also associated with nausea and sometimes vomiting. Patients often get relief from lying in a darkened room and say that bright light hurts their eyes during an attack of migraine. Classic migraine is three times more common in women than in men.

Common migraine. In common migraine, there is no prodromal phase (no aura); the headache may be one sided but both sides of the head may be affected and gastrointestinal (GI) symptoms such as nausea and vomiting may occur.

The International Headache Society has published diagnostic pointers for migraine.

International Headache Society's diagnostic pointers for migraine

Migraine without aura (common migraine)
   At least five previous episodes with
      Attacks lasting 4–72 h
   At least two of the following headache characteristics
      Pulsating/throbbing
      Pain of moderate-to-severe intensity
      Pain aggravated by movement
      Unilateral pain
   At least one associated symptom
      Nausea and/or vomiting
      Photophobia and phonophobia
Migraine with aura (classic migraine)
   At least three of the following characteristics
      One or more transient focal neurological aura symptoms
      Gradual development of aura symptoms up to 5 min or several symptoms
         in succession
      Aura symptoms lasting 5–60 min
      Headache following or accompanying aura within 60 min

Reproduced from *The International Classification of Headache Disorders* 2nd edition *Cephalalgia*, 2004; 24(Suppl. 1): 1–150. Reprinted with permission from Sage Publications.

Chronic daily headache

Chronic daily headache (CDH) is defined as headache that is present on most days, that is, more than 15 days a month, typically occurring over a 6-month period or longer, and it can be daily and unremitting. In some patients, an episode of chronic headache resolves in a much shorter time; it can occur in children and in the very old. Twice as many men have it compared to women. Chronic headache is characterised by a combination of background, low-grade muscle contraction-type symptoms, often with stiffness in the neck and superimposed migrainous symptoms. It is possible that daily use of simple analgesics and combinations containing codeine causes CDH. Any frequent headache needs referral to the general practitioner (GP) for assessment.

Cluster headaches (previously called migrainous neuralgia)

Cluster headaches involve, as their name suggests, a number of headaches one after the other. A typical pattern would be daily episodes of pain over 2–3 months, after which there is a remission for anything up to 2 years. The pain can be excruciating and often comes on very quickly even waking the sufferer from sleep. Each episode of pain can last from 0.5 to 3 h and the pain is usually experienced on one side of the head, in the eye, cheek or temple. A cluster headache is often accompanied by a painful, watering eye and a watering or blocked nostril on the same side as the pain. Any recurrent, persistent or severe headache needs referral to the GP for a diagnosis.

Sinusitis

Sinusitis may complicate a respiratory viral infection (e.g. cold) or allergy (e.g. hay fever), which causes inflammation and swelling of the mucosal lining of the sinuses. The increased mucus produced within the sinus cannot drain, a secondary bacterial infection develops and the pressure builds up, causing pain. The pain is felt behind and around the eye and usually only one side is affected. The headache may be associated with rhinorrhoea or nasal congestion. The affected sinus often feels tender when pressure is applied. It is typically worse on bending forwards or lying down.

Temporal arteritis

Temporal arteritis usually occurs in older patients; the arteries that run through the temples become inflamed. They may appear red and are painful and thickened to the touch. However, these signs are not always present. Any elderly patient presenting with a frontal or temporal headache that persists and is often associated with a general feeling of being unwell should be referred immediately. Temporal arteritis is a curable disease and delay in diagnosis and treatment may lead to blindness, because the blood vessels to the eyes are also affected by inflammation. Treatment usually involves high-dose steroids and is effective, provided the diagnosis is made sufficiently early.

Precipitating factors

Tension (psychogenic) headache and migraines may be precipitated by stress, for example, pressure at work or a family argument. Some migraine sufferers experience their attacks after a period of stress, for example, when on holiday or at weekends. Certain foods have been reported to precipitate migraine attacks, for example, chocolate and cheese. Migraine headaches may also be triggered by hormonal changes. In women, migraine attacks may be associated with the menstrual cycle.

Recent trauma or injury

Any patient presenting with a headache who has had a recent head injury or trauma to the head should be referred to the doctor immediately because bruising or haemorrhage may occur, causing a rise in intracranial pressure. The pharmacist should look out for drowsiness or any sign of impaired consciousness. Persistent vomiting after the injury is also a sign of raised intracranial pressure.

Recent eye test

Headaches associated with periods of reading, writing or other close work may be due to deteriorating eyesight and a sight test may be worth recommending to see whether spectacles are needed.

Medication

The nature of any prescribed medication should be established, since the headache might be a side effect of medication, for example, nitrates used in the treatment of angina.

It is also known now that headaches can occur because of medication overuse. Up to 4% of the population suffers from CDH. This is when headaches occur on more than 15 days per month. The headaches may be tension or sometimes associated with superimposed migraine. Sometimes the headaches may actually be caused by taking too much medication, as it is possible to develop tolerance and then rebound headaches. It is therefore important to determine what medication has been taken for headaches, in what dose and with what frequency. The NICE guideline (CG150) 'Headaches: diagnosis and management of headaches in young people and adults' states:

> 'Advise people to stop taking all overused acute headache medications for at least 1 month and to stop abruptly rather than gradually. Advise people that headache symptoms are likely to get worse in the short term before they improve and that there may be associated withdrawal symptoms, and provide them with close follow-up and support according to their needs'.

Contraceptive pill

Any woman taking the combined oral contraceptive (COC) pill and reporting migraine-type headaches, either for the first time or as an exacerbation of existing migraine, should be referred to the doctor, since this may be an early warning of cerebrovascular changes.

Occasionally, a headache is caused by hypertension but, contrary to popular opinion, such headaches are not common and occur only when the blood pressure is extremely high. Nevertheless, the pharmacist should consider the patient's medication carefully. In drug interactions which have led to a rise in blood pressure, for example, between a sympathomimetic such as pseudoephedrine and a monoamine oxidase inhibitor, a headache is likely to occur as a symptom.

The patient may already be taking a non-steroidal anti-inflammatory drug (NSAID) or other analgesic on prescription and duplication of treatments should be avoided, since toxicity may result. If OTC treatment has already been tried without improvement, referral is advisable.

Treatment timescale

If the headache does not respond to OTC analgesics within a day, referral is advisable.

Management

The pharmacist's choice of oral analgesic comprises three main agents: *paracetamol*, NSAIDs (ibuprofen and *diclofenac)* and *aspirin.* These may be combined with other constituents such as *codeine, dihydrocodeine, doxylamine* and *caffeine.* OTC analgesics are available in a variety of dosage forms and, in addition to traditional tablets and capsules, syrups, soluble tablets and sustained release dosage forms are available for some products. The peak blood levels of analgesics are achieved 30 min after taking a dispersible dosage form; after a traditional *aspirin* tablet, it may take up to 2 h for peak levels to be reached. The timing of doses is important in migraine where the analgesic should be taken at the first sign of an attack, preferably in soluble form, since GI motility is slowed during an attack and absorption of analgesics delayed. Combination therapy may sometimes be useful, for example, an analgesic and decongestant (systemic or topical) in sinusitis.

Sumatriptan 50 mg tablets can be used for acute relief of migraine with or without aura and where there is a 'clear diagnosis of migraine'.

Paracetamol

Paracetamol has analgesic and antipyretic effects but little or no anti-inflammatory action. The exact way in which *paracetamol* exerts its analgesic effect remains unclear, despite extensive research. However, the drug is undoubtedly effective in reducing both pain and fever. It is less irritating to the stomach than is *aspirin* and can therefore be recommended for those patients who are unable to take *aspirin* for this reason. Paracetamol can be given to children from 2 to 3 months old, depending on the product licence. Check the individual packs for doses, related to the child's age. A range of paediatric formulations, including sugar-free syrups, is available. Evidence for the effectiveness of *paracetamol* in the management of migraine is limited.

Liver toxicity

At high doses, *paracetamol* can cause liver toxicity and damage may not be apparent until a few days later. All overdoses of *paracetamol* should be taken seriously and the patient referred to a hospital casualty department.

NSAIDs (ibuprofen and diclofenac)

Ibuprofen and *diclofenac* have analgesic, anti-inflammatory and antipyretic activities and cause less irritation and damage to the stomach than does *aspirin*. The dose required for analgesic activity is 200–400 mg and that for anti-inflammatory action 300–600 mg (total daily dose of 1600–2400 mg). The maximum daily dose allowable for OTC use is 1200 mg and *ibuprofen* tablets or capsules should not be given to children under 12 years. *Ibuprofen* suspension 100 mg in 5 mL is available OTC. Differences in product licences mean that some ibuprofen suspensions can be used in children 3 months and over. Check individual product details for doses.

Diclofenac 12.5 mg tablets can be used in adults and children aged 14 years and over. Two tablets should be taken initially, then one or two tablets every 4–6 h as needed. The maximum daily dose is 75 mg. As a result of new safety information in 2013 diclofenac is now contraindicated in patients with cardiovascular disease. When responding to a request to buy OTC oral diclofenac or considering recommending it, pharmacists and their staff need to ask suitable questions to identify whether the patient has cardiovascular disease.

Indigestion

NSAIDs can be irritating to the stomach, causing indigestion, nausea and diarrhoea, but less so than *aspirin*. Gastric bleeding can also occur. For these reasons, it is best to advise patients to take NSAIDs with or after food, and they are best avoided in anyone with a peptic ulcer or a history of peptic ulcer. Elderly patients seem to be particularly prone to these effects. NSAIDs can increase the bleeding time due to an effect on platelets. This effect is reversible within 24 h of stopping the drug (whereas reversibility may take several days after stopping *aspirin)*.

Ibuprofen and *diclofenac* seem to have little or no effect on whole blood clotting or prothrombin time, but it is still not advised for patients taking anticoagulant medication for whom *paracetamol* would be a better choice.

Hypersensitivity

Cross-sensitivity between *aspirin* and NSAIDs occurs, so it would be wise for the pharmacist not to recommend them for anyone with a previous sensitivity reaction to *aspirin*. Since asthmatic patients are more likely to have such a reaction, the use of NSAIDs in asthmatic patients should be with caution.

Contraindications

Sodium and water retention may be caused by NSAIDs and they are therefore best avoided in patients with congestive heart failure or renal impairment and during pregnancy, particularly during the third trimester. Breastfeeding mothers may safely take *ibuprofen* and *diclofenac,* since it is excreted in only tiny amounts in breast milk.

Interactions

There is evidence of an interaction between NSAIDs and *lithium.* NSAIDs may inhibit prostaglandin synthesis in the kidneys and reduce *lithium* clearance. Serum levels of *lithium* are thus raised with the possibility of toxic effects. *Lithium* toxicity manifests itself as GI symptoms, polyuria, muscle weakness, lethargy and tremor.

Caution

NSAIDs are best avoided in *aspirin*-sensitive patients and should be used with caution in asthmatics. Adverse effects are more likely to occur in the elderly and *paracetamol* may be a better choice in these cases.

Aspirin

Aspirin is analgesic, antipyretic and also anti-inflammatory if given in doses greater than 4 g daily. About half of migraine sufferers show significant improvement in their headache 2 h after taking aspirin. It should not be given to children under 16 years because of its suspected link with Reye's syndrome. Reports indicate that some parents are still unaware of the contraindication in children under 16 years. Analgesics are often purchased for family use and it is worth reminding parents the minimum age for the use of aspirin. It has been suggested that in addition to its use in the symptomatic treatment of headaches, doses of *aspirin* on alternate days may be effective in the prophylaxis of migraine but evidence is limited.

Indigestion

Gastric irritation (indigestion, heartburn, nausea and vomiting) is sometimes experienced by patients after taking *aspirin,* and for this reason the drug is best taken with or after food. When taken as dispersible tablets, *aspirin* is less likely to cause gastric irritation. The local use of *aspirin,* for example, dissolving a soluble tablet near an aching tooth, is best avoided, since ulceration of the gums may result.

Bleeding

Aspirin can cause GI bleeding and should not be recommended for any patient who either currently has or has a history of peptic ulcer. *Aspirin* affects the platelets and clotting function, so bleeding time is increased, and it has been suggested that it should not be recommended for pain after tooth extraction for this reason. The effects of anticoagulant drugs are potentiated by *aspirin,* so it should never be recommended for patients taking these drugs.

Alcohol

Alcohol increases the irritant effect of *aspirin* on the stomach and also its effects on bleeding time. Concurrent administration is therefore best avoided.

Pregnancy

Aspirin is best avoided in pregnancy.

Hypersensitivity

Hypersensitivity to *aspirin* occurs in some people; it has been estimated that 4% of asthmatic patients have this problem and *aspirin* should be avoided in any patient with a history of asthma. When such patients take *aspirin,* they may experience skin reactions (rashes and urticaria) or sometimes shortness of breath, bronchospasm and even asthma attacks.

Codeine

Codeine is a narcotic analgesic; a systematic review of evidence from clinical trials showed that a dose of at least 15 mg is required for analgesic effect. *Codeine* is commonly found in combination products with *aspirin, paracetamol* or both. Constipation is a possible side effect and is more likely in elderly patients and others prone to constipation. *Codeine* can also cause drowsiness and respiratory depression, although this may be unlikely at OTC doses. Codeine-containing medicines should only be used in children over 12 years old to treat acute moderate pain, and only if it cannot be relieved by paracetamol or ibuprofen. Codeine should also not be used by breastfeeding mothers because it can pass to the baby through breast milk and potentially cause harm.

Dihydrocodeine

Dihydrocodeine is related to *codeine* and has similar analgesic efficacy. A combination product containing *paracetamol* and *dihydrocodeine* is available with a dose per tablet of 7.46 mg *dihydrocodeine*. The product is restricted to use in adults and children over 12 years. Side effects include constipation and drowsiness. Like *codeine,* the drug may cause respiratory depression at high doses.

Caffeine

Caffeine is included in some combination analgesic products to produce wakefulness and increased mental activity. It is probable that doses of at least 100 mg are needed to produce such an effect and that OTC analgesics contain 30–50 mg per tablet. A cup of tea or coffee would have the same action. Products containing *caffeine* are best avoided near bedtime because of their stimulant effect. It has been claimed that *caffeine* increases the effectiveness of analgesics but the evidence for such claims is not definitive. *Caffeine* has an irritant effect on the stomach.

Doxylamine succinate

Doxylamine is an antihistamine whose sedative and relaxing effects are probably responsible for its usefulness in treating tension headaches. Like other older antihistamines, *doxylamine* can cause drowsiness and patients should be warned about this. *Doxylamine* should not be recommended for children under 12 years.

Buclizine

Buclizine is an antihistamine and is included in an OTC compound analgesic for migraine because of its antiemetic action.

Sumatriptan

Sumatriptan 50 mg tablets can be used OTC for acute relief of migraine with or without aura and where there is a 'clear diagnosis of migraine'. It can be used by people aged between 18 and 65 years. A 50 mg tablet is taken as soon as possible after the migraine headache starts. A second dose can be taken at least 2 h after the first if symptoms come back. A second dose should be taken only if the headache responded to the first dose.

Practice guidance from Royal Pharmaceutical Society (RPS) suggests that if the patient has previously received sumatriptan on prescription and the pharmacy holds their patient medication record, then OTC supplies can be made, provided there has been no change in the condition. If the person has not used sumatriptan before, the pharmacist needs to determine their suitability for the treatment. They must have an established pattern of migraine and the pharmacist needs to identify any other symptoms or relevant medical conditions as well as any medication.

The following patients should be referred for medical assessment:

- Those aged under 18 years or over 65 years
- Those aged 50 years or over and experiencing migraine attacks for the first time. If a doctor confirms a diagnosis of migraine, they can be considered for OTC sumatriptan
- Patients who had their first ever migraine attack within the previous 12 months
- Patients who have had fewer than five migraine attacks in the past
- Patients who experience four or more attacks per month. The patient is potentially suitable for OTC sumatriptan but should be referred to a doctor for further evaluation and management
- If migraine headache lasts for longer than 24 h, the patient is potentially suitable for OTC sumatriptan but should be referred to a doctor for further evaluation and management
- Patients who do not respond to treatment
- Patients who have a headache (of any type) on 10 or more days per month
- Women with migraine who take the COC pill have an increased risk of stroke, so should be referred if the onset of migraine is within the previous 3 months, if migraine attacks are worsening or if they have a migraine with aura
- Patients who do not recover fully between attacks
- Pregnant or breastfeeding migraine sufferers
- Patients with three or more cardiovascular risk factors

(*Source*: Practice Guidance – OTC Sumatriptan. RPSGB, 2006.)

Cautions

People with three or more of the following cardiovascular risk factors are not suitable for OTC sumatriptan: men aged over 40 years; post-menopausal women; hypercholesterolaemia; regular smoker (10 or more daily); obesity – body mass index more than 30 kg/m^2; diabetes; family history of early heart disease – either father or brother had a heart attack or angina before the age of 55 years or mother or sister had a heart attack or angina before the age of 65 years.

Contraindications

Sumatriptan must not be used prophylactically. It should not be used in people with known hypertension, a previous myocardial infarction, ischaemic heart disease, peripheral vascular disease, coronary vasospasm/Prinzmetal's angina, cardiac arrhythmias (including Wolff–Parkinson–White syndrome), hepatic or renal impairment, epilepsy, a history of seizures, a history of cerebrovascular accident or transient ischaemic attack.

Adverse effects. Common adverse effects include nausea and vomiting, disturbances of sensation (including tingling), dizziness, drowsiness, flushing, warm sensation, feeling of weakness and fatigue and feelings of heaviness, pain or pressure in any part of the body.

Interactions

These include monoamine oxidase inhibitors (either current or within the last 2 weeks), ergot and St John's wort (may increase serotonin levels). It has been suggested that an interaction between sumatriptan and selective serotonin reuptake inhibitors or serotonin noradrenaline reuptake inhibitors may occur, causing 'serotonin syndrome' and a small number of cases have been reported in the United States.

Feverfew

Feverfew is a herb that has been used in the prophylaxis of migraine. Some clinical trials have been conducted to examine its effectiveness, but results have been conflicting. Adverse effects that have been reported from the use of feverfew include mouth ulceration involving the oral mucosa and tongue (which seems to occur in about 10% of patients), abdominal colic, heartburn and skin rashes. These effects occur both with feverfew leaves and when the herb is formulated in capsules. The herb has a bitter taste, which some patients cannot tolerate. Feverfew was used in the past as an abortifacient and it should not be recommended for pregnant women with migraine.

Topical headache treatments

These have a cooling action and can be used in children over 12 years and adults. They can be applied to the forehead, back of the neck and temples.

Headaches in practice

Patient perspectives

I have suffered from migraine for about 14 years now. At the beginning I didn't get much advice or medical help, but since then I've actively worked to find out what triggers my attacks. I have found that I have to eat at regular intervals; skipping meals can often trigger an attack. I need to drink at least 1.6 L of water a day and in the summer often much more. Caffeine was a trigger for me and I have stopped drinking coffee and tea now although I enjoy herbal teas. It is really worth experimenting with these as you will find one to your taste, eventually! I cut various things (cheese, red wine) out of my diet for a while to confirm if they were a problem. Other things that I know will set off an attack are lack of sleep and strong perfume.

Most people, when hearing the word 'migraine' think of headache. But people who get migraines know that these are not ordinary headaches. The pain associated with migraine can be debilitating, even disabling – but a lot of people, including healthcare professionals, still don't understand. Sometimes I wish people who think migraines are just a bad headache would have a migraine themselves so they'd know how mistaken they are. Just one migraine for every doctor and pharmacist who will ever treat a migraine patient.

Case 1

For several years Sandra Brown, a young mother, has purchased combination analgesics for migraine from your pharmacy every few months. She has suffered from migraine headaches since she was a child. Today she asks if you have anything stronger; the tablets do not seem to work like they used to. She is not taking any medicines on prescription. (You check whether she is taking the contraceptive pill and she is not.) Sandra tells you that she now suffers from migraines two or three times a month and they are making her life a misery. Nothing seems to trigger them and the pain is not more severe than before. She has read about feverfew and wonders whether she should give it a try.

The pharmacist's view

This woman has successfully used an OTC product to treat her migraines for a long time. Many patients who suffer migraines report that they get relief from OTC analgesics. Sandra's migraines have become more frequent for no apparent reason. Referral to the doctor is needed to exclude any serious cause of her headaches before considering further treatments.

The doctor's view

It makes sense for her to be reviewed by her GP as the headaches are so frequent and making her life a misery. It would be helpful to get more details of her experience of headaches and associated symptoms, for example, any preceding visual symptoms, nature and site of headache, duration; other useful information would include her understanding of migraine, any specific concerns she may have and what sort of treatment she would be prepared to try. There is some evidence that headaches improve more quickly if patients' expectations and concerns are addressed adequately in the consultation. It would also be useful to explore what level of stress she was experiencing. A limited examination would be usual, for example, blood pressure and fundoscopy to look for signs of raised intracranial pressure.

Prophylactic treatments (e.g. *propranolol*) for migraine are available and are worth considering in patients who report attacks more than four times a month. There is inconclusive evidence supporting the use of feverfew as a migraine prophylaxis. Sodium valproate has good evidence of efficacy in migraine prophylaxis but is not licensed for this indication. Although prophylactic treatments may reduce the frequency of migraine attacks, their adverse effects can make them unacceptable to some people. Valproate can cause fetal malformations and other problems if taken during pregnancy. $5HT_1$ agonists, for example, *sumatriptan, zolmitriptan* and *naratriptan,* are effective acute treatments for migraine, producing relief from a headache within 1 or 2 h for many patients. They are contraindicated in those with ischaemic heart disease or poorly controlled hypertension. Research evidence shows that about one of every three patients treated with oral *sumatriptan* will have his or her headache improved.

Case 2

Wei Lin, a woman aged about 30 years, has asked to speak to you. She tells you that she would like you to recommend something for the headaches that she has been getting recently. You ask her to describe the headache and she explains that the pain is across her forehead and around the back of the head. The headaches usually occur during the daytime and have been occurring several times a week, for several weeks. There are no associated GI symptoms and there is no nasal congestion. No medicines are being taken, apart from a compound OTC product containing *aspirin,* which she has been taking for her headaches. On questioning her about recent changes in lifestyle, she tells you that she has recently moved to the area and started a new job last month. In the past, she has suffered from occasional headache, but not regularly. This lady does not wear glasses and says she has not had trouble with her eyesight in the past. She confides that she has been worried that the headaches might be due to something serious.

The pharmacist's view

From the information obtained, it sounds as though this woman is suffering from tension headaches. The location of the pain and lack of associated symptoms lead towards this conclusion. The timing of the headaches indicates that this woman's recent move and change of employment are probably responsible for the problem. The pharmacist should obtain information about the current headaches in relation to the patient's past experience. This patient is worried that the headaches may signal a serious problem, but the evidence indicates that this would be unlikely. The pharmacist could recommend the use of *paracetamol, ibuprofen* or *diclofenac.* If the headaches do not improve within 1 week, she should see her doctor.

The pharmacist's assessment makes sense. A tension headache is the most likely explanation. If her symptoms do not settle within 1 week, it would be very reasonable to be reviewed by her GP. The most important aspect of the GP's assessment would be to determine what her concerns about the headache were; for example, many people with headaches become concerned that they might have a brain tumour. Hopefully, providing appropriate information and explanation will assist her in understanding and managing her headache.

Case 3

Monowarar Ahmed is a regular visitor to your shop. She is a young mother, aged about 25 years, and today she seeks your advice about headaches that have been troubling her recently. The headaches are of a migraine type, quite severe and affecting one side of the head. Mrs Ahmed had her second child a few months ago, and when you ask if she is taking any medicines she tells you that she recently started to take the COC pill. In the past, she has suffered from migraine-type headaches, but only occasionally and never as severe as the ones she has been experiencing during the past weeks. The headaches have been occurring once or twice a week for about 2 weeks. *Paracetamol* has given some relief, but Mrs Ahmed would like to try something stronger.

The pharmacist's view

Mrs Ahmed should be referred to her doctor immediately. Her history of migraine headaches associated with the COC is a cause for concern; in addition, you have established that she has suffered from migraine headaches in the past.

The doctor's view

The pharmacist should recommend referral to the doctor. Someone who develops a first migraine attack whilst taking the pill should be told to discontinue it. If there is a previous history of migraine, the pill may sometimes be used, but if the frequency, severity or nature (especially onset of focal neurological symptoms) of the migraines worsens on the pill, then once again the pill should be discontinued. The reason for this advice is that the migraine could herald a cerebral thrombosis (stroke), which could be prevented by stopping the pill.

Case 4

Ben Jones, a 35-year-old man, comes in asking whether he could have something stronger for his migraines. He tells you that he has had migraines since he was a teenager. The attacks are not that frequent but are quite disabling when they come on. He is particularly concerned that he travels a lot in his job as an IT consultant and cannot afford to be laid up when he is working away from home. Last year he saw his GP who encouraged him to continue with soluble paracetamol and also prescribed domperidone to reduce his nausea. The GP mentioned that he might benefit from a 'triptan' if this was not helping him enough.

Ben explains that his migraine starts with a small area of wavy vision in the centre of his visual field, which is then followed about half an hour later by a throbbing headache above his left eye with nausea and vomiting. He says he feels so bad that he has to lie down in a darkened room. He goes on to say that he usually falls asleep after an hour or so and then sleeps fitfully until the next day when he is better.

He is otherwise fit and well, plays regular sports, is a non-smoker and does not take any other medication.

He goes on to say, 'Can I buy the triptan or do I need to go back to the doctor?'

The pharmacist's view
This patient's history of migraines shows an established pattern and falls within the indications for OTC sumatriptan. Since he does not have any indication for referral to the GP, it would be reasonable for him to try sumatriptan. I would ask him to come back and let me know how the treatment went.

The doctor's view
The pharmacist's recommendation is reasonable since Ben is fit and healthy and has a long-established pattern of headaches previously diagnosed by his GP.

Musculoskeletal problems

Pharmacists are frequently asked for advice about muscular injuries, sprains and strains. Simple practical advice combined with topical or systemic OTC treatment can be valuable. Sometimes patients who are already taking prescribed medicines for musculoskeletal problems will ask for advice. Here a careful assessment of compliance with prescribed medicines and the need for referral is important.

What you need to know
Age
Child, adult, elderly
Symptoms
Pain, swelling, site, duration
History
Injury
Medical conditions
Medication

Significance of questions and answers

Age

Age will influence the pharmacist's choice of treatment, but other reasons make consideration of the patient's age important. In elderly patients, a fall is more likely to result in a fracture; elderly women are particularly at risk because of osteoporosis. Referral to the local casualty department for X-rays may be the best course of action in such cases.

Symptoms and history

Injuries commonly occur as a result of a fall or other trauma and during physical activity such as lifting heavy loads or taking part in sport. Exact details of how the injury occurred should be established by the pharmacist.

Symptoms in the Pharmacy: A Guide to the Management of Common Illness, Seventh Edition. Alison Blenkinsopp, Paul Paxton and John Blenkinsopp.
© 2014 John Wiley & Sons, Ltd. Published 2014 by John Wiley & Sons, Ltd.

Sprains and strains

Sprains. A sprain injury involves the overstretching of ligaments and/or the joint capsule, sometimes with tearing. The most common sprain involves the lateral ankle ligament. Referral is the best course of action, so that the family practitioner or casualty department doctor can examine the affected area and consider whether a complete tearing of ligaments has occurred, particularly for knee injuries. With a partial tear the knee is often swollen and the patient experiences severe pain on movement. A complete tear may involve the tearing of the capsule itself. If this occurs, any blood or fluid can leak out into the surrounding tissues, so the knee may not appear swollen.

Strains. Strains are injuries where the muscle fibres are damaged by overstretching and tearing. Sometimes the fibres within the muscle sheath are torn; sometimes the muscle sheath itself ruptures and bleeding occurs. Strains are most common in muscles that work over two joints, for example, the hamstring. When the strain heals, fibrosis can occur, and the muscle becomes shortened. The muscle is then vulnerable to further damage.

Early mobilisation, strengthening exercises and coordination exercises are all important after both sprains and strains. The return to full activity must occur gradually.

Muscle pain

Stiff and painful muscles may occur simply as a result of strenuous and unaccustomed work, such as gardening, decorating or exercise, and the resulting discomfort can be reduced by treatment with OTC medicines.

Bruising

Bruising as a result of injury is common and some products that minimise bruising are available OTC. The presence of bruising without apparent injury, or a description by the patient of a history of bruising more easily than usual, should alert the pharmacist to the possibility of a more serious condition. Spontaneous bruising may be symptomatic of an underlying blood disorder, for example, thrombocytopaenia or leukaemia, or may result from an adverse drug reaction or other cause.

Head injury

Pain occurring as a result of head injury should always be viewed with suspicion and such patients, particularly children, are best referred for further investigation.

Bursitis

Other musculoskeletal problems about which the pharmacist's advice might be sought include bursitis, which is inflammation of a bursa.

(This is the name given to tissues around joints and where bones move over one another. The function of a bursa is to reduce friction during movement.) Examples of bursitis are housemaid's knee and student's elbow.

Fibromyalgia refers to chronic widespread pain affecting the muscles but not the joints. Tender spots can be discovered in the muscles and the condition can be associated with a sleep disturbance. Brain wave studies often show a loss of deep sleep. This condition may be precipitated by psychological distress and physical trauma. The symptoms can be similar to those of myalgic encepalopathy (encephalomyelitis). Referral to the GP for assessment would be advisable. An empathetic approach from the doctor is important as many patients have felt rejected or that their problems have not been taken seriously by the health professional. Medication (e.g. tricyclics, NSAIDs and *gabapentin)* is of limited benefit in these situations.

Frozen shoulder

Frozen shoulder is a common condition where the shoulder is stiff and painful. It is more prevalent in older patients. The shoulder pain sometimes radiates to the arm and is often worse at night. Patients can sometimes relate the problem to injury, exertion or exposure to cold, but frozen shoulder may occur without apparent cause. The pain and limitation of movement are usually so severe that referral to the doctor is advisable.

Painful joints

Pain arising in joints (arthralgia) may be due to arthritis, for which there are many causes. The pain may be associated with swelling, overlying inflammation, stiffness, limitation of movement and deformity of the joint. A common cause of arthritis is osteoarthritis (OA), which is due to wear and tear of the joint. This often affects the knees and hips, especially in the older population. Another form of arthritis is rheumatoid arthritis (RA), which is a more generalised illness caused by the body turning its defences on itself. Other forms of arthritis can be caused by gout or infection, usually with signs of overlying inflammation and swelling. A joint infection is rare but serious and occasionally fatal. It is often difficult to distinguish between the different causes and it is therefore necessary to refer to the doctor except in mild cases.

Back pain

Lower back pain affects 60–80% of people at some stage in their lives and is often recurrent. Non-serious acute back problems need to be treated early, with mobilisation and exercise thought to be particularly important in the prevention of chronic low back pain. Acute back pain is generally regarded as lasting less than 6 weeks, subacute for 6–12 weeks and chronic longer than 12 weeks. The main cause is a strain of the muscles or other soft structures (e.g. ligaments and tendons) connected to the vertebrae. Sometimes it is the cushion between the bones (intervertebral disc) which is strained and which bulges out (herniates) and presses on the nearby nerves (as in sciatica). Lower back pain that is not too severe or debilitating and comes on after gardening, awkward lifting or bending may be due to muscular strain (lumbago) and appropriate advice may be given by the pharmacist.

Bed rest is not recommended for simple low back pain. The emphasis is on maintaining activity, supported by pain relief. There is evidence from RCTs that advice to stay active results in increased rate of recovery, reduced pain, reduced disability and reduced time off work compared with advice to rest. If there is no improvement within 1 week, referral is advisable.

Pain that is more severe, causing difficulty with mobility or radiating from the back down one or both legs, is an indication for referral. A slipped disc can press on the sciatic nerve (hence sciatica), causing pain and sometimes pins and needles and numbness in the leg. Low back pain associated with any altered sensation in the anal or genital area or bladder symptoms requires urgent referral to the GP.

Back pain that is felt in the middle to upper part of the back is less common, and if it has been present for several days, it is best referred to the doctor. Kidney pain can be felt in the back, to either side of the middle part of the back just below the ribcage (loin area). If the back pain in the loin area is associated with any abnormality of passing urine (discolouration of urine, pain on passing urine or frequency), then a kidney problem is more likely.

Repetitive strain disorder

Repetitive strain disorder covers several arm conditions, mainly affecting the forearm. Tenosynovitis is the term that has been used to refer to conditions around the wrist, which sometimes occur in computer operators. The condition presents as swelling on the back of the forearm. There may be crepitus (a creaking, grating sound) when the wrist is moved. Sometimes the symptoms disappear on stopping the job, but they may return when the work is restarted.

Whiplash injuries

Neck pain following a car accident can last for a long period – up to 2 years in some cases. Good posture is important and keeping both the back and the head straight has been shown to reduce pain and help recovery. A physiotherapist's advice would probably include the recommendation to sleep with only one pillow to facilitate extension of the neck.

Medication
Prescribed medication

Sufferers, for example, of RA or chronic back pain are likely to be taking painkillers or NSAIDs prescribed by their doctor. Although the recommendation of a topical analgesic would produce no problems in terms of drug interactions, if the patient is in considerable and regular pain despite prescribed medication, or the pain has become worse, referral back to the doctor would be appropriate.

Side effects. In elderly patients, it should be remembered that falls may occur as a result of postural hypotension, dizziness or confusion as adverse effects from drug therapy. Any elderly patient reporting falls should be carefully questioned about current medication, and the pharmacist should contact the doctor if an adverse reaction is suspected.

Self-medication

The pharmacist should also enquire about any preparations used in self-treatment of the condition and their degree of effectiveness.

When to refer
Suspected fracture
Possible adverse drug reaction: falls or bruising
Head injury
Medication failure
Arthritis
Severe back pain
Back pain (and/or pins and needles/numbness) radiating to leg
Back pain in the middle/upper back (especially in the older patient)

Treatment timescale

Musculoskeletal conditions should respond to treatment within a few days. A maximum of 5 days treatment should be recommended, after which patients should see their doctor.

Management

A wide range of preparations containing systemic and topical analgesics is available (see p. 199 for a discussion of systemic analgesics). The oral analgesic of choice would usually be an NSAID, such as *ibuprofen*, provided there were no contraindications. Taking the analgesic regularly is important to obtain full effect and the patient needs to know this. Topical formulations include creams, ointments, lotions, sticks and sprays.

Topical analgesics

There is a high placebo response to topical analgesic products. This is probably because the act of massaging the formulation into the affected area will increase blood flow and stimulate the nerves, leading to a reduction in the sensation of pain.

Counterirritants and rubefacients

Counterirritants and rubefacients cause vasodilatation, inducing a feeling of warmth over the area of application. Counterirritants produce mild skin irritation, and the term rubefacient refers to the reddening and warming of the skin. The theory behind the use of topical analgesics is that they bombard the nervous system with sensations other than pain (warmth and irritation) and this is thought to distract attention from the pain felt. Simply rubbing or massaging the affected area produces sensations of warmth and pressure and can reduce pain. Massage is known to relax muscles and it has also been suggested that massage may disperse some of the chemicals that are responsible for producing pain and inflammation by increasing the blood flow. The mode of action of topical analgesics is therefore twofold: one effect relying on absorption of the agent through the skin, while the other on the benefit of the massage. There is no published evidence on the effectiveness of counterirritants and rubefacients. This is not surprising as many of the active ingredients and formulations have been available for many years.

There are many proprietary formulations available, often incorporating a mixture of ingredients with different properties. Most pharmacists and customers have their own favourite product. For customers who live alone, a spray formulation, which does not require massage, can be recommended for areas such as the back and shoulders. Generally, patients can be advised to use topical analgesic products up to four times a day, as required.

Methyl salicylate

Methyl salicylate is one of the most widely used and effective counterirritants. Wintergreen is its naturally occurring form; synthetic versions are also available. A systematic review concluded that salicylates may be effective in acute pain but that the clinical trials were not of good quality. The agent is generally used in concentrations between 10% and 60% in topical analgesic formulations.

Nicotinates

Nicotinates (e.g. *ethyl nicotinate* and *hexyl nicotinate*) are absorbed through the skin and produce reddening of the skin, increased blood flow and an increase in temperature. *Methyl nicotinate* is used at concentrations of 0.25–1% to produce its counterirritant and rubefacient effects. There have been occasional reports of systemic adverse effects following absorption of *nicotinates*, such as dizziness or feelings of faintness, which are due to a drop in blood pressure following vasodilatation. However, systemic adverse effects are rare, seem to occur only in susceptible people and are usually due to use of the product over a large surface area.

Menthol

Menthol has a cooling effect when applied to the skin and acts as a mild counterirritant. Used in topical formulations in concentrations of up to 1%, *menthol* has antipruritic actions, but at higher concentrations it has a counterirritant effect. When applied to the skin in a topical analgesic formulation, *menthol* gives a feeling of coolness, followed by a sensation of warmth.

Capsaicin/capsicum

The sensation of hotness from eating peppers is caused by the excitation of nerve endings in the skin, body organs and airways. Capsicum preparations, for example, *capsaicin capsicum* and *capsicum oleoresin*, produce a feeling of warmth when applied to the skin. They do not cause reddening because they do not act on capillary or other blood vessels. *Capsaicin* (available on prescription) has been the subject of research in clinical trials as an analgesic for post-herpetic pain and this work is continuing. Studies in patients with arthritis have also shown effectiveness. *Capsaicin* has few side effects. A small amount needs to be rubbed well into the affected area. Patients should always wash their hands after use; otherwise they may inadvertently transfer the substance to the eyes, causing burning and stinging.

Topical anti-inflammatory agents

Topical gels, creams and ointments containing NSAIDs are widely used in the United Kingdom. Clinical trials have shown them to be as effective as oral NSAIDs in relieving musculoskeletal pain. There have been no comparative trials with counterirritants and rubefacients.

Ibuprofen, felbinac, ketoprofen and *piroxicam* are available in a range of cream and gel formulations. The drug is absorbed into the bloodstream and appears to become concentrated in the affected tissues. Topical NSAIDs (except *benzydamine*) should not be used by patients who experience adverse reactions to *aspirin*, such as asthma, rhinitis or urticaria. Because of the higher likelihood of *aspirin* sensitivity in patients with asthma, caution should be exercised when considering recommending a topical NSAID. Several reports of bronchospasm have been received following the use of these products. Rarely, GI side effects have occurred, mainly dyspepsia, nausea and diarrhoea.

Heparinoid and hyaluronidase

Heparinoid and *hyaluronidase* are enzymes that may help to disperse oedematous fluid in swollen areas. A reduction in swelling and bruising may therefore be achieved. Products containing *heparinoid* or *hyaluronidase* are used in the treatment of bruises, strains and sprains.

Glucosamine and chondroitin

There is some evidence that *glucosamine sulphate* and *chondroitin* improve the symptoms of OA in the knee and that *glucosamine* may have a beneficial structural effect on joints. The research shows that *glucosamine* may be as effective as NSAIDs in reducing pain. However, the quality of some trials is poor. Most trials used a daily dose of 1500 mg of *glucosamine*. Adverse effects are uncommon and include abdominal discomfort and tenderness, heartburn, diarrhoea and nausea. There is insufficient information about pharmaceutical quality and actual content of *glucosamine* to enable pharmacists to make informed choices between available products. Some are produced from natural sources (the shells of crabs and other crustaceans), while others are synthesised from glutamic acid and glucose. A licensed *glucosamine* product became available in 2007, initially limited to prescription use only. The 2008 NICE guideline suggested that patients wanting to try OTC glucosamine could be helped by advice on how to evaluate their pain before starting and to review at 3 months.

Acupuncture

There are no RCTs of acupuncture in acute low back pain and thus no evidence of effectiveness. For chronic low back pain, 8 of 11 RCTs found acupuncture to be no more effective than placebo.

In OA of the knee, acupuncture has been shown to be of benefit in pain relief and improvement in function. The effect size of acupuncture in OA knee is similar to NSAIDs and exercise.

Practical points

First-aid treatment of sprains and strains

The priority in treating sprains and soft tissue injuries is to apply compression, cooling and elevation immediately, and this combination should be maintained for at least 48 h. Although cooling has generally been the priority in the past, latest research evidence suggests that compression is the first priority. The aim of the treatment is to prevent swelling. If swelling is not minimised, the resulting pain and pressure will limit movement, lead to muscle wasting, cause pain and delay recovery. Ice packs by themselves will reduce metabolic needs of the tissues, reduce blood flow and result in less tissue damage and swelling, but will not prevent haemorrhage.

The area should be wrapped around with a cotton wool pad and held in place with a crepe bandage.

Once the injury has been protected and a compression bandage applied, an ice pack should be used. Its function is to produce vaso-constriction, thus preventing further blood flow into the injured area from the torn capillaries and, in turn, minimising further bruising and swelling. Proprietary cold packs are available, but in emergencies various items have been brought into service. For example, a bag of frozen peas is an excellent cold pack for the knee or ankle because it can be easily applied and wrapped around the affected joint.

The affected limb should be elevated to reduce blood flow into the damaged area by the effect of gravity. This will, in turn, reduce the amount of swelling caused by oedema. Finally, the injured limb should be rested to facilitate recovery. The acronym RICE is a useful aide-memoire for the treatment of sprains and strains.

R – Rest
I – Ice/cooling
C – Compression
E – Elevation

Heat

The application of heat can be effective in reducing pain. However, heat should never be applied immediately after an injury has occurred, because heat application at the acute stage will dilate blood vessels and increase blood flow into the affected area – the opposite effect to what is needed. After the acute phase is over (1 or 2 days after the injury), heat can be useful. The application of heat can be both comforting and effective in chronic conditions such as back pain.

Patients can use a hot-water bottle, a proprietary heat pack or an infrared lamp on the affected area. Heat packs contain a mixture of chemicals that give off heat and the packs are disposable. Keeping the joints and muscles warm can also be helpful and wearing warm clothing, particularly in thin layers that can retain heat, is valuable.

Prevention of recurrent back pain

Good posture, lifting correctly, a good mattress and losing excess weight can help. Paying attention to posture and body awareness is important, and classes to relearn good posture may help some patients (e.g. Feldenkrais method and Alexander technique). The additional pressure on the spine caused by excess weight may lead to structural compromise and damage (e.g. injury and sciatica). The lower back is particularly vulnerable to the effects of obesity, and lack of exercise leads to poor flexibility and weak back muscles.

Irritant effect of topical analgesics

Preparations containing topical analgesics should always be kept well away from the eyes, mouth and mucous membranes and should not be applied to broken skin. Intense pain and irritant effects can occur following such contact. This is due to the ready penetration of the irritant topical analgesics through both mucosal surfaces and direct access via the broken skin. When preparations are applied to thinner and more sensitive areas of the skin, irritant effects will be increased and hence, the restrictions on the use of topical analgesics in young children recommended by some manufacturers for their products. Therefore, the manufacturer's instructions and recommendations should be checked. Sensitisation to counterirritants can occur; if blistering or intense irritation of the skin results after application, the patient should discontinue use of the product.

Musculoskeletal problems in practice

Case 1

Charan Gogna, a regular customer in his late 20s, comes into your pharmacy. He asks what you would recommend for a painful lower back following his weekend football game; he thinks he must have pulled a muscle and says he has had the problem before in the same spot. On questioning, you find out that he has not taken any painkillers or used any treatment. He is not taking any other medicines.

The pharmacist's view

Mr Gogna could take an oral analgesic regularly until the discomfort subsides. A topical analgesic could also be useful if gently massaged into the affected area. Since the back is hard to reach, a spray formulation might be easier than a rub. Evidence shows that bed rest does not speed up recovery, and Mr Gogna should be advised to continue his usual daily routine.

The doctor's view

His low back pain should settle in a few days. As he has had recurrent bouts of pain he could be reviewed by his GP. A more detailed history of his problem describing his occupation would be useful with an examination of his back. Depending on the findings, he might be advised to see a physiotherapist or an osteopath. His posture and way of moving might be less than ideal and might be putting him at risk of future problems. If this is so, he might benefit from attending classes with an Alexander or Feldenkrais teacher.

Case 2

A middle-aged man comes into your shop. He is wearing a tracksuit and training shoes and asks what you can recommend for an aching back. On questioning, you find out that the product is, in fact, required for his wife, who was doing some gardening yesterday because the weather was fine and who now feels stiff and aching. The pain is in the lower back and is worse on movement. His wife is not taking any medicines on a regular basis but took two *paracetamol* tablets last night, which helped to reduce the pain.

The pharmacist's view

In this case it would have been very easy for the pharmacist to assume that the man in the shop was the patient whereas, in fact, he was making a request on his wife's behalf. This emphasises the importance of establishing the identity of the patient. The history described is of a common problem: muscle stiffness following unaccustomed or strenuous activity – in this case, gardening. The pharmacist might recommend a combination of systemic and topical therapy. If there were an adequate supply of *paracetamol* tablets at home, the woman could continue to take a maximum of two tablets four times daily until the pain resolved. Alternatively, an oral or topical NSAID or a topical rub or spray containing counterirritants could be advised. The woman should see her doctor if the symptoms have not improved within 5 days.

The doctor's view

The story is suggestive of simple muscle strain, which should settle with the pharmacist's advice within a few days. It would be helpful to enquire whether or not she has had backaches before and, if so, what happened. It would also be worth checking that she did not have pain or pins and needles radiating down her legs. If these symptoms were present, then she might have a slipped disc and referral to her doctor would be advisable.

Case 3

An elderly female customer who regularly visits your pharmacy asks what would be the best thing for 'rheumatic' pain, which is worse now that the weather is getting colder. The pain is in the joints, particularly of the fingers and knees. On further questioning, you find out that she has suffered from this problem for some years and that she sees her doctor quite regularly about this and a variety of other complaints. On checking your patient medication records, you find that she is taking five different medicines a day. Her regular medication includes a combination diuretic preparation, sleeping tablets and analgesics for her arthritis (*co-dydramol* plus an NSAID). The joint pains seem to have become worse during the recent spell of bad weather.

The pharmacist's view

It would be best for this customer to see her doctor. She is already taking several medicines, including analgesics for arthritis. It would therefore be inappropriate for the pharmacist to consider recommendation of a systemic anti-inflammatory or analgesic because of the possibilities of interaction or duplication. Indeed, the recent worsening of the symptoms indicates that consultation with the doctor would be wise. Perhaps this woman is not taking all her medicines; the pharmacist could explore any compliance problems with her before referring her back to the doctor.

The doctor's view

Referral to the doctor is advisable. She may have OA, RA or even some other form of arthritis and the doctor would be in the best position to advise further treatment. The GP is already likely to have made an assessment of her joint pains. OA most commonly affects the end joints of the fingers, whereas RA affects the other small joints of the fingers and knuckles. Knees can be affected by both OA and RA, whereas in the case of the hip, OA is most common. A feature of RA is morning joint stiffness. Blood tests and X-rays can assist the diagnosis. An appointment with the GP would also give an opportunity to review her medication. She may not have been taking her medicines regularly. It would be helpful to find out whether she is experiencing adverse effects and to renegotiate her treatment.

Women's Health

Cystitis

Cystitis is a term used to describe a collection of urinary symptoms including dysuria, frequency and urgency. The urine may be cloudy and strong smelling; these may be signs of bacterial infection. In 50% of cases, no bacterial cause is found. When infection is present, the common bacteria are *Escherichia coli* or *Staphylococcus saprophyticus,* and the source is often the gastrointestinal (GI) tract. About half of the cases will resolve within 3 days even without treatment. Cystitis is common in women but rare in men; it has been estimated that more than one in two women will experience an episode of cystitis during their lives. The pharmacist should be aware of the signs that indicate more serious conditions. Over-the-counter (OTC) products are available for the treatment of cystitis, but are recommended only when symptoms are mild, or for use until the patient can consult her doctor or nurse.

What you need to know

Age
  Adult, child
Male or female
Symptoms
  Urethral irritation
  Urinary urgency, frequency
  Dysuria (pain on passing urine)
  Haematuria (blood in the urine)
  Vaginal discharge
Associated symptoms
  Back pain
  Lower abdominal (suprapubic) pain
  Fever, chills
  Nausea/vomiting
Duration
Previous history
Medication

Symptoms in the Pharmacy: A Guide to the Management of Common Illness, Seventh Edition.
Alison Blenkinsopp, Paul Paxton and John Blenkinsopp.
© 2014 John Wiley & Sons, Ltd. Published 2014 by John Wiley & Sons, Ltd.

Significance of questions and answers

Age

Any child with the symptoms of cystitis should always be referred to the doctor for further investigation and treatment. Urinary tract infections (UTIs) occur in children, and damage to the kidney or bladder may result, particularly after recurrent infections.

Gender

Cystitis is much more common in women than in men for two reasons:

1 Cystitis occurs when bacteria pass up along the urethra and enter and multiply within the bladder. As the urethra is much shorter in females than in males, the passage of the bacteria is much easier. In addition, the process is facilitated by sexual intercourse.
2 There is evidence that prostatic fluid has antibacterial properties, providing an additional defence against bacterial infection in males.

Referral

Any man who presents with the symptoms of cystitis requires medical referral because of the possibility of more serious conditions such as kidney or bladder stones or prostate problems.

Pregnancy

If a pregnant woman presents with symptoms of cystitis, referral to the doctor is the best option, because bacteriuria (presence of bacteria in the urine) in pregnancy can lead to kidney infection and other problems.

Symptoms

Cystitis sufferers often report that the first sign of an impending attack is an itching or pricking sensation in the urethra. The desire to pass urine becomes frequent and women with cystitis may feel the need to pass urine urgently, but pass only a few burning, painful drops. This frequency of urine occurs throughout the day and night. Dysuria (pain on passing urine) is a classical symptom of cystitis. After urination, the bladder may not feel completely empty, but even straining produces no further flow. The urine may be cloudy and strong smelling; these may be signs of bacterial infection.

Chlamydial infection

Chlamydia is a sexually transmitted infection and is most commonly seen in women aged 16–24 years. About 1 in 10 women under the age of 25 years have it. Unfortunately, most women with it (about 80%) do not have any symptoms. Those that do can have symptoms of cystitis, an alteration in vaginal discharge or lower abdominal pain. Chlamydia can cause pelvic inflammatory disease (PID) and infertility. It is important that the infection be detected and treated. Screening programmes for chlamydia are now widespread. Women under 25 years attending health clinics (contraceptive clinics, general practice, young people's services, antenatal clinics, etc.) for any reason are offered screening and in some areas community pharmacies offer a screening (and sometimes treatment) service. Each woman is offered a urine test and given a vulvovaginal swab to self-collect. Women can choose how to receive their results, for example, phone, post, etc. Those with positive results are offered treatment with *azithromycin* and advised about informing their sexual partner(s). The use of condoms can prevent the infection from being spread.

Blood in urine

Haematuria (presence of blood in the urine) is an indication for referral to the doctor. It often occurs in cystitis when there is so much inflammation of the lining of the bladder and urethra that bleeding occurs. This is not serious and responds quickly to antibiotic treatment. Sometimes blood in the urine may indicate other problems such as a kidney stone. When this occurs, pain in the loin or between the loin and groin is the predominant symptom. When blood in the urine develops without any pain, specialist referral is required to exclude the possibility of a tumour in the bladder or kidney.

Vaginal discharge

The presence of a vaginal discharge would indicate local fungal or bacterial infection and would require referral.

Associated symptoms

When dealing with symptoms involving the urinary system, it is best to think of it as divided into two parts: the upper (kidneys and ureters) and the lower (bladder and urethra). The pharmacist should be aware of the symptoms that accompany minor lower UTI and those that suggest more serious problems higher in the urinary tract, so that referral for medical advice can be made where appropriate.

Upper UTI symptoms

Systemic involvement, demonstrated by fever, nausea, vomiting, loin pain and tenderness are indicative of more serious infection such as pyelitis or pyelonephritis, and patients with such symptoms require referral.

Other symptoms

Cystitis may be accompanied by suprapubic (lower abdominal) pain and tenderness.

Duration

Treatment with OTC preparations is reasonable for mild cystitis of short duration (less than 2 days).

Previous history

Women with recurrent cystitis should see their doctor. One in two episodes of cystitis is not caused by infection and the urethral syndrome is thought to be responsible for these non-infective cases. The anxiety produced by repeated occurrences of cystitis is itself thought to be a contributory factor.

An estimated one in ten cases of UTI is followed by relapse (the same bacterium being responsible) or reinfection (where a different organism may be involved). The remaining nine cases clear up without recurrence.

Diabetes

Recurrent cystitis can sometimes occur in diabetic patients and therefore anyone describing a history of increasing thirst, weight loss and a higher frequency of passing urine than normal should be referred.

Honeymoon cystitis

Sexual intercourse may precipitate an attack (honeymoon cystitis) due to minor trauma or resulting infection when bacteria are pushed along the urethra.

Other precipitating factors

Other precipitating factors may include the irritant effects of toiletries (e.g. bubble baths and vaginal deodorants) and other chemicals (e.g. spermicides and disinfectants). Lack of personal hygiene is not thought to be responsible, except in extreme cases.

Postmenopausal women

Oestrogen deficiency in postmenopausal women leads to thinning of the lining of the vagina. Lack of lubrication can mean the vagina and urethra are vulnerable to trauma and irritation and attacks of cystitis can occur. For such women, painful intercourse can also be a problem and this can be treated with OTC lubricants or prescribed products (e.g. oestrogen creams). Lubricant products are available OTC and newer formulations mean that a single application can remain effective for several days. Should this approach be unsuccessful, or if other troublesome symptoms are present, referral to the doctor would be advisable.

Medication
Cystitis can be caused by cytotoxic drugs such as *cyclophosphamide*.

When to refer
All men, children
Fever, nausea/vomiting
Loin pain or tenderness
Haematuria
Vaginal discharge
Duration of longer than 2 days
Pregnancy
Recurrent cystitis
Failed medication

The identity of any preparations already taken to treat the symptoms is therefore important. The pharmacist may then decide whether an appropriate remedy has been used. Failed medication would be a reason for referral to the doctor.

Treatment timescale

If symptoms have not subsided within 2 days of beginning the treatment, the patient should see her doctor.

Management

For pain relief, offer *paracetamol* or *ibuprofen* for up to 2 days. A high temperature will also be reduced, bearing in mind that a level above 38.5°C is more characteristic of pyelonephritis. The pharmacist can also recommend a product that will alkalinise the urine and provide symptomatic relief, although there is no good evidence of effectiveness. Other OTC preparations are of doubtful value. In addition to treatment, it is important for the pharmacist to offer advice about fluid intake (see 'Practical points' below). For women in whom cystitis is a recurrent problem, self-help measures can sometimes prevent recurrence. Signposting to relevant information is useful.

Potassium and sodium citrate
Potassium and sodium citrate work by making the urine alkaline. The acidic urine produced as a result of bacterial infection is thought to be responsible for dysuria; alkalinisation of the urine can therefore

provide symptomatic relief. While easing discomfort, alkalinising the urine will not produce an antibacterial effect, and it is important to tell patients that if symptoms have not improved within 2 days, they should see their doctor. Proprietary sachets are more palatable than *potassium citrate mixture.*

Contraindications

There are some patients for whom such preparations should not be recommended. For *potassium citrate,* these would include anyone taking potassium-sparing diuretics, aldosterone antagonists or angiotensin-converting enzyme inhibitors, in whom hyperkalaemia may result. Sodium citrate should not be recommended for hypertensive patients, anyone with heart disease or pregnant women.

Warning

Patients should be reminded not to exceed the stated dose of products containing *potassium citrate:* several cases of hyperkalaemia have been reported in patients taking *potassium citrate mixture* for relief from urinary symptoms.

Complementary therapies

Cranberry juice has been recommended as a folk remedy for years as a preventive measure to reduce UTI. A systematic review of evidence showed that drinking *cranberry juice* on a regular basis (300 mL per day) has a bacteriostatic effect. The mechanism for this is unknown and the full clinical implications have not been elucidated. Capsules containing 200 mg *cranberry extract* are available. *Cranberry juice* or capsules are unlikely to be effective in the treatment of acute cystitis. Patients taking *warfarin* should not take cranberry products.

Azithromycin and chlamydial infection

At the time of writing, it has been proposed that the antibiotic azithromycin should be deregulated from prescription-only medicine control for the treatment of asymptomatic chlamydial infection following a positive test result (nucleic acid amplification test (NAAT)). Two 500 mg tablets of azithromycin would be given as a single-dose treatment. Symptomatic cases of *Chlamydia* would be referred since they have an increased risk of complications. Some pharmacists already supply azithromycin for chlamydial infection via a patient group direction (PGD).

Practical points

1 There is little evidence to support much of the traditional advice that has been given to women with cystitis, and the list below can be discussed with the woman to consider acceptability.

(i) Drinking large quantities of fluids should theoretically help in cystitis because the bladder is emptied more frequently and completely as a result of the diuresis produced; this is thought to help flush the infecting bacteria out of the bladder. However, this may cause more discomfort where dysuria is severe and may be better as advice to prevent recurrence rather than to use during treatment. Drinking the normally recommended amount of fluids may be preferred.

(ii) During urination the bladder should be emptied completely by waiting for 20 seconds after passing urine and then straining to empty the final drops. Leaning backwards is said to help to achieve a complete emptying of the bladder than the usual sitting posture.

(iii) After a bowel motion wiping toilet paper from front to back may minimise transfer of bacteria from the bowel into the vagina and urethra.

(iv) Urination immediately after sexual intercourse will theoretically flush out most bacteria from the urethra but there is no evidence to support this.

2 Reduced intake of coffee and alcohol may help because these substances seem to act as bladder irritants in some people.

Cystitis in practice

Case 1

Mrs Anne Lawson, a young woman in her 20s, asks to have a quiet word with you. She tells you that she thinks she has cystitis. On questioning, you find that she is not passing urine more frequently than normal, but that her urine looks dark and smells unpleasant. Mrs Lawson has back pain and has been feeling feverish today. She is not taking any medicine from the doctor and has not tried anything to treat her symptoms.

The pharmacist's view

This woman has described symptoms that are not of a minor nature. In particular, the presence of fever and back pain indicates an infection higher in the urinary tract. Mrs Lawson should see her doctor as soon as possible.

The doctor's view

Referral is advisable. She may have a UTI, possibly in the kidney. However, there is insufficient information to make a definite diagnosis. It would be useful to know if she has pain on passing urine and the site and nature of her back pain. Her symptoms could, in fact, be accounted for by a flulike viral infection in which the backache is caused by muscular inflammation and the urine altered because of dehydration. The general practitioner (GP) is likely to check the urine in the surgery with a multistix test and also sends a sample (midstream specimen of urine) to the laboratory for miscroscopy and culture. If the multistix test were positive for leucocytes and nitrites, a urinary infection would be likely, and the patient would be started on antibiotics awaiting laboratory confirmation of the bacteria responsible. She may subsequently require further investigations of her renal tract, for example, an ultrasound of her kidneys and possibly an intravenous urogram. Severe cases of kidney infection require emergency hospital admission for intravenous antibiotics.

Case 2

A young man asks if you can recommend a good treatment for cystitis. In response to your questions, he tells you that the medicine is for him: he has been having pain when passing urine since yesterday. He otherwise feels well and does not have any other symptoms. No treatments have been tried already and he is not currently taking any medicines.

The pharmacist's view

This man should be referred to the doctor because the symptoms of cystitis are uncommon in men and may be the result of a more serious condition.

The doctor's view

Referral is necessary for accurate diagnosis. A urine sample will need to be collected for appropriate analysis. If it shows that he has a urinary infection, then treatment with a suitable antibiotic can be given and a referral to a specialist for further investigation made. The reason for referral is that urinary infection is relatively uncommon in men compared to women and may be caused by some structural problem within the urinary tract.

If in addition to discomfort on passing urine he develops a urethral discharge, he is most likely to be suffering from a sexually transmitted infection, such as *Chlamydia* (previously called non-specific urethritis) or gonorrhoea. *Chlamydia* is the more prevalent of the two and can be treated using *azithromycin* or *doxycycline*. *Chlamydia* can be complicated by an infection around the testis which becomes very painful swollen and red. It may also lead to reduced fertility. Another complication of *Chlamydia* is the development of a reactive arthritis (Reiters), which often affects the knees and feet often associated with conjunctivitis.

Case 3

It is Saturday afternoon and a young woman whom you do not recognise as a regular customer asks for something to treat cystitis. On questioning, you find out that she has had the problem several times before and that her symptoms are frequency and pain on passing urine. She is otherwise well and tells you that her doctor has occasionally prescribed antibiotics to treat the problem in the past. She is not taking any medicines.

The pharmacist's view

This woman represents a common situation in community pharmacy. She has had these symptoms before and is unlikely to be able to see her doctor before Monday. Antibiotic treatment without a urine culture is discouraged where symptoms are mild. She should see her doctor on Monday if the symptoms have not improved and the pharmacist could suggest that she take a urine sample with her, although in practice the GP may prescribe without test results if the symptoms are moderate or severe. In the meantime, she is experiencing considerable discomfort. It would be reasonable to recommend the use of an alkalinising agent, such as *sodium* or *potassium citrate,* over the weekend. You could advise her to drink plenty of fluids but with minimum consumption of tea, coffee and alcohol, all of which may cause dehydration and make the problem worse.

The doctor's view

The story is suggestive of cystitis. Symptomatic treatment with *potassium citrate* may help until after the weekend. It would be interesting to know how her infections usually resolve. If her symptoms did not ease with an alkalinising agent, she could be advised to speak to the on-call GP. If she had severe symptoms, it would be reasonable to start treatment with an antibiotic. If she brought a urine sample, the GP could test it immediately with a multistix dip test, which would determine the presence of protein, red blood cells, leucocytes and nitrite. Positive results for the latter two would be very suggestive of a bacterial infection. Changing patterns of resistance mean that first-line antibiotics vary according to local protocols.

Dysmenorrhoea

It has been estimated that as many as one in two women suffers from dysmenorrhoea (period pains). Up to one in ten of those affected will have severe symptoms, which necessitate time off school or work. Many of these women will try self-medication, seeking advice from their doctor only if this treatment is unsuccessful. Pharmacists should remain aware that discussing menstrual problems is potentially embarrassing for the patient and should therefore try to create an atmosphere of privacy.

What you need to know

Age
Previous history
Regularity and timing of cycle
Timing and nature of pains
Relationship with menstruation
Other symptoms
   Headache, backache
   Nausea, vomiting, constipation
   Faintness, dizziness, fatigue
   Premenstrual syndrome (PMS)
Medication

Significance of questions and answers

Age

The peak incidence of primary dysmenorrhoea occurs in women between the ages of 17 and 25 years. Primary dysmenorrhoea is defined as pain in the absence of pelvic disease, whereas secondary dysmenorrhoea refers to pain, which may be due to underlying disease. Secondary dysmenorrhoea is most common in women aged over 30 years and is rare in women aged under 25 years. Common causes of secondary dysmenorrhoea include endometriosis or PID. Primary dysmenorrhoea is uncommon after having children.

Symptoms in the Pharmacy: A Guide to the Management of Common Illness, Seventh Edition.
Alison Blenkinsopp, Paul Paxton and John Blenkinsopp.
© 2014 John Wiley & Sons, Ltd. Published 2014 by John Wiley & Sons, Ltd.

Previous history

Dysmenorrhoea is often not associated with the start of menstruation (menarche). This is because during the early months (and sometimes years) of menstruation, ovulation does not occur. These anovulatory cycles are usually, but not always, pain free and therefore women sometimes describe period pain that begins after several months or years of pain-free menstruation. The pharmacist should establish whether the menstrual cycle is regular and the length of the cycle. Further questioning should then focus on the timing of pains in relation to menstruation.

Timing and nature of pains

Primary dysmenorrhoea

Primary dysmenorrhoea classically presents as a cramping lower abdominal pain that often begins during the day before bleeding starts. The pain gradually eases after the start of menstruation and is often gone by the end of the first day of bleeding.

Mittelschmerz   Mittelschmerz is ovulation pain which occurs midcycle, at the time of ovulation. The abdominal pain usually lasts for a few hours, but can last for several days and may be accompanied by some bleeding.

Secondary dysmenorrhoea

The pain of secondary or acquired dysmenorrhoea may occur during other parts of the menstrual cycle and can be relieved or worsened by menstruation. Such pain is often described as a dull, aching pain rather than being spasmodic or cramping in nature. Often occurring up to 1 week before menstruation, the pain may get worse once bleeding starts. The pain may occur during sexual intercourse. Secondary dysmenorrhoea is more common in older women, especially in those who have had children. In pelvic infection, a vaginal discharge may be present in addition to pain. If, from questioning, the pharmacist suspects secondary dysmenorrhoea, the patient should be referred to her doctor for further investigation.

Endometriosis   Endometriosis mainly occurs in women aged between 30 and 45 years, but can occur in women in their 20s. The womb (uterus) has a unique inner lining surface (endometrium). In endometriosis, pieces of endometrium are also found in places outside the uterus. These isolated pieces of endometrium may lie on the outside of the uterus or ovaries, or elsewhere in the pelvis. Each section of endometrium is sensitive to hormonal changes occurring during the menstrual cycle and goes through the monthly changes of thickening, shedding and bleeding. This causes pain wherever the endometrial cells are found. The pain usually begins up to 1 week before menstruation and both lower abdominal and lower back pain may occur. The pain may also be non-cyclical and may occur with sexual intercourse (dyspareunia). Endometriosis may cause subfertility. Diagnosis can be confirmed by laparoscopy.

Pelvic inflammatory disease   Pelvic infection can occur and may be acute or chronic in nature. It is important to know whether or not an intrauterine contraceptive device (coil) is used. The coil can cause increased discomfort and heavier periods, but also may predispose to infection. Acute pelvic infection occurs when a bacterial infection develops within the fallopian tubes. There is usually severe pain, fever and vaginal discharge. The pain is in the lower abdomen and may be unrelated to menstruation. It may be confused with appendicitis.

Chronic PID may follow on from an acute infection. The pain tends to be less severe, associated with periods and may be experienced during intercourse. It is thought that adhesions that develop around the tubes following an infection may be responsible for the symptoms in some women. In others, however, no abnormality can be found and pelvic congestion is assumed to be the cause. In this situation, psychological factors are thought to be important.

Other symptoms

Women who experience dysmenorrhoea will often describe other associated symptoms. These include nausea, vomiting, general GI discomfort, constipation, headache, backache, fatigue, feeling faint and dizziness.

Premenstrual syndrome

The term premenstrual syndrome (PMS) describes a collection of symptoms, both physical and mental, whose incidence is related to the menstrual cycle. Symptoms are experienced cyclically, usually from 2 to 14 days before the start of menstruation. Relief from symptoms generally occurs once menstrual bleeding begins. The cyclical nature, timing and reduction in symptoms are all important in identifying PMS. Some women experience such severe symptoms that their working and home lives are affected.

Sufferers often complain of a bloated abdomen, increase in weight, swelling of ankles and fingers, breast tenderness and headaches. Women who experience PMS describe a variety of mental symptoms that may include any or all of irritability, tension, depression, difficulty in concentrating and tiredness.

If PMS is considered to be a possibility, advising the woman to keep a diary of symptoms recording when they occur and remit is useful, especially if the pharmacist later decides referral is needed.

Treatment of the symptoms of PMS is a matter for debate and there is a high placebo response to therapy of mood changes, breast discomfort and headaches when taken from 2 weeks before the period starts or throughout the cycle. There is some evidence that *pyridoxine* may reduce symptoms but the quality of clinical trials was poor and the evidence thus not definitive. The mechanism of action of *pyridoxine* in PMS is unknown. However, women should be advised to stick to the recommended dose; higher doses of *pyridoxine* are reported to have led to neuropathy. The *British National Formulary* states that 'prolonged use of pyridoxine in a dose of 10 mg daily is considered safe but the long-term use of pyridoxine in a dose of 200 mg or more daily has been associated with neuropathy. The safety of long-term pyridoxine supplementation with doses above 10 mg daily has not been established'.

Evening primrose oil has been used to treat breast tenderness associated with PMS. However, there are no good-quality trials to support its use and therefore is of unknown effectiveness. The mechanism of action of *evening primrose oil* in such cases is thought to be linked to effects on prostaglandins, particularly in increasing the level of prostaglandin E, which appears to be depleted in some women with PMS. The active component of *evening primrose oil* is *gamma-linolenic (gamolenic) acid,* which is thought to reduce the ratio of saturated to unsaturated fatty acids. The response to hormones and prolactin appears to be reduced by *gamma-linolenic acid.*

Medication

The pain of dysmenorrhoea is thought to be linked to increased prostaglandin activity, and raised prostaglandin levels have been found in the menstrual fluids and circulating blood of women who suffer from dysmenorrhoea. Therefore, the use of analgesics that inhibit the synthesis of prostaglandins is logical. It is important, however, for the pharmacist to make sure that the patient is not already taking a non-steroidal anti-inflammatory drug (NSAID).

Women taking oral contraceptives usually find that the symptoms of dysmenorrhoea are reduced or eliminated altogether and so any woman presenting with the symptoms of dysmenorrhoea and who is taking the pill is probably best referred to the doctor for further investigation.

When to refer

Presence of abnormal vaginal discharge
Abnormal bleeding
Symptoms suggest secondary dysmenorrhoea
Severe intermenstrual pain (mittelschmerz) and bleeding

> Failure of medication
> Pain with a late period (possibility of an ectopic pregnancy)
> Presence of fever

Treatment timescale

If the pain of primary dysmenorrhoea is not improved after two cycles of treatment, referral to the doctor would be advisable.

Management

Simple explanation about why period pains occur, together with sympathy and reassurance, is important. Treatment with simple analgesics is often very effective in dysmenorrhoea.

NSAIDs (Ibuprofen, *diclofenac* and *naproxen*) (see also p. 200)

NSAIDs can be considered the treatment of choice for dysmenorrhoea provided they are appropriate for the patient (i.e. the pharmacist has questioned the patient about previous use of *aspirin*, and history of GI problems and asthma). NSAIDs inhibit the synthesis of prostaglandins and thus have a rationale for use. Most trials have studied the use of NSAIDs at the onset of pain. One small study compared treatment started premenstrually against treatment from onset of pain: both strategies were equally effective. Sustained-release formulations of *ibuprofen* are also available.

Doses for *ibuprofen* and *diclofenac* are on p. 200. Diclofenac is contra-indicated in patients with cardiovascular disease. When responding to a request to buy OTC oral diclofenac or considering recommending it, pharmacists and their staff need to ask suitable questions to identify whether the patient has cardiovascular disease. *Naproxen* 250 mg tablets can be used by women aged between 15 and 50 years for primary dysmenorrhoea only. Two tablets are taken initially, then one tablet 6–8 h later if needed. Maximum daily dose is 750 mg and maximum treatment time is 3 days.

Contraindications

Care should be taken when recommending NSAIDs which can cause GI irritation and should not be taken by anyone who has or has had a peptic ulcer. All patients should take NSAIDs with or after food to minimise GI problems (see also p. 200).

NSAIDs should not be taken by anyone who is sensitive to *aspirin* and should be used with caution in anyone who is asthmatic, because such patients are more likely to be sensitive to NSAIDs. The pharmacist can check if a person with asthma has used an NSAID before. If they have done so without problems, they can continue.

Aspirin

Aspirin also inhibits the synthesis of prostaglandins but is less effective in relieving the symptoms of dysmenorrhoea than is *ibuprofen*. One review found the number needed to treat was 10 for *aspirin* compared with 2.4 for *ibuprofen*. *Aspirin* can cause GI upsets and is more irritant to the stomach than NSAIDs. For those who experience symptoms of nausea and vomiting with dysmenorrhoea, *aspirin* is probably best avoided. Soluble forms of *aspirin* will work more quickly than traditional tablet formulations and are less likely to cause stomach problems. Patients should be advised to take *aspirin* with or after meals. The pharmacist should establish whether the patient has any history of *aspirin* sensitivity before recommending the drug.

Paracetamol

Paracetamol has little or no effect on the levels of prostaglandins involved in pain and inflammation and so it is theoretically less effective for the treatment of dysmenorrhoea than either NSAIDs or *aspirin*. However, *paracetamol* is a useful treatment when the patient cannot take NSAIDs or *aspirin* because of stomach problems or potential sensitivity. *Paracetamol* is also useful when the patient is suffering with nausea and vomiting as well as pain, since it does not irritate the stomach. The pharmacist should remember to stress the maximum dose that can be taken.

Hyoscine

Hyoscine, a smooth muscle relaxant, is marketed for the treatment of dysmenorrhoea on the theoretical basis that the antispasmodic action will reduce cramping. In fact, the dose is so low (0.1-mg *hyoscine)* that such an effect is unlikely. The anticholinergic effects of *hyoscine* mean that it is contraindicated in women with closed-angle glaucoma. Additive anticholinergic effects (dry mouth, constipation and blurred vision) mean that *hyoscine* is best avoided if any other drug with anticholinergic effects (e.g. tricyclic antidepressants) is being taken.

Caffeine

There is some evidence (from a trial comparing combined *ibuprofen* and *caffeine* with *ibuprofen* alone and *caffeine* alone) that *caffeine* may enhance analgesic effect. OTC products contain 15–65 mg of *caffeine* per tablet. A similar effect could be achieved through drinking tea, coffee or cola. A cup of instant coffee usually contains about 80 mg of *caffeine*; a cup of freshly brewed coffee, about 130 mg; a cup of tea, 50 mg and a can of cola drink, about 40–60 mg.

Non-drug treatments

A systematic review of evidence found that high-frequency transcutaneous electrical nerve stimulation (TENS) may be of benefit. It seems to work by altering the body's ability to receive or perceive pain signals. High-frequency TENS has pulses of 50–120 Hz at low intensity and, when compared with placebo in seven small randomised controlled trials, was found to be effective for pain relief in primary dysmenorrhoea. Low-frequency TENS is also available and has pulses of 1–4 Hz delivered at high intensity. Although low-frequency TENS was better than placebo, the evidence is less convincing than for high frequency.

Acupuncture may be helpful and was found in a small, but well-designed, study to be more effective than its placebo equivalent (sham acupuncture, where the needles are positioned away from the 'real' acupuncture sites). The treatments were given once a week for 3 weeks per month over a 3-month period. Women receiving 'real' acupuncture gained significant pain relief. While further research is needed to confirm this effect, some women may want to try it.

Locally applied low-level heat may also help pain relief. Results from one study showed that the time to noticeable pain relief was significantly reduced when *ibuprofen* was combined with locally applied heat, as compared with *ibuprofen* alone.

Fish oil (omega-3 fatty acids) compared with placebo in one study showed the use of additional pain relief to be significantly lower in the treatment group. There were significantly more adverse effects in the women treated with fish oil, but these were not serious.

Pyridoxine alone and combined with magnesium showed some benefit in reducing pain, compared with placebo.

Practical points

1 Exercise during menstruation is not harmful and may well be beneficial, since it raises endorphin levels, reducing pain and promoting a feeling of well-being. There is some evidence that moderate aerobic exercise can improve symptoms of PMS.

2 There is some evidence that a low-fat, high-carbohydrate diet reduces breast pain and tenderness.

3 Advice for women taking analgesics for dysmenorrhoea is as follows.

(i) Take the first dose as soon as your pain begins or as soon as the bleeding starts, whichever comes first. Some doctors advise to start taking the tablets on the day before your period is due. This may prevent the pain from building up.

(ii) Take the tablets regularly, for 2–3 days each period, rather than 'now and then' when pain builds up.

(iii) Take a strong enough dose. If your pains are not eased, ask your doctor or pharmacist whether the dose that you are taking is the maximum allowed. An increase in dose may be all that you need.

(iv) Side-effects are uncommon if you take an anti-inflammatory for just a few days at a time, during each period. (But read the leaflet that comes with the tablets for a full list of possible side-effects.)

Dysmenorrhoea in practice

Case 1

Linda Bailey is a young woman aged about 26 years, who asks your advice about painful periods. From your questioning, you find that Linda has lower abdominal pain and sometimes backache, which starts several days before her period begins. Her menstrual cycle used to be very regular, but now tends to vary; sometimes she has only 3 weeks between periods. The pain continues throughout menstruation and is quite severe. She has tried taking *aspirin,* which did not have much effect.

The pharmacist's view

This woman sounds as though she is experiencing secondary dysmenorrhoea. The pain begins well before her period starts and continues during menstruation. Her periods, which used to be regular, are no longer so and she has tried *aspirin* which has not relieved the pain. She should be referred to her doctor.

The doctor's view

Referral does seem appropriate in this situation. Further information needs to be gathered from history taking (how long overall has she experienced pain and what it is like, the effect on her life, any pregnancies, does she use contraception, any history of pelvic infection, her concerns and ideas about her problem, the sort of help is she expecting, etc.), examination and preliminary investigations. It is quite possible that the patient has endometriosis and referral to a gynaecologist may be indicated. The diagnosis of endometriosis can be confirmed by a laparoscopy. The range of treatment options includes other NSAIDs, hormone treatments and surgery. The hormonal treatments that can be used are progestogens, antiprogestogens, combined oral contraceptives and gonadotropin-releasing hormone analogues (GnRH). GnRH preparations such as *goserelin* work by suppressing the hormones to create an artificial menopause. They can be used for up to 6 months (not to be repeated) and may have to be used with hormone replacement therapy to offset menopausal-like symptoms.

Case 2

Jenny Simmonds is a young woman aged about 18 years who looks rather embarrassed and asks you what would be the best thing for period pains. Jenny tells you that she started her periods about 5 years ago and has never had any problem with period pains until recently. Her periods are regular – every 4 weeks. They have not become heavier, but she now gets pain, which starts a few hours before her period. The pain is usually gone by the end of the first day of menstruation and Jenny has never had any pain during other parts of the cycle. She says she has not tried any medicine yet, is not taking any medicines from the doctor and can normally take *aspirin* without any problems.

The pharmacist's view

From the results of questioning, it sounds as though Jenny is suffering from straightforward primary dysmenorrhoea. She could be advised to take an NSAID. She could be recommended to follow this regimen for 2 months and invited back to see if the treatment has worked.

The doctor's view

Jenny's pain is most likely due to primary dysmenorrhoea. An explanation of this fact would probably be very reassuring. The treatment recommended by the pharmacist is sensible. If her pain was not helped by an NSAID, she could be advised to discuss further management with her GP. Sometimes the combined oral contraceptive pill (OCP) can be helpful in reducing painful periods.

Menorrhagia

Menorrhagia is excessive (heavy) menstrual blood loss which occurs over several consecutive cycles and can be treated OTC with tranexamic acid. One in three women describes periods as being 'heavy' and although the technical definition of menorrhagia is blood loss of 60–80 mL or more per period (compared with average loss of 30–40 mL), this definition is not useful in practice. A more useful description is of heavy menstrual blood loss which, in the woman's view, interferes with her quality of life (physical, emotional, social). In most cases, where women present with symptoms of menorrhagia, there is no underlying pathology. Careful history-taking is needed to support the decisions about whether to treat or refer.

What you need to know

Age
    Menstrual cycle – length, number of days of menstruation
    Symptoms – bleeding pattern; impact on quality of life
    Duration – how long have the periods been heavy?
    Previous history – previous nature of periods

Age

Most patients with menorrhagia are aged over 30. The most common cause of heavy periods in women aged under 30 is anovulatory cycles and bleeding does not occur at regular intervals in such cases.

Menstrual cycle

A normal cycle is between 21 and 35 days in duration and with no more than 3 days' variation in the length of individual cycles. If a patient's period was previously regular and this has changed, pathology must be ruled out.

Symptoms in the Pharmacy: A Guide to the Management of Common Illness, Seventh Edition. Alison Blenkinsopp, Paul Paxton and John Blenkinsopp.
© 2014 John Wiley & Sons, Ltd. Published 2014 by John Wiley & Sons, Ltd.

Symptoms

A description of the symptoms is needed, and of how they are affecting the woman's life. Specific questions can check for the presence of other symptoms that may suggest an underlying condition:

- Fibroids – dysmennorrhoea, pelvic pain
- Endometriosis – dysmenorrhoea, pain on intercourse (dyspareunia), pelvic pain
- Pelvic inflammatory disease/pelvic infection – fever, vaginal discharge, pelvic pain, intermenstrual and/or postcoital pain
- Endometrial cancer – postcoital bleeding, intermenstrual bleeding, pelvic pain

Tranexamic acid has been available OTC in Sweden for over a decade and there has been no increase in the reported incidence of endometrial carcinoma.

When to refer
Presence of abnormal vaginal discharge
Intermenstrual and/or postcoital bleeding
Pelvic pain
Pain on intercourse (dyspareunia)
Dysmenorrhoea
Presence of fever

Treatment timescale

If menorraghia is not improved after three cycles of treatment, referral to the doctor would be advisable.

Management

There is one treatment available over the counter, tranexamic acid.

Tranexamic acid

Oral *tranexamic acid* reduces the volume of menstrual blood loss by about half through its antifibrinolytic effect which increases blood clotting. It can be used in women aged 18–45 whose cycle is regular (21–35 day cycles with no more than 3 days variation in the length of individual cycles). The treatment can be taken for up to 4 days per cycle, starting on the first day of the period. The usual dose is 1 g (2 × 500 mg tablets) taken three times a day, this can be increased to four times a day if the bleeding is particularly heavy (maximum daily dose 4 g).

Contraindications

Tranexamic acid should not be taken by women with current or previous thromboembolic disease, those with a family history of such problems or those taking anticoagulants or oral contraception. Excretion of tranexamic acid is almost exclusively by the kidney; therefore, the treatment is not advised for women with mild-to-moderate renal insufficiency. Haematuria (blood in the urine) from upper urinary tract pathology is a contraindication because clotting may cause obstruction in the ureter. Risk factors for endometrial cancer include obesity, diabetes, nulliparity, family history, polycystic ovary syndrome, unopposed oestrogen treatment or tamoxifen, and OTC tranexamic acid is therefore not recommended in these circumstances.

Cautions

Breastfeeding women should only take tranexamic acid on the advice of their doctor because the drug passes into breast milk.

Side effects

Nausea, vomiting and diarrhoea may occur; reducing the dose may help. Any patient who expriences visual disturbances while taking tranexamic acid should be referred to the doctor.

Other advice

There is no evidence that menorrhagia can be reduced by exercise or dietary changes.

Vaginal thrush

Women often seek to buy products for feminine itching and may be embarrassed to seek advice or answer what they see as intrusive questions from the pharmacist. Vaginal pessaries, intravaginal creams containing *imidazole* antifungals and oral *fluconazole* are effective treatments. Before making any recommendation it is vital to question the patient to identify the probable cause of the symptoms. Advertising of these treatments direct to the public means that a request for a named product may be made. It is important to confirm its appropriateness.

What you need to know
Age
Child, adult, elderly
Duration
Symptoms
Itch
Soreness
Discharge (colour, consistency, odour)
Dysuria
Dyspareunia
Threadworms
Previous history
Medication

Significance of questions and answers

Age

Vaginal candidiasis (thrush) is common in women of childbearing age, and pregnancy and diabetes are strong predisposing factors. This infection is rare in children and in postmenopausal women because of the different environment in the vagina. In contrast to women of childbearing age, where vaginal pH is generally acidic (low pH) and contains glycogen, the vaginal environment of children and menopausal women tends to be alkaline (high pH) and does not contain large amounts of glycogen.

Symptoms in the Pharmacy: A Guide to the Management of Common Illness, Seventh Edition.
Alison Blenkinsopp, Paul Paxton and John Blenkinsopp.
© 2014 John Wiley & Sons, Ltd. Published 2014 by John Wiley & Sons, Ltd.

Oestrogen, present between adolescence and the menopause, leads to the availability of glycogen in the vagina and also contributes to the development of a protective barrier layer on the walls of the vagina. The lack of oestrogen in children and postmenopausal women means this protective barrier is not present, with a consequent increased tendency to bacterial (but not fungal) infection.

In the United Kingdom, the Commission on Human Medicines (CHM) recommends that women under 16 or over 60 years complaining of symptoms of vaginal thrush should be referred to their doctor. Child abuse may be the source of vaginal infection in girls, making referral even more important. Vaginal thrush is rare in older women and other causes of the symptoms need to be excluded.

Duration

Some women delay seeking advice from the pharmacist or doctor because of the embarrassment about their symptoms. They may have tried an OTC product or a prescription medicine already (see 'Medication' below).

Symptoms

Itch (pruritus)

Dermatitis Allergic or irritant dermatitis may be responsible for vaginal itch. It is worth asking whether the patient has recently used any new toiletries (e.g. soaps, bath or shower products). Vaginal deodorants are sometimes the source of allergic reactions. Women sometimes use harsh soaps, antiseptics and vaginal douches in an overenthusiastic cleansing of the vagina. Regular washing with warm water is all that is required to keep the vagina clean and maintain a healthy vaginal environment.

Candidiasis (thrush) The itch associated with thrush is often intense and burning in nature. Sometimes the skin may be excoriated and raw from scratching when the itch is severe.

Discharge

In women of childbearing age, the vagina naturally produces a watery discharge and cervical mucus is also produced, which changes consistency at particular times of the menstrual cycle. Such fluids may be watery or slightly thicker, with no associated odour. Some women worry about these natural secretions and think they have an infection.

The most common infective cause of vaginal discharge is candidiasis. Vaginal candidiasis may be (but is not always) associated with a discharge. The discharge is classically cream-coloured, thick and curdy in appearance but, alternatively, may be thin and rather watery. Other vaginal infections may be responsible for producing discharge but are markedly different from that caused by thrush. The discharge associated with candidal infection does not usually produce an unpleasant odour, in contrast to that produced by bacterial infection. Infection leading to discharge described as yellow or greenish is more likely to be bacterial in origin, for example, bacterial vaginosis, chlamydia or gonorrhoea.

Partner's symptoms

Men may be infected with *Candida* without showing any symptoms. Typical symptoms for men are an irritating rash on the penis, particularly on the glans.

Dysuria (pain on urination)

Dysuria may be present and scratching the skin in response to itching might be responsible, although dysuria may occur without scratching. Sometimes the pain on passing urine may be mistaken for cystitis by the patient. If a woman complains of cystitis, it is important to ask about other symptoms (see p. 225). The CHM advises that lower abdominal pain and dysuria are indications for referral because of their possible link with kidney infections.

Dyspareunia (painful intercourse)

Painful intercourse may be associated with infection or a sensitivity reaction where the vulval and vaginal areas are involved.

Threadworms

Occasionally, threadworm infestation can lead to vaginal pruritus and this has sometimes occurred in children. The patient would also be experiencing anal itching in such a case. The pharmacist should refer girls under the age of 16 years to the doctor in any case of vaginal symptoms.

Previous history

Recurrent thrush is a problem for some women, often following antibiotic treatment (see below). Recurrent infections are defined as 'four or more episodes of symptomatic candidosis annually'. The CHM advice is that any woman who has experienced more than two attacks of thrush during the previous 6 months should be referred to the doctor. Repeated thrush infections may indicate an underlying problem or altered immunity and further investigation is needed.

Pregnancy

During pregnancy almost one in five women will have an episode of vaginal candidiasis. This high incidence has been attributed to hormonal changes with a consequent alteration in the vaginal environment leading to the presence of increased quantities of glycogen. Any pregnant woman with thrush should be referred to the doctor.

Diabetes

It is thought that *Candida* is able to grow more easily in diabetic patients because of the higher glucose levels in blood and tissues. Sometimes recurrent vaginal thrush can be a sign of undiagnosed diabetes or, in a patient who has been diagnosed, of poor diabetic control.

Sexually transmitted diseases

In the United Kingdom, the CHM insists that women who have previously had a sexually transmitted infection should not be sold OTC treatments for thrush. The thinking behind this ruling is that with a previous history of sexually transmitted disease (STD), the current condition may not be thrush or may include a dual infection with another organism.

Pharmacists may be concerned about how patients will respond to personal questions. However, it should be possible to enquire about previous episodes of these or similar symptoms in a tactful way, for example, by asking 'Have you ever had anything like this before?' and if 'Yes', 'Tell me about the symptoms. Were they exactly the same as this time?' and about the partner, 'Has your partner mentioned any symptoms recently?'

Oral steroids

Patients taking oral steroids may be at increased risk of candidal infection.

Immunocompromised patients

Patients with HIV or AIDS are prone to recurrent thrush infection because the immune system is unable to combat them. Patients undergoing cancer chemotherapy are also at risk of infection.

Medication

Oral contraceptives

It has been suggested that the OCP is linked to the incidence of vaginal candidiasis; however, oral contraceptives are no longer considered a significant precipitating factor.

Antibiotics

Broad-spectrum antibiotics wipe out the natural bacterial flora (lactobacilli) in the vagina and can predispose to candidal overgrowth. Some women find that an episode of thrush follows every course of antibiotics they take. The doctor may prescribe an antifungal at the same time as the antibiotic in such cases.

Local anaesthetics

Vaginal pruritus may actually be caused by some of the products used to relieve the symptom. Creams and ointments advertised for 'feminine' itching often contain local anaesthetics – a well-known cause of sensitivity reactions. It is important to check what, if any, treatment the patient has tried before seeking your advice.

When to refer
The UK CHM list:
First occurrence of symptoms
Known hypersensitivity to imidazoles or other vaginal antifungal products
Pregnancy or suspected pregnancy
More than two attacks in the previous 6 months
Previous history of STD
Exposure to partner with STD
Patient under 16 or over 60 years
Abnormal or irregular vaginal bleeding
Any blood staining of vaginal discharge
Vulval or vaginal sores, ulcers or blisters
Associated lower abdominal pain or dysuria
Adverse effects (redness, irritation or swelling associated with treatment)
No improvement within 7 days of treatment

Management

Single-dose intravaginal and oral *azole* preparations are effective in treating vaginal candidiasis and give 80–95% clinical and mycological cure rates. A Cochrane review found them to be equally effective. Topical preparations give quicker initial relief, probably due to the vehicle. They may sometimes exacerbate burning sensations initially, and oral treatment may be preferred if the vulva is very inflamed. Oral therapies are effective, but it may be 12–24 h before symptoms improve. Some women find oral treatment more convenient. Patients find single-dose products very convenient and compliance is higher than with treatments involving several days' use. The patient can be asked whether she prefers a pessary, vaginal cream or oral formulation. Some experts argue that oral antifungals should be reserved for resistant cases. Pharmacists will use their professional judgement together with patient preference in making the decision on treatment.

The pharmacist should make sure that the patient knows how to use the product. An effective way to do this is to show the patient the manufacturer's leaflet instructions. Where external symptoms are also a problem, an *azole* cream *(miconazole or clotrimazole)* can be useful in addition to the intravaginal or oral product. The cream should be applied twice daily, morning and night.

The azoles can cause sensitivity reactions but these seem to be rare. Oral *fluconazole* interacts with some drugs: anticoagulants, oral sulphonylureas, ciclosporin (cyclosporin), phenytoin, rifampicin and theophylline.

The effects of single-dose *fluconazole* rather than continuous therapy with the drug in relation to interactions are not clear. Theoretically, single-dose use is unlikely to cause problems but in a small study of women taking warfarin the prothrombin time was increased.

Reported side-effects from oral *fluconazole* occur in some 10% of patients and are usually mild and transient. They include nausea, abdominal discomfort, flatulence and diarrhoea. Oral *fluconazole* should not be recommended during pregnancy or for nursing mothers because it is excreted in breast milk.

Practical points
Privacy

Patients seeking advice about vaginal symptoms may be embarrassed, fearing that their conversation with the pharmacist will be overheard. It is therefore important to try and ensure privacy. Requests for a named product may be an attempt to avoid discussion. However, a careful response is needed to ensure that the product is appropriate.

Treatment of partner

Men may be infected with *Candida* without showing any symptoms. Typical symptoms for men are an irritating rash on the penis, particularly on the glans. While expert opinion is that male partners without symptoms should not be treated, this remains an area of debate. Symptomatic males with candidal balanitis (penile thrush) and whose female partner has vaginal thrush should be treated. An azole cream can be used twice daily on the glans of the penis, applied under the foreskin for 6 days. Oral *fluconazole* can also be used.

'Live' yoghurt

Live yoghurt contains lactobacilli, which are said to alter the vaginal environment, making it more difficult for *Candida* to grow. It has been suggested that women prone to thrush should regularly eat live yoghurt to increase the level of lactobacilli in the gut. However, data are inconclusive as to the effectiveness of *Lactobacillus*-containing yoghurt, administered either orally or vaginally, in either treating or preventing thrush. Direct application of live yoghurt onto the vulval skin and into the vagina on a tampon has been recommended as a treatment for thrush. This process is messy and some women have reported stinging on application, which is not surprising if the skin is excoriated and sore. It is otherwise harmless, although evidence of effectiveness is lacking.

Prevention

Thrush thrives in a warm environment. Women who are prone to attacks of thrush may find that avoiding nylon underwear and tights and using cotton underwear instead may help to prevent future attacks.

The protective lining of the vagina is stripped away by foam baths, soaps and douches and these are best avoided. Vaginal deodorants can themselves cause allergic reactions and should not be used. If the patient wants to use a soap or cleanser, an unperfumed, mild variety is best.

Since *Candida* can be transferred from the bowel when wiping the anus after a bowel movement, wiping from front to back should help to prevent this.

Vaginal thrush in practice

Case 1

Julie Parker telephones your pharmacy to ask for advice because she thinks she might have thrush. She tells you she didn't want to come to the pharmacy as she was concerned that the conversation might be overheard. When you ask why she thinks she may have thrush, she tells you that she was recently prescribed a week's course of *metronidazole*. She had her first baby about 6 months ago and has had some skin irritation following an episiotomy. When she went back to the GP after taking the *metronidazole,* she was prescribed a second course of *metronidazole* plus a course of *amoxicillin* for 1 week and a swab was taken. She didn't hear anything further for about 2 weeks until the surgery rang her and asked if she had been told the results of the swab (she hadn't). She was asked to go and collect a prescription from the surgery. She hasn't brought it in yet to be dispensed but it is for a pessary.

The pharmacist's view

This sort of query is difficult to deal with because the pharmacist does not have access to diagnosis or test results. It sounds as though there may have been a communication problem initially and a delay in the test results being dealt with. I would ask what the name of the pessary on the prescription is and then explain what it's used for. I would explain that thrush sometimes happens after a course of antibiotics and that the pessary is likely to cure it.

It would probably be best for Julie Parker to go back and see her GP who has already given her two courses of treatment and taken a swab. She needs to find out exactly what the GP has been treating her for, what the swab result is and to be able to explain to her GP what her current symptoms are. *Metronidazole* is often prescribed for bacterial vaginosis. It could be that she has also developed thrush especially as she has been taking *amoxycillin*. It is always important for patients to know how and when they can get their results. Often patients understandably assume that if they don't hear from their doctors' surgery, the result is negative or normal. This is potentially dangerous and it is always important for the person taking laboratory samples to explain clearly how and when the results will be available and agree this with their patient. In this situation it is also important for the prescriber to explain the need for the prescription that has been left out at the surgery.

Case 2

Helen Simpson is a student at the local university. She asks one of your assistants for something to treat thrush and is referred to you. You walk with Helen to a quiet area of the shop where your conversation will not be overheard. Initially, Helen is resistant to your involvement, asking why you need to ask all these personal questions. After you have explained that you are required to obtain information before selling these products and that, in any case, you need to be sure that the problem is thrush and not a different infection, she seems happier.

She has not had thrush or any similar symptoms before but described her symptoms to a flatmate who made the diagnosis. The worst symptom is itching, which was particularly severe last night. Helen has noticed small quantities of a cream-coloured discharge. The vulval skin is sore and red. Helen has a boyfriend, but he hasn't had any symptoms. She is not taking any medicines and does not have any existing illnesses or conditions. Since arriving at the university a few months ago she has not registered with the university's health centre and has therefore come to the pharmacy hoping to buy a treatment.

The pharmacist's view

The key symptoms of itch and cream-coloured vaginal discharge make thrush the most likely candidate here. Helen has no previous history of the condition and, unfortunately, the regulations preclude the recommendation of an intravaginal azole product or oral *fluconazole* in such a case. An azole cream would help to ease the itching and soreness of the vulval skin. As her boyfriend is not experiencing symptoms he does not need treatment. However, because external treatment alone is unlikely to prove effective in eradicating the infection, it would be best for Helen to see a doctor.

She would be well advised to register at the university health centre. You can explain to her that she can seek treatment on a temporary resident basis but that it would be best to get proper medical cover.

The doctor's view
The history is very suggestive of thrush and treatment should include an appropriate intravaginal preparation. The case history highlights some of the difficulties of asking personal questions about genitalia and sexual activity. These difficulties are also likely to occur in the doctor's surgery. It is important for the doctor to carefully explore the patient's ideas, understanding, concerns and preconceptions of her condition. Many doctors would prescribe without an examination with such a clear history and examine and take appropriate microbiology samples only if treatment fails.

Emergency hormonal contraception

Dealing with requests for emergency hormonal contraception (EHC) requires sensitive interpersonal skills from the pharmacist. Enabling privacy for the consultation is essential and the wider availability of consultation areas and rooms has improved this. Careful thought needs to be given to the wording of questions. Some 20% of women will go to a pharmacy other than their regular one because they want to remain anonymous.

What you need to know

Age
> Why EHC is needed – confirmation that unprotected sex or contraceptive failure has occurred
> When unprotected sex/contraceptive failure occurred
> Could the woman already be pregnant?
> Other medicines being taken

Significance of questions and answers

Age
> EHC can be supplied OTC as a P medicine for women aged 16 years and over. For women under 16 years the pharmacist can refer to the doctor or family planning service. In the National Health Service (NHS), EHC may be supplied under PGDs according to a locally agreed-upon protocol. Some of these schemes include community pharmacies and if the PGD so states, supply can be made to a woman under 16 years.

Why EHC is needed
> The most common reasons for EHC to be requested are failure of a barrier contraceptive method (e.g. condom that splits), missed contraceptive pill(s) and unprotected sexual intercourse (UPSI). In the case of missed pills the pharmacist should follow the guidance of the Faculty of Family Planning and Reproductive Health Care Clinical Effectiveness

---

Symptoms in the Pharmacy: A Guide to the Management of Common Illness, Seventh Edition.
Alison Blenkinsopp, Paul Paxton and John Blenkinsopp.
© 2014 John Wiley & Sons, Ltd. Published 2014 by John Wiley & Sons, Ltd.

Unit (*Emergency Contraception: Guidance,* updated January 2012 at www.ffprhc.org.uk).

Recommendations for use of EHC (FFPRHC 2012)	
Combined pills	If *two or more* active ethinyloestradiol pills have been missed in the first week of pill taking (i.e. days 1–7) and UPSI occurred in week 1 or the pill-free week
Progestogen-only pills (POPs)	If *one or more* POPs have been missed or taken >3 h late (>12 h late for desogestrel) *and* UPSI has occurred in the 2 days following this
Progestogen-only injectable	If the contraceptive injection is late (>14 weeks from the previous injection for medroxyprogesterone acetate or >10 weeks for norethisterone enantate) *and* UPSI has occurred
Barrier methods	If there has been failure of a barrier method

When unprotected sex/contraceptive failure occurred

EHC needs to be started within 72 h of unprotected intercourse. The sooner it is started, the higher is its efficacy. If unprotected sex took place between 72 h and 5 days ago, the woman can be referred to have an intrauterine device (IUD) fitted as a method of emergency contraception.

Requests are sometimes made for EHC to be purchased for use in the future (advance requests, for example, to take on holiday just in case). This is considered below.

Could the woman already be pregnant?

Any other episodes of unprotected sex in the current cycle are important. Ask whether the last menstrual period was lighter or later than usual. If in doubt, the pharmacist can suggest that the woman has a pregnancy test. EHC will not work if the woman is pregnant. There is no evidence that EHC is harmful to the pregnancy.

Other medicines being taken

Medicines that induce specific liver enzymes have the potential to increase the metabolism of *levonorgestrel* and thus to reduce its efficacy. Women taking the following medicines should be referred to an alternative source of supply of EHC:

Anticonvulsants *(carbamazepine, phenytoin, primidone, phenobarbital (phenobarbitone))*
Rifampicin and *rifabutin*
Griseofulvin

Ritonavir
St John's wort

There is an interaction between *ciclosporin* and *levonorgestrel*. Here, the progestogen inhibits the metabolism of *ciclosporin* and increases levels of the latter. A woman requesting EHC who is taking *ciclosporin* should be referred.

Treatment timescale

EHC must be started within 72 h of unprotected intercourse.

When to refer
Age under 16 years
Longer than 72 h since unprotected sex
Taking a medicine that interacts with EHC
Requests for future use

Management

Dosage
Levonorgestrel EHC is taken as a dose of one 1.5-mg tablet as soon as possible after unprotected intercourse.

Side-effects
The most likely side effect is nausea, which occurred in about 14% of women during clinical trials of *levonorgestrel* EHC. Far fewer women (1%) actually vomited. Although the likelihood of vomiting is small, absorption of *levonorgestrel* could be affected if vomiting occurs within 3 h of taking the tablet. Another dose is needed as soon as possible.

Women who should not take EHC
The product licence for the P medicine states that it should not be taken by a woman who is pregnant (because it will not work), has severe hepatic dysfunction or has severe malabsorption (e.g. Crohn's disease).

Advice to give when supplying EHC
1 Take the tablet as soon as possible.
2 About one in seven women feels sick after taking *levonorgestrel* EHC but only one in every hundred is actually sick.
3 If the woman is sick within 3 h of taking the tablet, she should obtain a further supply.

4 The next period may start earlier, on time or later than usual. If it is lighter, shorter or more than 3 days later than usual, the woman should see her doctor or family planning adviser to have a pregnancy test.

5 If the woman takes the combined oral contraceptive (COC), she and her partner should use condoms in addition to continuing the pill, until she has taken it for 7 consecutive days.

6 EHC does not equate to ongoing contraception, nor does it offer protection against STD.

Practical points

1 A PGD is available in many areas for pharmacists to supply EHC on the NHS. The PGD was introduced to enable quicker access for EHC to women who are not covered by the OTC product licence (e.g. those under 16 years) and to overcome the difficulties faced by some women in relation to the cost of OTC EHC (around £25). Pharmacists supplying under a PGD undertake additional training, follow a closely defined protocol and keep records of their supplies.

In some areas the pharmacy PGD includes ulipristal acetate (UPA, EllaOne®), the progesterone receptor modulator, which blocks the action of progestogen and is licensed for use up to 5 days (120 h) after UPSI. Ulipristal is more effective than levonorgestrel in women of body mass index (BMI) over 30 and for women presenting in their fertile period. There are differences between ulipristal and levonorgestrel in drug interactions.

2 Pharmacists need to know local sources of family planning services and their opening hours so that they can refer if, for some reason, it is not appropriate for the pharmacy emergency hormonal contraception (P EHC) to be supplied. Knowledge of local services is also important for advice to women who may wish to obtain regular contraception and information about STDs.

3 EHC can be used on more than one occasion within the same menstrual cycle but this is likely to disrupt the cycle. There are no safety concerns about repeated use of EHC but a woman doing so would find it difficult to keep track of her cycle because of the changes EHC can cause. Some women may believe that repeated courses of EHC are a substitute for other contraceptive methods. EHC used in this way is less effective than other methods of contraception and the risk of becoming pregnant is higher.

4 On advance supply of EHC, the Faculty of Family Planning and Reproductive Health Care (FFPRHC) guidance states that 'Health professionals may consider advance provision on an individual basis for women who may be at risk (e.g. women relying on barrier methods or travelling abroad)'. Research shows, however, that women can be reluctant to ask for advance supply of EC due to concerns about being

judged, and thus FFPRHC recommends that 'professionals should be more proactive in providing women with information about the use of EC'. Royal Pharmaceutical Society (RPS) guidance states that 'if faced with a request for advanced supply of EHC the pharmacist should use their professional judgement to decide the clinical appropriateness of the supply'. The RPS suggests the following:

> Declining repeated requests for advance supply and advising clients to seek more reliable methods of contraception
> Providing reminders to ensure that any prospective use of EHC is safe, effective and appropriate

The following points are suggested for inclusion in counselling:

(a) Read the patient information leaflet (PIL) again before taking the product to ensure that it is still suitable for you.
(b) EHC efficacy (levonorgestrel) decreases with time and will be effective only if taken within 72 h (3 days) of unprotected sex/intercourse or failure of a contraceptive method.
(c) IUDs can be fitted up to 120 h (5 days) after unprotected sex or within 5 days of expected ovulation.
(d) Pregnancy is a contraindication for EHC. If you have had unprotected sex which was more than 72 h ago, and since your last period, you may already be pregnant and the treatment won't work. Refer to your doctor or pharmacist for advice.

In a trial of wider access to EHC involving over 2000 women, those who had advance supplies at home were more likely to use EHC when required, without compromising regular contraceptive use or increasing risky sexual behaviour.

EHC in practice

Case 1

A customer whom you recognise as a regular comes into the pharmacy and asks to speak to the pharmacist. She says that she thinks she needs EHC and you move to a quiet area of the pharmacy. On questioning, you find out that she takes the POP but was away from home on business earlier this week and missed one pill, as she forgot to take them with her. The packet says that other contraception will be needed for 7 days. She had sex last night and says she had not had the chance to get any condoms. She is not taking any medicines other than the pill and is not taking any herbal remedies. Her last period was normal and there have been no other episodes of unprotected sex.

The pharmacist's view

Many of the women who request EHC are aged between 20 and 30 years and are regular users of contraception but something has gone wrong. This woman needs to take EHC and the pharmacist can go through the PIL with her to advise on timing of doses and what to do about side-effects should they occur. The pharmacist can also sell condoms/spermicide and reinforce the advice about continuing other contraceptive methods until the pill has been taken for 7 consecutive days as well as taking her POP.

The doctor's view

The pharmacist's approach is appropriate. It is likely that the consultation was made easier because the pharmacist already had a professional relationship with the patient and it would have easier for her to seek advice in the first place. It would be useful for the customer to review the appropriateness of her POP and whether she has missed pills before. She could be advised to have a follow-up with her pill prescriber.

Case 2

It is a Saturday afternoon about 4.30 p.m. A young woman comes into your pharmacy, asks your counter assistant for EHC and is referred to you. You move to consultation area of the pharmacy and in response to your questions she tells you that she had intercourse with her boyfriend last night for the first time. No contraception was used. She is not taking any medicines or herbal remedies. Her periods are fairly regular about every 30 days. You think the woman may be under 16 years.

The pharmacist's view

This woman had unprotected sex 12–18 h ago. If she is under 16 years, the use of P EHC would be outside the terms of the product licence and the pharmacist could ask her age. Some pharmacies can supply EHC on the NHS to under-16s through a PGD. If the area does not have a PGD, the pharmacist will have to consider what other methods of access are available. A walk-in centre, GP out-of-hours centre or Accident and Emergency Department might be available and the timescale for use of ulipristal is up to 120 hours, so an appointment on Monday to access it would still be within this. If all other avenues proved unfeasible, the pharmacist might have to weigh the benefits and risks of referral versus supplying outside the terms of the OTC licence. While there is time for it to be started within 72 h of unprotected sex, the earlier EHC is taken, the more likely it is to be effective. The pharmacist should tactfully suggest that she could get advice on regular contraception and discuss whether she would prefer to get this from her GP or local family planning service.

The doctor's view

Referral does depend on her age, which can be difficult to assess, and whether or not there is a local PGD. One of the problems here is the day and time of presentation. It is unlikely that the local family planning service would be open late on a Saturday. She could wait until Monday but that would be getting close to the 72-h deadline for levonorgestrel although it would be OK for ulipristal. Clearly, it would be better to take the EHC as soon as possible. Her best option would be to phone the on-call GP service. This could probably be done in the pharmacy and she could discuss what to do with the duty GP or nurse. If she turns out to be under age, the GP has a duty to encourage her to discuss this with her parents. The General Medical Council guidance is that the GP can prescribe contraceptives to young people under 16 years without parental consent or knowledge, provided that:

(a) They understand all aspects of the advice and its implications.
(b) You cannot persuade the young person to tell their parents or to allow you to tell them.
(c) In relation to contraception and sexually transmitted infections, the young person is very likely to have sex with or without such treatment.
(d) Their physical or mental health is likely to suffer unless they receive such advice or treatment.
(e) It is in the best interests of the young person to receive the advice and treatment without parental knowledge or consent.

Case 3

A woman asking for EHC is referred to you. She thinks that she may be pregnant as she takes the combined OCP and missed one pill 2 days ago during the second week of the packet. Her brand of pill contains 20 μg ethinyloestradiol. She had sex last night. Her last period was normal.

The pharmacist's view

The Faculty of Family Planning Guidelines state that EHC is not needed unless the woman has missed two or more pills during the first week of taking it. The woman should use an additional contraceptive method such as condoms until pills have been taken on 7 consecutive days. The pharmacist should discuss this with the woman. If she continues to be concerned and still wants to take EHC, the pharmacist could supply it as there are no safety concerns. The timing of the next period may be disrupted. The pharmacist should also suggest that she buys some condoms and spermicide.

The doctor's view

The pharmacist's advice is appropriate. It would be useful to know if she has had similar problems before. If she has, she may benefit from discussion with her GP or adviser at the contraceptive clinic whether or not she decides to take EHC this time.

Case 4

It was the week before I was due to go travelling in South America with my boyfriend for 6 months during my gap year. We're used to using condoms but I'm worried in case one splits while we're away. So I'm going to a pharmacy to see if I can buy the emergency contraception pill to take with me. I don't want to go to the doctors to ask for it.

This woman is now in your pharmacy asking to purchase EHC. Use the chart below to use your professional judgement and decide how to deal with the request.

Potential harm to patient from not supplying	Potential harm to patient from supplying	Potential benefit to patient from supplying	Consequences for pharmacist of supplying/ not supplying	What would I do if the patient were me/my spouse/my parent/my child? Is this decision different from the one I have reached for the patient? Why?

Common symptoms in pregnancy

Constipation (see p. 102)

Constipation can occur in pregnancy because of the effect of hormonal changes. These changes reduce the contractility of the intestines, slowing down the transit of waste products. This in turn allows more fluid to be extracted through the bowel wall drying and hardening the faecal matter. Some women are also taking oral iron preparations for anaemia, which can aggravate constipation. It makes sense to try to prevent this problem by attention to diet (fruit, vegetables and wholegrain cereal, lentils and pulses) and increased fluid intake. If the constipation is aggravated by iron tablets, it may be worthwhile discussing a change of preparation with the GP.

Haemorrhoids (see p. 132)

Haemorrhoids can be aggravated by constipation, and in pregnancy relaxation of the muscles in the anal veins can lead to dilation and swelling of the veins (haemorrhoids or piles). The venous dilatation occurs under the influence of the pregnancy hormones. Later in pregnancy, as the baby's head pushes down into the pelvis, further pressure is exerted on these veins aggravating piles.

In the management of haemorrhoids it is important to avoid constipation, take regular exercise to improve circulation, avoid standing for long periods and discuss with the pharmacist, midwife or GP an appropriate OTC treatment.

Backache

As pregnancy progresses the ligaments of the lower back and pelvis become softer and stretch. Posture also changes leading to an increased forward curve in the lumbar (lower) spine, which is called a lordosis. The change in the ligaments and the lordosis can lead to low backache.

Common-sense techniques avoiding heavy lifting, awkward bending and twisting are advisable, as is a good supportive mattress. Further

Symptoms in the Pharmacy: A Guide to the Management of Common Illness, Seventh Edition. Alison Blenkinsopp, Paul Paxton and John Blenkinsopp.
© 2014 John Wiley & Sons, Ltd. Published 2014 by John Wiley & Sons, Ltd.

help may be gained from an obstetric physiotherapist and chiropractor or osteopath.

Cystitis (see p. 225; reason for referral)

Increased frequency of urination is common in pregnancy and, although inconvenient, is medically unimportant. When it is associated with any signs of cystitis such as discomfort on urination, discolouration or offensive smell of urine, referral to the GP is important. When cystitis occurs in pregnancy, the infection can move upwards from the bladder to the kidneys, causing a much more serious infection. If there is any doubt about cystitis being present, it is important to have the urine sent for analysis.

Headache

Headaches can be a common problem for some women in pregnancy. It is best to have a balance of exercise, rest and relaxation. Occasional *paracetamol* can be taken but it is generally best to avoid medication during pregnancy. Occasionally persistent or severe headaches are due to raised blood pressure. It is important to get the midwife or GP to check for this.

Heartburn (see p. 76)

Heartburn is caused by the relaxation of the muscles in the lower oesophagus, allowing the acid stomach contents to regurgitate upwards. This acid reflux causes inflammation of the oesophagus and heartburn. It is aggravated as pregnancy progresses by pressure on the stomach from the growing baby. It can be reduced by raising the head of the bed, eating small meals and not eating prior to going to bed. A glass of milk may help. If treatment is to be recommended, the pharmacist will need to consider the sodium content and avoid any medicine with a high sodium level.

Nausea/vomiting (morning sickness)

Nausea and vomiting is very common, especially in early pregnancy: nausea affects 70% and vomiting 60%. It is sometimes misleadingly called morning sickness as it actually can occur anytime during the day. Vomiting ceases by the sixteenth week in 90% of women. It may be caused by the change in hormone levels. It is important to take plenty of rest and get up in the mornings slowly, drink plenty of fluids, avoid food and smells that aggravate and eat bland foods. Ginger may be helpful. There are some trials which suggest that ginger reduces nausea and vomiting but they all involve small numbers of people. One crossover trial assessed 27 women with severe nausea during pregnancy. Women were given ginger 250 g four times daily or placebo for 4 days. Nausea was significantly reduced in the ginger group compared to the placebo one. The evidence for P6 acupressure is at present inconclusive, with some trials showing benefit and others that it is less effective than placebo. A recent trial suggests that acupuncture is effective, although the numbers involved were too small to draw firm conclusions.

Vaginal discharge

Vaginal discharge occurs in most women during pregnancy. Providing the discharge is clear and white and non-offensive, it is a normal response to pregnancy. If, however, the discharge has an unpleasant odour, is coloured or is associated with symptoms such as soreness or irritation, referral to the midwife or GP is advised. The most common infection is thrush and is usually managed with topical and intravaginal azoles.

Irritation

Mild skin irritation is common in pregnancy. It is caused by increased blood flow to the skin and by the stretching of the abdominal skin. Wearing loose clothing may help as may perhaps the use of an emollient/moisturising cream. Rarely if the itching is severe, a more serious cause may be revealed, that is, obstetric cholestasis. This condition may be associated with jaundice and can have a deleterious effect on the baby. It is important to refer patients who complain of severe itching.

Men's Health

Benign prostatic hyperplasia

Benign prostatic hyperplasia (BPH) is enlargement of the prostate and is a common condition which is estimated to affect a quarter of men over the age of 40. The cause is unknown, but ageing and long-term exposure to testosterone (and particularly dihydrotestosterone) are important. Symptoms can affect the quality of life of both the sufferer and their family but many men perceive their symptoms as being an inevitable part of growing older and do not seek help. Tamsulosin is available OTC and can be used for up to 6 weeks, with a medical diagnosis required before any further treatment. Pharmacists should follow the guidance on OTC tamsulosin from the National Institute of Health and Care Excellence (NICE).

What you need to know

Age
  Nature of the symptoms
  Urinary symptoms – hesitancy, weak stream, urgency
  Duration
  Previous history
  Other symptoms
  Medication

Significance of questions and answers

Age
  BPH is a condition affecting men who are aged over 40.

Nature of the symptoms
  The enlarged prostate puts pressure on the bladder and urethra leading to lower urinary tract symptoms (LUTS). Common symptoms include the following.

  • A weak urine flow
  • Needing to urinate more often, especially at night
  • A feeling that the bladder has not emptied properly

Symptoms in the Pharmacy: A Guide to the Management of Common Illness, Seventh Edition.
Alison Blenkinsopp, Paul Paxton and John Blenkinsopp.
© 2014 John Wiley & Sons, Ltd. Published 2014 by John Wiley & Sons, Ltd.

- Difficulty starting to pass urine
- Dribbling urine
- Urgency – needing to rush to the toilet

The International Prostate Symptom Score (IPSS) is helpful in assessing the symptoms of BPH. It includes seven urinary symptoms (incomplete emptying/frequency/intermittency/urgency/weak stream/straining/nocturia) and one quality of life question, all graded in severity from one to five. 'Mild' refers to an IPSS of 0–7, 'moderate' refers to an IPSS of 8–19 and 'severe' refers to an IPSS of 20–35. Severity of LUTS should ideally be assessed using a validated scoring system such as the IPSS and it is good practice to use a questionnaire to elicit information.

Duration
Men may present with symptoms that have lasted for months or even years.

Previous history
A typical history would describe gradual onset of the symptoms covered by the IPSS over a period of time, with symptoms slowly increasing.

Other symptoms
BPH comprises a well-defined set of symptoms. Men who are experiencing other urinary symptoms – pain on micturition, blood in the urine, cloudy urine, fever or incontinence – need to see their GP.

Medication
Tamsulosin should not be recommended for patients taking antihypertensive medicines with significant alpha$_1$-adrenoceptor antagonist activity; for example, doxazosin, indoramin, prazosin, terazosin or verapamil.

When to refer

'Red flag' warning symptoms (urgent referral)

- Pain on urination in the last 3 months
- Fever that might be related to a UTI
- Bloody or cloudy urine in the last 3 months (could indicate possible UTI)
- Urinary incontinence (leaking of urine may indicate chronic urinary retention)

Treatment timescale

If urinary symptoms have not improved within 14 days of starting treatment, or are getting worse, the patient should be referred to the doctor.

Management

Mild symptoms may be managed through lifestyle changes. Tamsulosin can be used OTC to treat BPH.

Tamsulosin

Tamsulosin is an alpha$_1$-adrenoceptor antagonist ('alpha$_1$-blocker') which relaxes smooth muscle resulting in increased urinary flow. OTC tamsulosin is indicated for treatment of functional symptoms of BPH in males aged 45–75 years. The dose is one 400 μg capsule swallowed whole after the same meal each day. Symptoms may start to improve within a few days and it may take at least a month to see the full effect. The more severe the symptoms, the greater the absolute reduction in symptom scores.

Medical review is required to confirm the diagnosis of BPH, and exclude that of prostatic cancer. All patients must see their doctor within 6 weeks of starting treatment, for assessment of their symptoms and the confirmation that they may continue to take OTC tamsulosin from their pharmacist. The GP will:

- assess the man's general medical history, comorbidities and review current medication to identify possible causes of the LUTS
- offer a physical examination
- assess baseline symptoms to allow assessment of subsequent symptom changes
- offer urine dipstick, prostate-specific antigen and serum creatinine testing as appropriate (see the guideline for further details)
- refer the man for specialist assessment in some cases

Pharmacy staff will assess eligibility for an initial supply of tamsulosin (up to 6 weeks initial treatment: 14 tablets followed by a further 28 tablets if appropriate) whilst the GP confirms diagnosis and suitability for longer-term OTC treatment. Before making any further OTC supplies the pharmacist needs to check with the patient that the doctor has carried out a clinical assessment and confirmed that OTC treatment can continue. For patients taking tamsulosin longer-term, the pharmacist should advise seeing their doctor annually for a clinical review.

Contra-indications

Tamsulosin should not be supplied if the LUTS are of recent duration (less than 3 months). Any patient who has had prostate surgery, problems with liver/kidney/heart or unstable or undiagnosed diabetes should not take OTC tamsulosin. Patients who suffer from fainting, dizziness or weakness when standing (postural hypotension) should not be recommended tamsulosin. Planned cataract surgery or recent blurred/cloudy vision that has not been examined by a GP or optometrist (may be indicative of unrecognised cataracts) are also contra-indications.

Side effects

Dizziness is a common side effect (affects between 1 in 10 and 1 in 100 people). Uncommon side effects (affects between 1 in 100 and 1 in 1000 people) are: headache, palpitations, postural hypotension, rhinitis, constipation, diarrhoea, nausea, vomiting, rash, pruritus, urticaria, abnormal (dry) ejaculation, asthenia (weakness). As with other alphablockers, drowsiness, blurred vision, dry mouth or oedema can occur.

Cautions

Tamsulosin can, in some individuals, cause a reduction in blood pressure. Signs of orthostatic hypotension are dizziness and weakness on standing. If this occurs, the patient should sit or lie down straight away. A rare problem that has occurred during cataract surgery in some patients taking (or who have previously taken) tamsulosin is 'Intraoperative Floppy Iris Syndrome' (IFIS). Therefore, tamsulosin is not recommended for patients who are due to have cataract surgery.

Herbal remedies

Some men find that herbal remedies, such as saw palmetto and red stinkwood (African plum) help to control their BPH symptoms. However, research into these remedies has shown differing results. Some studies have shown that they may improve symptoms for an average of 2 months. Other studies have shown that they have no effect on symptoms.

Lifestyle advice

Mild symptoms may be relieved by making some lifestyle changes.

(a) Avoiding alcohol and caffeine. Alcoholic drinks or drinks containing caffeine, such as tea, coffee or cola, can irritate the bladder and result in needing to pass urine more often.

(b) Drinking less in the evening. Reducing the volume of fluid drunk in the evening and avoiding drinking liquids for 2 h before bedtime. This will reduce the chance of needing to get up in the night to pass urine. It is still important to drink enough fluid earlier on during the day.

(c) Emptying the bladder. Going to the toilet before long journeys or in situations where a toilet cannot easily be reached.

(d) Double voiding. This involves waiting a few moments after finishing passing urine and then trying to go again. It can help to empty your bladder more completely.

(e) Avoid constipation that can put pressure on the bladder. Increasing the amount of fruit and fibre eaten helps.

(f) Cold and allergy medicines containing decongestants and antihistamines can affect the bladder muscles and might be best avoided.

Hair loss

The two major types of hair loss are diffuse hair loss and localized patches of hair loss (alopecia areata). Alopecia androgenetica (male pattern baldness, sometimes known as common baldness because it can affect women) is the most common cause of diffuse hair loss. Other causes of diffuse hair loss include telogen effluvium, hypothyroidism, severe iron deficiency and protein deficiency. Occasionally, diffuse hair loss is seen after pregnancy, in chronic renal failure and with certain drugs and chemical agents.

Alopecia androgenetica may be treatable, but there are currently no treatments that the pharmacy can offer for alopecia areata. Although hair loss has been largely regarded as a cosmetic problem, the psychological effects on sufferers can be substantial. A sympathetic approach is therefore essential.

What you need to know
Male or female
History and duration of hair loss
Location and size of affected areas
Other symptoms
Influencing factors
Medication

Significance of questions and answers

Male or female

Men and women, both may suffer from alopecia androgenetica or alopecia areata. Alopecia areata can affect people at any age.

History and duration of hair loss

Alopecia androgenetica is characterised by gradual onset. In men, the pattern of hair loss is recession of the hairline at the front and/or loss of hair on the top of the scalp. In women, the hair loss is generalised and there is an increase in the parting width. Another pattern of hair loss in women in the 20+ age group is increased shedding of hair but

Symptoms in the Pharmacy: A Guide to the Management of Common Illness, Seventh Edition.
Alison Blenkinsopp, Paul Paxton and John Blenkinsopp.
© 2014 John Wiley & Sons, Ltd. Published 2014 by John Wiley & Sons, Ltd.

without any increase in the parting width. This latter pattern is not due to alopecia androgenetica and it is thought that the cause may be nutritional. Hair loss in women is increasingly recognised as a problem.

Alopecia areata may be sudden and results in patchy hair loss. The cause of alopecia areata remains unknown but it is thought that the problem may be autoimmune in origin.

Telogen effluvium usually occurs 2–3 months after significant physical or emotional stress. The rate of hair loss increases significantly for a period of time before resolving spontaneously and returning to normal. Typically this can occur following a major surgery or illness.

Location and size of affected area

If the affected area is less than 10 cm in diameter in alopecia androgenetica, then treatment may be worth trying.

Other symptoms

Coarsening of the hair and hair loss can occur as a result of hypothyroidism (myxoedema) where other symptoms might include a feeling of tiredness or being run down, a deepening of the voice and weight gain.

Inflammatory conditions of the scalp such as ringworm infection (tinea capitis) can cause hair loss. Other symptoms would be itching and redness of the scalp with an advancing reddened edge of the infected area. Referral would be needed in such cases.

In women, excessive bleeding during periods (menorrhagia) could lead to iron deficiency and anaemia, which in turn could cause diffuse hair loss or aggravate alopecia androgenetica. Absent or very infrequent periods are sometimes due to polycystic ovary disease or elevated prolactin levels, which in both cases can result in alopecia androgenetica.

Influencing factors

Hormonal changes during and after pregnancy mean that hair loss is common both during pregnancy and after the baby is born. While this is often distressing for the woman concerned, it is completely normal and she can be reassured that the hair will grow back. Treatment is not appropriate.

Medication

Cytotoxic drugs are well known for causing hair loss. Anticoagulants (*coumarins*), lipid-lowering agents (*clofibrate*) and vitamin A (in overdose) have also been associated with hair loss. Such cases should be referred to the doctor. Other medications include *allopurinol*, beta-blockers, *bromocriptine, carbamazepine, colchicine, lithium* and *sodium valproate*.

Treatment timescale

Treatment with *minoxidil* may take up to 4 months to show full effect.

Management

Minoxidil

The only treatment licensed for use in hair loss is *minoxidil*, available as a 2% or 5% lotion with the drug dissolved in an aqueous alcohol solution. *Propylene glycol* is included to enhance absorption. The mechanism of action of *minoxidil* in baldness is unknown. The earlier *minoxidil* is used in balding, the more likely it is to be successful. Treatment is most likely to work where the bald area is less than 10 cm in diameter, where there is still some hair present and where the person has been losing hair for less than 10 years. The manufacturers of *minoxidil* say that the product works best in men with hair loss or thinning at the top of the scalp and in women in a generalised thinning over the whole scalp – both manifestations of alopecia androgenetica. Up to one in three users in such circumstances report hair regrowth of non-vellus (normal) hair and stabilisation of hair loss. A further one in three are likely to report some growth of vellus (fine, downy) hair. The final third will not see any improvement.

It is important that patients understand the factors that make successful treatment more or less likely and believe that their expectations are realistic. Some patients may still want to try the treatment, even where the chances of improvement are less.

After 4–6 weeks, the patient can expect to see a reduction in hair loss. It will take 4 months for any hair regrowth to be seen, and some dermatologists suggest continuing use for 1 year before abandoning treatment. Initially, the new hair will be soft and downy but it should gradually thicken to become like normal hair in texture and appearance.

Application

The lotion should be applied twice daily to the dry scalp and lightly massaged into the affected area. The hair should be clean and dry and the lotion should be left to dry naturally. The hair should not be washed for at least 1 h after using the lotion.

Caution

Irritant and allergic reactions to the *alcohol/propylene glycol* vehicle sometimes occur. A small amount (approximately 1.5%) of the drug is absorbed systemically and there is the theoretical possibility of a hypotensive effect, but this appears to be unlikely in practice. *Minoxidil* is also known to cause a reflex increase in heart rate. While this is a theoretical risk, where such small amounts of the drug are involved, tachycardia and palpitations have occasionally been reported. The manufacturers advise against the use of minoxidil in anyone with hypertension, angina or heart disease without first checking with the patient's doctor. Although no specific problems have been reported, the manufacturers advise against the use when pregnant or breast-feeding.

It is important to explain to patients that they will need to make a long-term commitment to the treatment should it be successful. Treatment must be continued indefinitely; new hair growth will fall out 2–3 months after the treatment is stopped. One year's treatment costs about £350.

Minoxidil should not be used in alopecia areata or in hair loss related to pregnancy.

Eye and Ear Problems

Eye problems: the painful red eye

Conjunctivitis is one cause of a painful red eye. There are other serious causes of painful red eyes and there are several causes of conjunctivitis. Accurate diagnosis of these causes is of vital importance and requires specific knowledge and skills. Notes on some of the causes of painful red eyes are provided below.

What you should know

Causes of painful red eye
  Conjunctivitis
  Infective
  Allergic
  Corneal ulcers
  Keratitis
Other causes
  Iritis/uveitis
  Glaucoma
One or both eyes affected?
  What is the appearance of the eye?
  What are the symptoms – pain, gritty feeling, photophobia?
  Is vision affected?
  Any discharge from the eye(s) – purulent, watery?
  Does the patient wear contact lenses?

Significance of questions and answers

Conjunctivitis

The term *conjunctivitis* implies inflammation of the conjunctiva, which is a transparent surface covering the white of the eye. It can become inflamed due to infection, allergy or irritation.

Infective conjunctivitis

Both bacteria and viruses can cause conjunctivitis. The symptoms are a painful gritty sensation and a discharge. The discharge is sticky and purulent in bacterial infections and more watery in viral infections.

Symptoms in the Pharmacy: A Guide to the Management of Common Illness, Seventh Edition. Alison Blenkinsopp, Paul Paxton and John Blenkinsopp.
© 2014 John Wiley & Sons, Ltd. Published 2014 by John Wiley & Sons, Ltd.

It nearly always affects both eyes. Conjunctivitis occurring in only one eye suggests the possible presence of a foreign body or another condition accounting for the red eye.

Management. Acute infective conjunctivitis is frequently self-limiting. A systematic review found that 65% of cases resolved within 2–5 days when treated with placebo. Gentle cleansing of the affected eye(s) with cotton wool soaked in water can be recommended regardless of whether treatment is also being suggested.

There is some evidence that infective conjunctivitis treated with antibacterial eye drops and ointment resolves more quickly. *Chloramphenicol eye drops* 0.5% every 2 h for the first 24 h and then four times daily or *chloramphenicol eye ointment* 1% can be used over the counter (OTC) for the treatment of acute bacterial conjunctivitis in adults and children aged 2 years or over.

People with infective conjunctivitis or those treating someone who is infected should wash their hands regularly and avoid sharing towels and pillows. Contact lenses should not be worn until the infection has completely cleared and until 24 h after any treatment has been completed.

Medical advice is urgently needed if the eye(s) become markedly painful, there is photophobia, marked redness or vision is affected. NHS Clinical Knowledge Service advises that if symptoms persist for longer than 2 weeks, further investigation is needed.

Other conditions with similar symptoms
Allergic conjunctivitis
This produces irritation, discomfort and a watery discharge. It typically occurs in the hay fever season. It is sometimes difficult to differentiate between infection and allergy and therefore referral is important if there is any doubt.

Management. In seasonal allergic conjunctivitis, decongestant and antihistamine drops can be helpful and *sodium cromoglicate (sodium cromoglycate) eye drops* is an effective, safe treatment. Mast cell stabilisers help to prevent the onset of allergic reactions by blocking the attachment of immunoglobulin/allergen complexes to mast cells. They do not provide the rapidity of relief associated with topical antihistamines but are effective when used for longer periods of time. In recurrent seasonal allergies, it is appropriate to use a mast cell stabiliser for 4 weeks before the start of an allergy season.

If there is prolonged exposure to allergens in perennial allergic conjunctivitis, then the continued use of a topical antihistamine becomes inappropriate and it is better to recommend drops containing a mast cell stabiliser such as *Sodium cromoglicate. Sodium cromoglicate* 2% eye drops can be recommended OTC for the treatment of both seasonal and perennial allergic conjunctivitis. A number of proprietary brands are available. Warn patients that they might experience a mild transient burning or stinging sensation after administering these products.

A more chronic form of allergic conjunctivitis is called vernal kerato-conjunctivitis. It usually occurs in atopic individuals. It is an important diagnosis to make, as leaving it untreated can lead to corneal scarring. It would normally be managed by an ophthalmologist. Steroid drops may be used in the management of more severe cases.

Blepharitis may present with similar symptoms to allergic conjunctivitis. However, it is often the case that pruritus (itching) is less prominent with blepharitis. This is also the case with dry eye syndrome (keratoconjunctivitis sicca). Blepharitis is an infection along the lid margin. Its management usually requires removal of the crusty matter from between the lashes with a cotton wool bud.

Corneal ulcers

These may be due to an infection or a traumatic abrasion. The main symptom is that of pain. There may be surrounding conjunctival inflammation. An abrasion can be caused by wearing contact lenses. Early diagnosis is important as the cornea can become permanently scarred, with loss of sight. If a corneal ulcer is suspected, the eye is examined after instilling *fluorescein drops,* which will colour and highlight an otherwise invisible ulcer. The cornea is the transparent covering over the front of the eye and early ulcers are not visible.

Keratitis (inflammation or infection of the cornea) often presents with a unilateral, acutely painful red eye and the patient complaining of photophobia. It may be caused by herpes simplex virus or, occasionally, a bacterial infection. *Acanthamoeba keratitis* is commoner in soft contact lens wearers and is associated with poor lens hygiene, extended wear and swimming whilst wearing lenses. Both these conditions need to be referred.

Management. This is obviously determined by the cause of the ulcer. Specialist referral is invariably required.

Other causes
Iritis/uveitis

Iritis is inflammation of the iris and surrounding structures. It may occur in association with some forms of arthritis, sarcoidosis or tuberculosis. It may occur as an isolated event with no obvious cause. The inflammation causes pain, which is felt more within the eye than is the superficial gritty pain of conjunctivitis, and there is no discharge. The affected eye is red and the pupil is small and possibly irregular. Urgent specialist referral is necessary for accurate diagnosis. Treatment is with topical steroids to reduce inflammation.

Glaucoma

Glaucoma occurs when the pressure of the fluids within the eye becomes abnormally high. This may either happen suddenly or develop slowly and insidiously; two different abnormalities are involved. It is the sudden onset type (acute closed-angle glaucoma) that causes a painful red eye. Emergency hospital referral is necessary in order to prevent permanent loss of sight. The pain of acute glaucoma is severe and may be felt in and around the eye. There may be associated vomiting. As the pressure builds up, the cornea swells, becoming hazy, causing impaired vision and a halo appearance around lights. Treatment involves an operation to lower the pressure to prevent it from developing again. Acute closed-angle glaucoma is rare, whereas 2% of people over 40 years suffer from primary open-angle glaucoma (chronic simple glaucoma). This condition starts slowly and insidiously, without warning symptoms. As the intraocular pressure builds up, the optic nerve is damaged, which leads to loss of visual field and blindness if not treated. Chronic glaucoma can be detected by an examination at the optician. Regular check-ups are advised if there is a family history of glaucoma, especially in those over 40 years of age. Free eye tests are available to those over the age of 40 years who have a close relative with glaucoma.

Contact lenses

There are two main types of lens: hard (gas-permeable) and soft (hydrogel). Soft lenses are the most popular because of their comfort. One-day disposable lenses, which are worn once and require no maintenance or storage, are becoming increasingly popular. However, this can lead to patients keeping lenses in for longer periods of time. Extended wear involves much greater risks and increases the chances of complications such as ulcerative keratitis, *Acanthamoeba keratitis* and papillary conjunctivitis.

Contact lenses should not be worn if the patient has conjunctivitis or is using eye drops. Soft contact lenses can absorb the preservative benzalkonium chloride used in eye drops. Consequently, soft lenses should not be worn within 24 h of instilling eye drops containing this preservative.

Dry eye

Dry eye is a common problem, particularly in older adults. Tears are needed to maintain a healthy eye surface and for enabling clear vision and have three layers: oil, water and mucus. The oily layer helps to prevent evaporation of the water layer, and the mucin layer spreads the tears evenly over the surface of the eye. In dry eye, the quantity or the composition of tears changes. Tears may evaporate too quickly or they may not spread evenly over the cornea. Tear production diminishes with age and is affected by female hormones. Hence the problem is more common in women.

What you should know
Causes of dry eye
Environment
Medical conditions
Medication
What are the symptoms – pain, gritty feeling, photophobia?
Is vision affected?
Does the patient wear contact lenses?

Significance of questions and answers

Environment – windy, dry climates increase tear evaporation. Long periods of time spent working at a computer screen are associated with dry eye because blinking tends to be less frequent thus redistribution of the tear film happens less often.

Medical conditions – patients with rheumatoid arthritis, diabetes or thyroid problems are more likely to experience dry eyes.

Medication – antihistamines, beta-blockers, chemotherapy, diuretics, HRT, oral contraceptives, selective serotonin reuptake inhibitors (SSRIs), tricyclic antidepressants (TCAs) may affect the quantity and composition of tears. Preservatives in topical treatments may also contribute to dry eyes.

Symptoms – people with dry eyes may report irritated, gritty, scratchy or burning eyes, a feeling of something in their eyes, excess watering and blurred vision.

Vision – patients with dry eyes may report experiencing some blurring of vision when they first wake up in the morning.

Contact lenses – individuals who wear contact lenses are more likely to experience dry eyes.

When to refer

Most cases of mild-to-moderate dry eyes can be managed by the patient using self-care. Severe symptoms or those that do not improve with self-care should be referred to the general practitioner (GP) or optometrist.

Management

Treatments for dry eyes aim to restore or maintain the normal amount of tears in the eye to minimise dryness. There are two main treatments: lubricant eye preparations and treatments that replenish the oily layer and reduce the evaporation of tears. The former include a range of drops, gels and ointments. Patients who wear contact lenses should use a preservative-free preparation. Preparations to replenish the oily layer include eye drops containing synthetic guar gum or a spray containing liposomes. A liposomal eye spray is applied onto the closed eyelids. When the eyes open, the liposomes spread across the surface of the eye, creating a new oily film.

Practical advice. Using a humidifier at home and work can help keep the air moist. Opening windows, even for a short time, will also help to refresh and moisten the air. Wearing sunglasses (especially of a wraparound style) outside will protect the eyes from the drying effects of sun and wind.

Eye problems in practice

Case 1

Paul Greet is a man in his 40s who comes into your pharmacy on his way home from work wanting treatment for a stye. He asks to speak to the pharmacist. It is Friday night and you are just about to close. Your pharmacy is in the city centre. He asks if you would make him an emergency supply of *chloramphenicol eye ointment,* which his doctor usually prescribes for him. OTC chloramphenicol is licensed only for the treatment of acute bacterial conjunctivitis. What would you do?

Pharmacist's view

This sort of dilemma sometimes happens. Unless this man's GP surgery is open in the morning, he will not be able to get a prescription until Monday, by which time his stye may have worsened. In areas where community pharmacies can supply *chloramphenicol eye ointment* through a patient group direction, the pharmacist can, following a protocol, supply treatment for a stye (hordeolum) where appropriate. In areas that have an NHS walk-in centre, he could be directed there for treatment. If his GP surgery is open in the morning, he could be seen then.

As for making an emergency supply, it is up to the pharmacist to decide whether this constitutes an emergency, which requires the pharmacist to satisfy him or herself that 'there is an immediate need for the POM requested to be sold or supplied and it is impracticable in the circumstances to obtain a prescription without undue delay'. Patients' and pharmacists' views of what constitutes an emergency do not always coincide. A possible framework for making such decisions is shown below.

Potential harm to patient from not supplying	Potential harm to patient from supplying	Potential benefit to patient from supplying	Consequences for pharmacist of supplying/ not supplying	What would I do if the patient were me/my spouse/my parent/my child? Is this decision different from the one I have reached for the patient? Why?

However, the pharmacist will take into account the consequences of not making a supply, including suffering and any potential harm from delayed treatment. If, in the pharmacist's view, the circumstances constitute an emergency, the requirements for emergency supplies are set out in *Medicines, Ethics and Practice* (Royal Pharmaceutical Society).

The doctor's view

Most styes are self-limiting. A stye can be an external one: a localised infection of the hair follicles of the eyelid margin; or an internal stye, an infection of meibomian glands on the inner surface of the lid.

Staphylococcus aureus is the infection responsible in nearly all cases. If left untreated, the stye will point and discharge and resolve spontaneously. The stye can be encouraged to point by the regular application of heat. A way of doing this would be to dip a cotton wool bud in hot water and then gently press it against the stye. Often *chloramphenicol ointment* is prescribed more to protect the eye from any discharge rather than actually treat the stye. It would probably help Paul Greet to understand the natural course of styes; although if he has used *chloramphenicol ointment* in the past, he is not likely to be happy without a further supply this time. It would be useful for his GP to review him as the styes have been recurrent. Sometimes recurrent styes can be associated with blepharitis, diabetes or raised lipids.

If there is inflammation surrounding the stye on the eyelid, then this would be a reason for referral to the GP, as systemic antibiotics may be indicated. Very occasionally, styes need incision and drainage to speed up their resolution.

Case 2

Kate Cosattis is a mum in her late 30s who wants advice about a problem with her daughter's eyes. Both of Ellie's eyes were sticky in the morning with 'yellow stuff' yesterday and today. The child is 18 months old and her eyes seem to be bothering her because she has been rubbing them.

Pharmacist's view

I couldn't recommend *chloramphenicol* for this child because she's under 2 years. In any case I'm not convinced that it offers any benefit in infective conjunctivitis in children. So I explained to Kate that if she gently bathed the eyes to keep them clean over the next few days it was likely that the infection would go by itself. She wanted to get some treatment, so I referred her to the GP.

The doctor's view

I agree with the pharmacist's opinion. The available evidence suggests that there is no advantage in prescribing *chloramphenicol eye drops* compared to placebo drops even in those who are subsequently shown to have bacterial infections on laboratory testing. In other words, most infections resolve spontaneously. In Ellie's situation it would be important to find out her mum's ideas, concerns and expectations about conjunctivitis and its management. She may be very insistent on a prescription and many GPs would be persuaded by her wishes and issue one, especially given the time pressures of a consultation. If possible, time spent listening to her concerns and addressing them could avoid a prescription and a rerun of this scenario in the future.

The parent's view

I wasn't happy with the pharmacist. I come here a lot for advice and usually he's really good. But this time he told me that the infection would probably go away by itself without treatment. And in any case he said he couldn't sell me anything and I would have to take Ellie to the doctor. I was worried that the infection might get worse or even damage Ellie's eyesight for the future. Anyway the doctor gave me some eye ointment and the infection cleared up in a few days. I don't see why the pharmacist couldn't have done the same.

Common ear problems

Although the treatment of common ear problems is straightforward, it does depend on accurate diagnosis and may require a prescription. It is not always possible to determine the problem from the story. A key issue for the pharmacist is the potential risk from not examining the inside of the ear and seeing how the ear looks. Unless the pharmacist is trained in clinical examination of the ear, diagnosis is best made by the doctor, who can examine the ear with an auriscope or otoscope. Referral to the doctor is therefore advisable for ear problems. Ear problems that commonly present are described below.

What you need to know

Wax
Otitis externa (OE)
Otitis media
Glue ear
One or both ears affected?
Symptoms – pain, itching
Is there any hearing loss?

Significance of questions and answers

Wax

Symptoms

Wax blocking the ear is one of the commonest causes of temporary deafness. It may also cause a discomfort and a sensation that the ear is blocked.

Management

Ear drops. The ear can be unblocked by using ear drops such as olive oil and various proprietary drops containing urea and hydrogen peroxide. A systematic review found that oil-based and water-based preparations are equally effective at clearing ear wax and for softening ear wax before syringing. The drops should be warmed before use (ideally to body temperature). With the head inclined, five drops should be

Symptoms in the Pharmacy: A Guide to the Management of Common Illness, Seventh Edition. Alison Blenkinsopp, Paul Paxton and John Blenkinsopp.
© 2014 John Wiley & Sons, Ltd. Published 2014 by John Wiley & Sons, Ltd.

instilled. A cotton wool plug should be applied to retain the fluid and be kept in for at least 1 h or overnight. This procedure should be repeated at least twice a day for 3–5 days. The use of these drops can worsen the deafness initially and appropriate warning should be given. Cotton wool buds should not be poked into the ear as wax is just pushed further in and it is possible to damage the eardrum.

Ear irrigation. If any wax remains despite this treatment, referral to the doctor or nurse is advisable. An electronic ear irrigator is used, which directs a pressurized flow of water into the ear. Metal ear syringes were used in the past but these sometimes triggered an infection (OE). The use of drops for 3–5 days to soften the wax prior to syringing the ears is recommended to make the procedure more effective.

Otitis externa

OE involves inflammation and infection of the skin in the ear canal (meatus). One in ten people experiences it at some time in their life. OE may be localised or diffuse. In the former (due to a furuncle or boil), the main symptom is ear pain and, in the latter, a combination of some or all of pain, itching, hearing loss and discharge. Sometimes it is a site of eczema, which may become secondarily infected.

OE can be precipitated by ear trauma (scratching, foreign bodies and use of cotton buds), swimming (especially in polluted water), chemicals (hairspray, hair dyes, shampoo and ceruminolytics) and skin conditions (eczema, seborrhoeic dermatitis and psoriasis). OE is five times more common in swimmers than in non-swimmers. It is more frequent in hot and humid environments and is 10 times more common in summer than winter.

Symptoms

The symptoms of OE are usually pain and discharge. Referral to the doctor may be necessary for accurate diagnosis. It is possible that the same symptoms can arise from a middle ear infection (otitis media) with a perforated eardrum. In such a situation, which usually involves a child, the middle ear infection is likely to be associated with an upper respiratory tract infection. As the middle ear infection develops, so does the pain. It is often intense and remains so until the drum perforates alleviating the pressure and pain and leading to a discharge.

Management

A good history is essential, including questions about any previous OE and recent foreign travel (association with swimming pools). Patients with OE should be referred to their local surgery, where they may be seen by a GP or a nurse. Some surgeries have a policy of taking a swab to enable treatment with an antibiotic to which the responsible bacterium is sensitive, rather than treating on a trial-and-error basis, which may lengthen time to healing. Thorough cleansing of the external ear canal is needed in many cases of OE. This is performed under direct vision using microsuction or dry swabbing.

Acute localised otitis externa

Acute localised OE is caused by a boil in the outer third of the external auditory meatus. If there is spreading cellulitis associated, then systemic antibiotics should be started and *flucloxacillin* would be the treatment of choice. Regular analgesics help and effective pain relief can be achieved using *paracetamol*. This can be combined with *codeine* when the pain is more severe, although the evidence of benefit is not definitive. Applying heat by holding a hot flannel against the ear can help to relieve pain.

Diffuse otitis externa

Approximately 90% of diffuse OE cases are bacterial. *Pseudomonas* infections account for two-thirds and *Staphylococcal* are the next most common. The remaining 10% of infections are fungal and *Aspergillus* is the most common form. Topical treatments containing an antibiotic alone or in combination with a corticosteroid are effective.

For people who are prone to recurrent OE, the following advice is helpful:

• Try not to let soap or shampoo get into your ear canal. While having a shower, you can do this by placing a piece of cotton wool coated in soft white paraffin (e.g. Vaseline) in the outer ear.
• Silicone rubber earplugs may be helpful to keep the ears dry whilst you swim.
• Do not use corners of towels or cotton buds to dry any water that does get in the ear canal. This will push things further in. Let it dry naturally.
• Try not to scratch or poke the ear canal with fingers, cotton wool buds, towels, etc.
• Do not clean the ear canal with cotton buds. They may scratch and irritate, and push wax or dirt further into the ear. The ear cleans itself, and bits of wax will fall out now and then.

Otitis media

Otitis media is an infection of the middle ear compartment. The middle ear lies between the outer ear canal and the inner ear. Between the outer ear and the middle is the eardrum (tympanic membrane). The middle ear is normally an air-containing compartment that is sealed from the outside apart from a small tube (the Eustachian tube), which connects to the back of the throat. Within the middle ear are tiny bones that transmit the sound wave vibrations of the eardrum to the inner ear.

An infection typically starts with a common cold, especially in children, which leads to blockage of the Eustachian tube and fluid formation within the middle ear. The fluid can then be secondarily infected by a bacterial infection.

Symptoms

The symptoms of otitis media are pain and temporary deafness. Sometimes the infection takes off so quickly that the eardrum perforates, releasing the infected fluid. When this occurs, a discharge will also be present and be associated with considerable lessening of pain.

As with OE, referral is usually necessary so that the eardrum can be examined. Treatment may involve a course of oral antibiotics (e.g. *amoxicillin (amoxycillin) or erythromycin)*. However, the use of antibiotics is being increasingly questioned. It appears that many cases of otitis media settle spontaneously and the effect of taking antibiotics possibly provides some benefit in symptoms after the first 24 h only when symptoms are already resolving. A meta-analysis of the research done on the value of antibiotics shows the number needed to successfully treat one patient is seven. In other words, six of every seven children treated for otitis media do not need antibiotics or show no response to them. Pharmacists can explain this to parents. Other concerns with the use of antibiotics are increasing bacterial resistance and adverse effects, such as diarrhoea, which occurs in about 10% of cases. Research has shown that it is reasonable to delay starting antibiotics for 72 h and starting only if symptoms persist at that time. 'Delayed prescriptions' are used where either the patient is given a postdated prescription which is 'cashed' only if needed or the patient can return to the surgery after a specified length of time to collect a prescription if needed. Sometimes topical or oral decongestants are used in addition to antibiotics. These can be useful if air travel is to be undertaken after such an infection. If the Eustachian tube is still blocked during a flight, pain can be experienced due to the change in air pressure. Decongestants would make this less likely.

Glue ear

Some children who are subject to recurrent otitis media develop glue ear. This occurs because the fluid that forms in the middle ear does not drain out completely. The fluid becomes tenacious and sticky. One method of dealing with this common problem is a minor operation in which the fluid is sucked out through the eardrum. After this, it is usual to insert a small grommet into the hole in the drum. The grommet has a small hole in the middle, which allows any further fluid forming to drain from the middle ear. The grommet normally falls out within a few months and the small hole in the drum closes over. The long-term effectiveness of this procedure is debatable.

Earplugs. Some children are advised not to get water into the ear after the insertion of a grommet. One method is to use earplugs that can be purchased from the pharmacy. However, this is often unnecessary and bathing and swimming can be undertaken without using plugs, although it is sensible to avoid deep diving as water may enter the middle ear under pressure, which will impair hearing and may predispose to infection.

Ear problems in practice

Case 1

Sue Moorhouse is a woman in her 20s. She and her parents have been regular customers for years and you know, she recently went to Kenya on holiday. It is Saturday afternoon and Sue tells you that her ear problem has returned. She has had antibiotics to treat it on four previous occasions during the last 3 years. She tells you she recognises the signs. Her face started to swell this morning. Her outer ear now feels swollen and her jaw is painful when she moves it. She knows from experience that if she can take some antibiotics within 24 h, the ear infection will not be so bad. In the past, the doctor has had trouble inserting the otoscope because the inside of her ear had been so swollen and painful. The problem causes a feeling of intense pressure inside the ear and she then has a discharge from the ear, which seems to ease the pain. When you check your patient medication record, you find that you have dispensed four courses of *erythromycin* for Sue in the last 3 years.

The pharmacist's view

It is typical that a problem like this happens on a Saturday afternoon when it is less easy to refer to the doctor. I could send Sue to the walk-in centre (if there is one) or to accident and emergency (A&E) department. Using the framework used in other parts of this book, I can think about possible actions I could take. There is no way I would consider leaving her to see the doctor on Monday.

Potential harm to patient from not supplying	Potential harm to patient from supplying	Potential benefit to patient from supplying	Consequences for pharmacist of supplying/ not supplying	What would I do if the patient were me/my spouse/my parent/my child? Is this decision different from the one I have reached for the patient? Why?

The doctor's view

Sue needs referral to the emergency on-call GP service or, failing that, to the local A&E department. It sounds like she has recurrent OE with cellulitis. She is likely to need high-dose antibiotic treatment. As this is her fifth episode in the last 3 years, she would need some follow-up, possibly with an ENT surgeon. If on resolution of this infection there were exudate and debris present in the outer ear canal, she could benefit from cleaning of the ear using microsuction. This would reduce the possibility of recurrence.

Childhood Conditions

Illnesses affecting infants and children up to 16 years

Childhood problems understandably create significant parental anxiety. This can affect the interchange with the pharmacist. If the pharmacist has children, this will be well understood. Whether the pharmacist is confident about childhood problems or not, the most important method of dealing with this is to listen well, not just to the presenting complaints but also to the specific concerns of the parent. Sometimes people will be more open with their concerns and sometimes it will be necessary to ask them about their concerns more than once. Just sharing a concern can literally diminish the perceived problem and make the rest of the consultation with the pharmacist more effective.

Common childhood rashes

Most childhood rashes are associated with self-limiting viral infections. Some of these rashes fit well-described clinical pictures (e.g. measles) and are described below. Others are more difficult to label. They may appear as short-lived, fine, flat (macular) or slightly raised (papular) red spots, often on the trunk. The spots blanch with pressure (erythematous). There is usually associated cold, cough and raised temperature. These relatively minor illnesses occur in the first few years of life and settle without treatment. Any rash in early childhood, particularly during the first year, can be alarming and frightening for parents. Advice, reassurance and referral are needed as appropriate.

What you need to know

When did it start?
Where did it start?
Where did it spread?
Any other symptoms?
Infectious diseases
    Chickenpox
    Measles

Symptoms in the Pharmacy: A Guide to the Management of Common Illness, Seventh Edition.
Alison Blenkinsopp, Paul Paxton and John Blenkinsopp.
© 2014 John Wiley & Sons, Ltd. Published 2014 by John Wiley & Sons, Ltd.

Roseola infantum
Fifth disease
German measles
Meningitis
Rashes that do not blanch

Chickenpox (also known as varicella)

This is most common in children under 10 years. It can occur in adults but is unusual. The incubation time (i.e. time between contact and development of the rash) is usually about 2 weeks (11–21 days). Sometimes the rash is preceded by a day or so of feeling unwell with a temperature. The rash is characteristic and difficult to diagnose when only very few spots are present. Typically it starts with small red lumps that rapidly develop into minute blisters (vesicles). The vesicles then burst, forming crusted spots over the next few days. The spots mainly occur on the trunk and face but may involve the mucous membranes of the mouth. They tend to come out in crops for up to 5 days. The rash is often irritating. Once the spots have all formed crusts, the individual is no longer contagious. NHS Clinical Knowledge Summaries (CKS) advises that exclusion from school or work is not necessary after 6 days from the onset of the rash. The whole infection is usually over within 1 week but it may be longer and more severe in adults. Sometimes the spots can become infected after scratching, so it can be helpful to advise cutting the child's fingernails short to reduce the chance of this possibility.

Measles

This is now a less common infection in the more developed countries but a significant cause of childhood mortality on a large scale in developing countries. A combined measles, mumps, rubella (MMR) vaccine is given between the ages of 12 and 15 months. The uptake of MMR in England was about 85% in 2006. The ideal is 95%. In England and Wales, the provisional number in 2012 for confirmed cases of measles was 2030 (www.hpa.org.uk). Many of these occurred in unvaccinated children, which included some in the travelling communities (see Table 1 for the nature and risk of complications from measles). At the time of introduction of the MMR, there were about 86 000 cases per year.

Measles has an incubation period of about 10 days. The measles rash is preceded by 3–4 days of illness with symptoms of cold, cough, conjunctivitis and fever. After the first 2 days of this prodromal phase, small white spots (Koplik spots), like grains of salt, can be seen on the

Table 1 Nature and risk of complications of measles.

Complications	Risk
Diarrhoea	1 in 6
Ear infection	1 in 20
Pneumonia/chest infection	1 in 25
Fits	1 in 200
Meningitis/encephalitis	1 in 1000
Death	1 in 2500–5000
Serious brain complication years later (subacute sclerosing panencephalitis)	1 in 8000 (of children who have measles under 2 years)

Source: From www.medinfo.co.uk.

inner cheek and gums. The measles rash then follows. It starts behind the ears, spreading to the face and trunk. The spots are small, red patches (maculae) that will blanch if pressed. Sometimes there are so many spots that they merge together to form large red areas.

In most cases the rash fades after 3 days, at which time the fever also subsides. If, however, the fever persists, the cough becomes worse or there is a difficulty in breathing or earache, then medical attention should be sought as complications may be developing. Someone with measles is infectious for about 5 days after the rash appears.

Roseola infantum

Roseola infantum is a viral infection occurring most commonly in the first year of life (but also between 3 months and 4 years of age). It can be confused with a mild attack of measles. There is a prodromal period of 3–4 days of fever followed by a rash similar to measles but which is mainly confined to the chest and abdomen. Once the rash appears there is usually an improvement in symptoms, in contrast to measles, and it lasts only about 24 h.

Fifth disease (erythema infectiosum)

Fifth disease is another viral infection (parvovirus B_{19}) that usually affects children. It does not often cause systemic upset but may cause fever, headache and, rarely, painful joints. The rash characteristically starts on the face. It particularly affects the cheeks and gives the appearance that the child has been out in a cold wind. Fifth disease is sometimes called 'slapped cheek' disease because of the appearance of reddened cheeks. The rash then appears on the limbs and trunk as small red spots that blanch with pressure. The infection is usually short-lived.

Fifth disease can have adverse effects in pregnancy. If the infection occurs in the first 20 weeks of gestation, there is an increased chance of miscarriage and a small chance the developing baby will become anaemic.

German measles (rubella)

German measles is a viral infection that is generally very mild, its main significance being the problems caused to the fetus if the mother develops the infection in early pregnancy. The incubation time for German measles is 12–23 days. The rash is preceded by mild catarrhal symptoms and enlargement of glands at the back of the neck. It usually starts on the face and spreads to the trunk and limbs. The spots are very fine and red. They blanch with pressure. They do not become confluent as in measles. In adults, rubella may be associated with painful joints. The rubella rash lasts for 3–5 days.

Meningitis

Meningitis is a very serious infection that can be caused by bacterial, viral or fungal infections. The bacterial causes, which are much more serious than viral causes, include meningococcus, *Haemophilus* and pneumococcus infections. In the United Kingdom, there are now vaccines routinely given for meningococcus C, *Haemophilus influenzae* B, and pneumococcus. A meningococcus B vaccine is also available but not for routine use yet. Meningococcus can cause a septicaemia (infection spreading throughout the body in the blood) in addition to meningitis alone, causing a typical rash. Meningococcal septicaemia usually presents with flu-like symptoms that may rapidly worsen (see Table 2). There may be an associated rash that appears as tiny purplish red blotches or bruises. (Very small bruises are called petechiae and larger ones, purpura and ecchymoses). These bruises do not blanch with pressure. The spots will start as a few tiny pinpricks and progress to widespread larger ones which coalesce together. The tumbler or glass test can be used to determine whether or not the rash is serious. The side of a glass tumbler should be pressed firmly against the skin. If the spots are the small bruises of septicaemia, they will not fade when the tumbler is pressed against the skin. Any suspicion of this condition requires emergency medical help.

Rashes that do not blanch

As a general rule all rashes that do not blanch when pressed (use glass tumbler test described in section on meningitis) ought to be referred to a doctor. These rashes are caused by blood leaking out of a capillary,

Table 2 Warning symptoms.

Meningitis symptoms in babies	Meningitis symptoms in children and adults
High temperature, fever, possibly with cold hands and feet	High temperature, fever, possibly with cold hands and feet
Vomiting or refusing feeds	Vomiting, sometimes diarrhoea
High-pitched moaning, whimpering cry	Neck stiffness (unable to touch chin to chest)
Blank, staring expression	Joint or muscle pains, sometimes stomach cramps
Pale blotchy complexion	Dislike of bright lights
May be floppy, may dislike being handled, may be fretful	Drowsiness
Difficult to wake or lethargic	Fits
Fontanelle (soft spot) may be tense or bulging	Confusion or disorientation
May have rash	May have rash

Source: Data from the Meningitis Trust website (http://www.meningitis-trust.org/). (There is no particular order for these symptoms to occur, not all have to be present and there may be others not mentioned.)

which may be caused by a blood disorder. It could be the first sign of leukaemia or a much less serious condition. Blanching is not a concept that parents are familiar with. It is important to explain what is meant by blanching and how parents can check for it.

When to refer

Suspected meningitis (see Table 2)
- Flu-like symptoms
- Vomiting
- Headache
- Neck stiffness
- Rash
- Small widespread spots or bruises that do not blanch when pressed
- Rashes that do not blanch when pressed

Management

Fever

Moderate fever (raised temperature up to 40°C from normal 36.5°C to 37.5°C) is usually not harmful and some experts believe it could even have beneficial effects in some illnesses. The question of whether and when an antipyretic medicine should be given remains a matter of debate. The National Institute for Health and Care Excellence Guideline on Feverish Illness in Children advises against routine use of antipyretic to solely reduce temperature if the child is otherwise well and recommends:

paracetamol or ibuprofen be considered when a feverish child is in distress, but not for the sole purpose of reducing body temperature. When using either medicine in children with fever:

1 continue only as long as the child appears distressed
2 consider changing to the other agent if the child's distress is not alleviated
3 do not give both agents simultaneously
4 only consider alternating these agents if the distress persists or recurs before the next dose is due

Parents often want to reduce a child's temperature when there is a fever. There is no clear evidence that reducing a raised temperature is harmful and doing so may reduce the child's discomfort and distress.

Sponging with lukewarm water used to be recommended as a method of reducing fever but can cause goosebumps and shivering and is now viewed as potentially causing discomfort to the child.

Paracetamol or *ibuprofen* can be used if a high temperature is present.

Many babies develop a raised temperature after immunisation. Some preparations containing *paracetamol* or *ibuprofen* can be used over the counter (OTC) to reduce post-immunisation fever. Product licences vary, so check the labels.

Itching

The itching caused by childhood rashes such as chickenpox can be intense, and the pharmacist is in a good position to offer an antipruritic cream, ointment or lotion. *Crotamiton cream* or *lotion* may help to soothe itchy skin. *Calamine lotion* has been used traditionally but it is now thought that the powdery residue it leaves may further dry and irritate itchy dry skin. If itching is very severe, *chlorpheniramine* can be effective in providing relief, can be given to children of 1 year and over and is licensed for use OTC in chickenpox rash. Such treatment would be likely to make the child drowsy but may be useful at nighttime. A medical device is available comprising an osmotic gel containing glycerol which has the effect of drawing water from the dermis to the skin surface creating a cooling effect. There are no published studies of efficacy.

Colic

The cause of colic is unknown and it may affect between one in twenty and one in five babies. Although infantile colic is not harmful, it is stressful for both the baby and parents. It generally begins in the first few weeks after the baby is born and resolves by the time the baby is 3–4 months old.

> **What you need to know**
>
> Age
>   Symptoms
>   Feeding
>   Does the mother smoke?
>   Any advice already sought?

Age

Colic generally starts in the early weeks and may last up to the age of 3–4 months.

Symptoms

Mothers usually describe crying that occurs in the late afternoon and evening, where the baby cannot be comforted, becomes red in the face and may draw the knees up. Passing wind and difficulty in passing stools may also occur.

It is important to be aware that colic is not the only cause of crying and discomfort. If a baby becomes inconsolable and cannot be comforted, the parent should be advised to consult the general practitioner (GP). Rarely, problems such as volvulus (twisting of the intestines) can occur and cause incessant and loud crying.

Feeding

Establish whether the baby is bottle- or breast-fed (or a combination) and the type of formula milk being used.

Symptoms in the Pharmacy: A Guide to the Management of Common Illness, Seventh Edition. Alison Blenkinsopp, Paul Paxton and John Blenkinsopp.
© 2014 John Wiley & Sons, Ltd. Published 2014 by John Wiley & Sons, Ltd.

Does the mother smoke?

There does seem to be an association between maternal smoking and colic in the baby.

Any advice already sought?

It is useful to ask whether advice has been sought already either from health professionals or from lay sources. The pharmacist can assess the relevance and appropriateness of advice already received.

Management

There is no good evidence to support any of the commonly tried approaches to management. It is important to reassure parents that colic is not their fault and that the baby will 'grow out of it'.

Simethicone

Simethicone has been commonly used to treat infantile colic and is included in several proprietary preparations. However, only three small trials were found in systematic reviews, and the evidence of benefit is uncertain. A trial of *simethicone drops for 1 week* could be suggested if other strategies are unsuccessful and the parents would like to try treatment.

Feeding

For breastfed infants, it may be worth the mother considering the exclusion of cow's milk from her diet. There is a theoretical ratio-nale for this in that breast milk contains intact cow's milk proteins. However, there is no good evidence of benefit. A trial of cow's milk exclusion for 1 week could be suggested. This means that the mother needs to stop eating all forms of dairy produce. If there appears to be some improvement, referral to the health visitor for further advice on diet is appropriate.

Where the baby is being bottle-fed and symptoms are severe and persistent, the mother might consider trying hypoallergenic formula (*caseinogen (casein) hydrolysate*) milk. Studies indicate that this may reduce crying by over 20%. A trial of such milk for 1 week could be suggested. If there appears to be a response, referral for further advice on diet from the health visitor is appropriate. Evidence is less strong for whey hydrolysate formula. There is limited evidence of effectiveness of soya milk in reducing crying. There is no evidence to support the use of low-lactose or fibre-enriched milk.

Complementary therapies

A study of herbal tea in colic showed a large reduction in crying but there are concerns over the study design. Furthermore, the safety of herbal teas in infants has been questioned, probably because of issues around standardisation of ingredients and questions about the possible presence of other ingredients.

Behavioural approaches

In the past, it was thought that overstimulation of the baby might be a cause of colic. Therefore, there have been studies to test avoiding carrying or holding the baby unnecessarily and not intervening too rapidly when the baby cries. These studies did not show a significant effect.

Baby massage

Although baby massage seems to have become more popular as a method of managing colic, the evidence of benefit is uncertain.

Other health professionals

Health visitors can advise and support families on infant feeding and other problems.

Teething

Teething can start as early as 3 months and continue up to 3 years. The association of discomfort and physical change associated with teething is a matter of some debate. Some health professionals and parents incorrectly associate symptoms of agitation, fever and diarrhoea with teething. A study showed that the number of symptoms ascribed to teething was paediatricians (2.8), dentists (4.4), GPs (6.5), pharmacists (8.4) and nurses (9.8). The more contemporary view of teething is that it is a local phenomenon that may account for symptoms such as dribbling, drooling, reddened cheeks, inflamed gums, biting objects and increase in general irritability but is not itself a cause of infection. One theory is that bottle-fed babies receive fewer antibodies than those who are breastfed, and this may result in an association between teething and systemic symptoms. An important point about associating systemic problems with teething is that a more serious underlying cause may be overlooked.

The appropriate management of teething is local discomfort relief using application of cold and the use of analgesics *(paracetamol suspension)* or topical gels. There is a homoeopathic teething product available as granules, and some parents may prefer complementary therapies. Parents should be encouraged to clean their baby's teeth from their first appearance using a baby toothbrush. Dummies should be avoided, but if used then it is important not to dip them or teething rings into honey, fruit juices or syrups. Further advice on prevention of teething problems can be obtained from the health visitor.

Symptoms in the Pharmacy: A Guide to the Management of Common Illness, Seventh Edition.
Alison Blenkinsopp, Paul Paxton and John Blenkinsopp.

Napkin rash

Most babies will have napkin (nappy) rash at some stage during their infancy. Contributory factors include contact of urine and faeces with the skin, irritant effect of soaps/detergents/bubble baths and wetness and maceration of skin due to infrequent nappy changes and inadequate skin care. Advice from the pharmacist is important in both treating and preventing recurrence of the problem.

> **What you need to know**
>
> Nature and location of rash
> > Severity
> > Broken skin
> > Signs of infection
> > Duration
> > Previous history
> > Other symptoms
> > Precipitating factors
> > Skin care and hygiene
> > Medication

Significance of questions and answers

Nature and location of rash

Nappy rash, sometimes called napkin dermatitis, appears as an erythematous rash on the buttock area. Other areas of the body are not involved, in contrast to infantile seborrhoeic dermatitis, where the scalp may also be affected (cradle cap). In infantile eczema, other body areas are usually involved. The initial treatment of nappy rash would be the same in each case.

Severity

In general, if the skin is unbroken and there are no signs of secondary bacterial infection, treatment may be considered. The presence of bacterial infection could be signified by weeping or yellow crusting. Secondary fungal infection is common in napkin dermatitis and the

Symptoms in the Pharmacy: A Guide to the Management of Common Illness, Seventh Edition. Alison Blenkinsopp, Paul Paxton and John Blenkinsopp.
© 2014 John Wiley & Sons, Ltd. Published 2014 by John Wiley & Sons, Ltd.

presence of satellite papules (small, red lesions near the perimeter of the affected area) would indicate such an infection. Referral to the doctor would be advisable if bacterial infection were suspected, since topical or systemic antibiotics might be needed. Secondary fungal infection could be treated by the pharmacist using one of the azole topical antifungal preparations that are available.

Duration

If the condition has been present for longer than 2 weeks, the pharmacist might decide that referral to the doctor would be the best option, depending on the nature and severity of the rash.

Previous history

The pharmacist should establish whether the problem has occurred before and, if so, what action was taken, for example, treatment with OTC products.

Other symptoms

Napkin dermatitis sometimes occurs during or after a bout of diarrhoea, when the perianal skin becomes reddened and sore. The pharmacist should therefore enquire about current or recent incidence of diarrhoea. Diarrhoea may occur as a side effect of antibiotic therapy and this may be the cause. Sometimes thrush in the nappy area may be associated with oral thrush that causes a sore mouth or throat (see p. 323). If this is suspected, referral to the doctor is advisable.

Precipitating factors

Skin care and hygiene

At one time napkin dermatitis was thought to be a simple irritant dermatitis due to ammonia, produced as a breakdown product of urine in soiled nappies. However, other factors are now known to play a part. These include irritant substances in urine and faeces, sensitivity reactions to soaps and detergents and antiseptics left in reusable nappies after inadequate rinsing and sensitivity reactions to ingredients in some topical preparations, for example, in baby wipes. The major factor thought to influence the incidence of nappy rash is the constant wetting and rewetting of the skin when left in contact with soiled nappies. Maceration of the skin ensues, leading to enhanced penetration of irritant substances through the skin and the breakdown of the skin. Wearing occlusive plastic pants exacerbates this effect. Frequent changes of nappy together with good nappy-changing routine and hygiene are essential (see 'Practical points' below).

Medication

The identity and effectiveness of any preparations used for the current or any previous episode, either prescribed or purchased OTC, should be ascertained by the pharmacist. The possibility of a sensitivity reaction to an ingredient in a topical product already tried should be considered by the pharmacist, especially if the rash has worsened.

When to refer

Broken skin, severe rash
Signs of infection
Other body areas affected

Treatment timescale

A baby with nappy rash that does not respond to skin care and OTC treatment within 1 week should be seen by the doctor.

Management

Treatment and the prevention of further episodes can be achieved by a combination of OTC treatment and advice on care of the skin in the nappy area.

Emollient preparations

Emollient preparations are the mainstay of treatment. The inclusion of a water repellent such as *dimethicone* is useful in theory but there is no convincing evidence that such products are more effective. The choice of individual preparation may sometimes depend on customer preference and many preparations are equally effective. Most pharmacists will have a particular favourite that they usually recommend. Some of the ingredients included in preparations for the treatment and prevention of nappy rash and their uses are described below.

Zinc

Zinc acts as a soothing agent.

Lanolin

Lanolin hydrates the skin. It can sometimes cause sensitivity reactions, although the high grades of purified lanolin used in many of today's products should reduce the problem.

Castor oil/cod liver oil

Castor oil and cod liver oil provide a water-resistant layer on the skin.

Antibacterials (e.g. chlorhexidine gluconate)
These may be useful in reducing the number of bacteria on the skin. Some antibacterials have been reported to produce sensitivity reactions.

Antifungals
Secondary infection with *Candida* is common in napkin dermatitis and the azole antifungals would be effective. *Miconazole* or *clotrimazole* applied twice daily could be recommended by the pharmacist with advice to consult the doctor if the rash has not improved within 5 days. If an antifungal cream is advised, treatment should be continued for 4 or 5 days after the symptoms have apparently cleared. An emollient cream or ointment can still be applied over the antifungal product.

Practical points
1 Nappies should be changed as frequently as necessary. Babies up to 3 months old may pass urine as many as 12 times a day.
2 Nappies should be left off wherever possible so that air is able to circulate around the skin, helping the affected skin to become and remain dry. Laying the baby on a terry nappy or towel with a waterproof sheet underneath will prevent the soiling of furniture or bedding.
3 At each nappy change the skin should be cleansed thoroughly by washing with warm water or using a proprietary lotion or wipes. The skin should then be carefully and thoroughly dried. The use of talcum powder can be helpful, but the clumping of powder can sometimes cause further irritation. Talcum powder should always be applied to dry skin and should be dusted lightly over the nappy area. The regular use of an emollient cream or ointment, applied to clean dry skin, can help to protect the skin against irritant substances.

Napkin rash in practice

Case 1
Jane Simmonds, a young mother, asks you to recommend a good cream for her baby daughter's nappy rash. The baby (Sarah) is 3 months old and Mrs Simmonds tells you that the buttocks are covered in a red rash. The skin is not broken and there is no weeping or yellow matter present. On further questioning, you find that the rash is also affecting the upper back and neck and there are signs of its appearance around the wrists. The rash seems to be itchy, as Sarah keeps trying to scratch the affected areas. Mrs Simmonds uses disposable nappies, which she changes frequently, and *zinc* and *castor oil cream* is applied at each nappy change, after cleansing the skin. The baby has no other symptoms and is not taking any medicines.

The pharmacist's view

Mrs Simmonds' nappy-changing and skin-care routine seems to be adequate, but the baby has nappy rash and the rash has affected other areas of the body. It is possible that Sarah has infantile eczema and referral to the doctor would be the best course of action.

The doctor's view

It is quite likely that Sarah does have eczema, which could be the cause of her nappy rash. It is also possible that an eczematous rash can be complicated by a secondary infection. Referral to the doctor or health visitor for further assessment would be wise. Such skin problems can be upsetting for the mother and it is important that Mrs Simmonds should be given an opportunity to air her understanding and concerns about the problem and, in return, that the doctor offer an appropriate explanation. The management would be to reinforce all the above practical points and possibly prescribe a weak topical steroid, such as 1% *hydrocortisone,* with or without an antifungal or antibacterial agent.

Case 2

Mrs Lesley Tibbs is worried about her baby son's nappy rash, which, she tells you, seems to have appeared over the last few days. The skin is quite red and looks sore and she has been using a proprietary cream, but the rash seems to be even worse. The baby has never had nappy rash before and is about 5 months old. Mrs Tibbs is using reusable nappies and recently changed the washing powder she uses, on a friend's recommendation. The rash affects only the napkin area and the baby has no other symptoms.

The pharmacist's view

The history gives two clues to the possible cause of the problem. This baby has not had nappy rash before and this episode has coincided with a change in detergent, so it is possible that a sensitivity reaction is occurring due to residues of detergent in the nappies after washing. The second factor is the cream that Mrs Tibbs has been using to treat the problem, with no success. The ingredients of the product should be carefully considered by the pharmacist to see if any might be potential sensitizers.

Initial advice to Mrs Tibbs might be to revert to her original detergent and to use a different treatment. Advice on nappy-changing routine could be given and if the rash has not started to resolve within 1 week, or has become worse, referral to the doctor should be indicated.

The doctor's view

The advice given by the pharmacist should clear up the problem quickly. It would be quite reasonable to refer Mrs Tibbs and her baby to the health visitor for further advice if the rash does not settle down.

Head lice

Head lice infection is common in young children. Effective treatments are available, but treatment failure may occur if products are not used correctly. It is therefore important for the pharmacist to explain how products should be used, since more patients are now being directed to pharmacies to obtain treatment. The pharmacist has a valuable health education role in explaining how to check children's hair for lice and in discouraging prophylactic use of insecticides. Parents are often embarrassed to seek advice, particularly if the child has head lice. Pharmacists can reassure parents that the condition is common and does not in any way indicate a lack of hygiene. The term infection is preferred to infestation because of the unpleasant image associated with infestation.

What you need to know
Age
Child, adult
Signs of infection
Live lice
Checking for infection
Nits
Scalp itching
Previous infection
Medication
Treatments used

Significance of questions and answers

Age

Head lice infection is most commonly found in children, particularly at around 4–11 years, with girls showing a higher incidence than boys. Older children and adults seem to be less prone to infection. Adult women occasionally become infected, but head lice infection is rare in adult men because, as men lose hair through male pattern baldness, the scalp offers less shelter to lice.

Symptoms in the Pharmacy: A Guide to the Management of Common Illness, Seventh Edition. Alison Blenkinsopp, Paul Paxton and John Blenkinsopp.
© 2014 John Wiley & Sons, Ltd. Published 2014 by John Wiley & Sons, Ltd.

Signs of infection

Unless infection has been confirmed by a nurse or doctor who has conducted wet combing of the hair or inspected the scalp, the pharmacist should ask whether any check has been made to confirm the presence of head lice. Parents often worry that their children may catch lice and want the pharmacist to recommend prophylactic treatment. Insecticides should never be used prophylactically, since this may accelerate resistance. Treatment should be reserved for infected heads.

Checking for infection

Wet combing of the hair is a more reliable detection method than scalp inspection. Parents can easily check for infection by combing the child's hair over a piece of white- or light-coloured paper, using a fine-toothed comb (tooth spacing of less than 0.3 mm). The hair should be damp or wet to make the combing process easier and less painful. Also, dry hair can produce static that causes lice to be repelled from the comb, making detection less likely. After each stroke the comb should be wiped on a white tissue or cloth. The hair should be combed one section at a time. The hair at the nape of the neck and behind the ears should be thoroughly checked. These spots are preferred by lice because they are warm and relatively sheltered. Such a check should be carried out regularly, say once a week, and perhaps more often when infection is known to have occurred in other children at school or playgroup.

If live lice are present, some will be combed out of the hair and onto the paper, where they will be seen as small beige, black, greyish or brown-coloured specks. Cast shells are discarded as the louse grows and appear yellowish in colour. Louse faeces may be seen as small blackish specks on pillows and collars.

Nits

The presence of empty eggshells – the cream- or white-coloured nits attached to the hair shafts – is not necessarily evidence of current infection unless live lice are also found. Parents sometimes think that treatment has failed because nits can still be seen in the hair. It is therefore important for the pharmacist to explain that the empty shells are firmly glued to the hair shaft and will not be removed by the lotion used in treatment. A fine-toothed comb can be used to remove the nits after treatment.

Itching

Contrary to popular belief, itching is not experienced by everyone with a head lice infection. In fact, as few as one in five cases present with itching, perhaps because detection now occurs at an earlier stage than used to be the case. Where it occurs, itching of the scalp is an allergic response to the saliva of the lice, which is injected into the scalp in small amounts each time the lice feed. Sensitisation does not occur immediately and it may take weeks for itching to develop. It has been estimated that thousands of bites from the lice are required before the reaction develops. The absence of itching does not mean that infection has not occurred. In someone who has previously been infected and becomes reinfected, itching may quickly begin again.

Previous infection

The pharmacist should establish whether the child has been infected before. In particular, it is important to know whether there has been a recent infection, as reinfection may have occurred from other family members if the whole family was not treated at the same time. Head-to-head contact, between family members and also among young children while playing, is responsible for the transmission of head lice from one host to the next. The pharmacist could ask whether the parent was aware of any contact with infected children, for example, if there is currently a problem with head lice at the child's school.

Medication

While it is possible that treatment failure may occur, this is unlikely if a recommended insecticide has been used (see 'Management' below) correctly. Careful questioning will be needed to determine whether treatment failure has occurred. The identity of any treatment used and its method of use should be elicited.

Management

Having established that infection is present, the pharmacist can go on to recommend an appropriate treatment. Only those individuals in whom a live head louse has been found should be treated, and all those affected in the same household should be treated on the same day. Depending on the parent's preference and on the treatment history, treat with:

dimethicone or isopropyl myristate/cyclomethicone solutionwet combing ('Bug Busting')
coconut, anise, and ylang ylang spray
malathion 0.5% aqueous liquid.

Dimethicone and isopropyl myristate/cyclomethicone

There is evidence of efficacy from randomised clinical trials for dimethicone which is thought to coat the lice and prevent the insects from excreting excess water. It is applied to dry hair and scalp, left for 8 h and then rinsed off. A second application is used after 7 days.

Detection combing at day 4 and again at 8–10 days is recommended. Dimethicone has a good safety profile. Adverse effects are not common and include itchy or flaky scalp and irritation if it gets into the eyes. It can be used for people with eczema or asthma. Isopropyl myristate/cyclomethicone solution also has a physical effect on the lice. It is applied to dry hair and washed out after 10 min.

Wet combing (Bug Busting) method
The effectiveness of this method is dependent on repeated use over a period of 2 weeks. The procedure is:

wash the hair as normal;
apply conditioner liberally (This causes the lice to lose their grip on the hair);
comb the hair through with a normal comb first;
with a fine-toothed nit comb, comb from the roots along the complete length of the hair and after each stroke check the comb for lice and wipe it clean. Work methodically over the whole head for at least 30 min;
rinse the hair as normal;
repeat every 3 days for at least 2 weeks (Wet combing should be continued until no fully grown lice have been seen for three consecutive sessions)
(*Source:* NHS Clinical Knowledge Summaries)

Coconut, anise and ylang ylang spray
The spray can be used in children aged over 2 and is left on the hair for 15 min. The hair is then washed using shampoo to remove the spray, and then systematically combed with a fine-toothed comb to remove lice. A second application is used 7 days later. The preparation is not suitable for those with asthma or skin conditions such as eczema.

Malathion
Malathion liquid is applied to dry hair and scalp and left for a minimum contact time of 12 h (or overnight). A repeat application 7 days after the initial treatment should be recommended. This second application will kill any lice that have emerged from the eggs in the meantime. Eggs take around 7 days to hatch. A detection comb should be used at day 4 and again at 8–10 days.

Malathion is available as alcoholic and aqueous lotions. Alcohol-based formulations are not suitable for all patients because they can cause two types of problems. Firstly, alcohol can cause stinging when applied to scalps with skin broken as a result of scratching, for example, in eczema. Secondly, in patients with asthma, it is thought that alcohol-based lotions are best avoided, as the evaporating alcohol might irritate the lungs and cause wheezing, perhaps even precipitating an attack of asthma. Such reactions are likely to be extremely rare, but caution is still advised.

Malathion should be rubbed gently into dry hair and care should be taken to ensure that the scalp is thoroughly covered; the wet hair is then combed. The most effective method of application is to sequentially part sections of the hair and then apply a few drops of the treatment, spreading it along the parting into the surrounding scalp and along the hair. Approximately 50–55 mL of lotion should be sufficient for one application, although people with very thick or long hair may need more. A towel or cloth can be placed over the eyes and face to protect them from the liquid. When applying the product, particular attention should be paid to the areas at the nape of the neck and behind the ears, where lice are often found. The hair should then be left to dry naturally. A hair drier should not be used because malathion is inactivated by heat. Where an alcoholic lotion is used, the hair should be kept away from naked flames.

A residual effect from malathion lotion can occur. It takes several hours of contact to develop and the level of residual action varies from person to person. Once established, the effect may last for several weeks. Contact with chlorinated water during swimming will reduce any residual effect, as will the application of heat via hairdryers.

Complementary therapies

Herbal treatments (e.g. tea tree oil) and aromatherapy have been tried but there is little evidence of their effectiveness.

Other points

1 Teamwork between pharmacists, GPs and nurses (particularly those involved in prescribing for head lice) is important to ensure consistency of messages and treatment information. Pharmacists can also liaise with health visitors and school nurses to communicate with schools in the area and ensure the accuracy and currency of information given to parents and children.

Head lice in practice

Case 1

A young mother, who often comes into your pharmacy to ask for advice and buy medicines for her children, asks for a product to prevent head lice. Her children have not got head lice but she wants to use a treatment 'just to be on the safe side'. On questioning, you find out that the children are aged 5 and 7 years and that there are no signs of infection such as itching scalps. The children's heads have not been checked for lice. She is not sure how to go about making such a check.

There has not been any communication from the children's school to indicate that head lice is a current problem at the school. This lady explains that she is very hygiene conscious and would hate her children to get nits.

The pharmacist's view

Treatment should not be used unless there is evidence of infection. From what this mother has said, it seems unlikely that her children have head lice and there is no evidence of a current problem at school. However head lice are easily transferred from one head to another, particularly among schoolchildren and the pharmacist can explain how to make weekly checks for lice using wet combing with a fine-toothed comb and a light-coloured sheet of paper. It would also be helpful to explain that head lice and hygiene are not linked. If any live lice are found, treatment can be recommended.

The doctor's view

The advice given by the pharmacist is very helpful. It would have certainly been a lot quicker and more convenient, but inappropriate, to have sold a treatment. Hopefully, the information given by the pharmacist will allay her anxiety regarding hygiene and lice. This demonstrates an important role of health education that can be provided in the pharmacy.

Threadworms (pinworms)

Infection with threadworms *(Enterobius vermicularis)* is common in young children, and parents may seek advice from the pharmacist. As with head lice infections, many parents feel embarrassed about discussing threadworms and feel ashamed that their child is infected. Pharmacists can give reassurance that this is a common problem. In addition to recommending OTC antihelminthic treatment, it is essential that advice be given about hygiene measures to prevent reinfection.

What you need to know
Age
Signs of infection
Perianal itching
Appearance of worms
Other symptoms
Duration
Recent travel abroad
Other family members affected
Medication

Significance of questions and answers

Age

Threadworm infection is very common in schoolchildren.

Signs of infection

Usually the first sign that parents notice is the child scratching his or her bottom. Perianal itching is a classic symptom of threadworm infection and is caused by an allergic reaction to the substances in and surrounding the worms' eggs that are laid around the anus. Sensitisation takes a while to develop. So in someone infected for the first time, itching will not necessarily occur.

Itching is worse at night, because at that time the female worms emerge from the anus to lay their eggs on the surrounding skin. The eggs are secreted together with a sticky irritant fluid onto the perianal

Symptoms in the Pharmacy: A Guide to the Management of Common Illness, Seventh Edition. Alison Blenkinsopp, Paul Paxton and John Blenkinsopp.
© 2014 John Wiley & Sons, Ltd. Published 2014 by John Wiley & Sons, Ltd.

skin. Persistent scratching may lead to secondary bacterial infection. If the perianal skin is broken and there are signs of weeping, referral to the doctor for antibiotic treatment would be advisable.

Loss of sleep due to itching may lead to tiredness and irritability during the day. Itching without the confirmatory sighting of threadworms may be due to other causes, such as an allergic or irritant dermatitis caused by soaps or topical treatments used to treat the itching. In some patients, scabies or fungal infection may produce perianal itching.

Appearance of worms

The worms themselves can be easily seen in the faeces as white- or cream-coloured thread-like objects, about 10 mm in length and less than 0.5 mm in width. Males are smaller than females. The worms can survive outside the body for a short time and hence may be seen to be moving. Sometimes the worms may be seen protruding from the anus itself.

Other symptoms

In severe cases of infection, diarrhoea may be present and, in girls, vaginal itch.

Duration

If a threadworm infection is identified, the pharmacist needs to know how long the symptoms have been present and to consider this information in the light of any treatments tried.

Recent travel abroad

If any infection other than threadworm is suspected, patients should be referred to their doctor for further investigation. If the person has recently travelled abroad, this information should be passed on to the doctor so that other types of worm can be considered.

Other family members

The pharmacist should enquire whether any other member of the family is experiencing the same symptoms. However, the absence of perianal itching and threadworms in the faeces does not mean that the person is not infected; it is important to remember that during the early stages, these symptoms may not occur.

Medication

The pharmacist should enquire about the identity of any treatment already tried to treat the symptoms. For any antihelminthic agent, correct use is essential if treatment is to be successful. The pharmacist should therefore also ask how the treatment was used, in order to establish whether treatment failure might be due to incorrect use.

Management

When recommending treatment for threadworms, it is important that the pharmacist emphasise how and when the treatment is to be used. In addition, advice about preventing recurrence can be given, as described under 'Practical points' below. The BNF states that mebendazole is the choice of treatment for patients of all ages. If symptoms do not remit after correct use of an appropriate preparation, patients should see their doctor.

Mebendazole

Mebendazole is the preferred treatment for threadworms and is an effective, single-dose treatment. It is also active against whipworm, roundworm and hookworm. Compliance with therapy is high because of the single dose. The drug is formulated as a suspension or a tablet that can be given to children aged 2 years and over and to adults. Reinfection is common and a second dose can be given after 2–3 weeks. Occasionally, abdominal pain and diarrhoea may occur as side effects. Mebendazole is not recommended for pregnant women.

Piperazine

Piperazine is effective against threadworm and roundworm. It is available in granular form in sachets. The mode of action of piperazine seems to be paralysis of the threadworms in the gut. The incorporation of a laxative (senna) in the sachet preparation helps to ensure that the paralysed worms are then expelled with the faeces.

Instructions

One dose is followed by another 2 weeks later to destroy any worms that might have hatched and developed after the first dose. Only two doses are required.

Side effects

Side effects of piperazine include nausea, vomiting, diarrhoea and colic but these are uncommon. Adverse effects on the central nervous system include headaches and dizziness but these are rare.

Contraindications
Piperazine can be recommended OTC for children from 3 months onwards. It should not be recommended for pregnant women because, although a direct causal relationship has not been established, some cases of fetal malformations have been reported. Its use is contraindicated in epileptic patients since it has been shown to have the potential to induce fits in patients with grand mal epilepsy. In some European countries, piperazine has been removed from the market because of the concern about adverse effects. The most common adverse effects are gastrointestinal with nausea, vomiting and diarrhoea.

Non-drug treatment   Some parents may prefer not to use a drug treatment. Measures to physically remove the eggs include washing the perianal area first thing in the morning, and during the day washing or wet-wiping. Ideally this would be at 3-hour intervals but twice a day is probably more realistic.

Practical points
1 Parents are often anxious and ashamed that their child has a threadworm infection, thinking that lack of hygiene is responsible. The pharmacist can reassure parents that threadworm infection is extremely common and that any child can become infected; infection does not signify a lack of care and attention.
2 All family members should be treated at the same time, even if only one has been shown to have threadworms. This is because other members may be in the early stages of infection and thus asymptomatic. If this policy is not followed, reinfection may occur.
3 Transmission and reinfection by threadworms can be prevented by the following practical measures:

(a) Cutting fingernails short to prevent large numbers of eggs being transmitted. Hands should be washed and nails should be brushed after going to the toilet and before preparing or eating food, since hand-to-mouth transfer of eggs is common. Eggs may be transmitted from the fingers while eating food or onto the surface of food during preparation. Eggs remain viable for up to 1 week.
(b) Children wearing pyjamas to reduce the scratching of bare skin during the night. Underpants can be worn under pyjama bottoms.
(c) Affected family members having a bath or shower each morning to wash away the eggs that were laid during the previous night.

Oral thrush

Thrush (candidosis) is a fungal infection that occurs commonly in the mouth (oral thrush), in the nappy area in babies and in the vagina (see p. 246). Oral thrush in babies can be treated by the pharmacist.

Significance of questions and answers

Age

Oral thrush is most common in babies, particularly in the first few weeks of life. Often, the infection is passed on by the mother during childbirth. In older children and adults, oral thrush is rarer, but may occur after antibiotic or inhaled steroid treatment (see 'Medication' below). In this older group it may also be a sign of immunosuppression and referral to the doctor is advisable.

Affected areas

Oral thrush affects the surface of the tongue and the insides of the cheeks.

Appearance

Oral thrush

When candidal infection involves mucosal surfaces, white patches known as plaques are formed, which resemble milk curds; indeed, they may be confused with the latter by mothers when oral thrush occurs in babies. The distinguishing feature of plaques due to *Candida* is that they are not so easily removed from the mucosa, and when the

Symptoms in the Pharmacy: A Guide to the Management of Common Illness, Seventh Edition.
Alison Blenkinsopp, Paul Paxton and John Blenkinsopp.
© 2014 John Wiley & Sons, Ltd. Published 2014 by John Wiley & Sons, Ltd.

surface of the plaque is scraped away, a sore and reddened area of mucosa will be seen underneath, which may sometimes bleed.

Napkin rash

In the napkin (nappy) area, candidal infection presents differently with characteristic red papules on the outer edge of the area of nappy rash, so-called satellite papules. Another feature is that the skin in the folds is nearly always affected. Candidal infection is thought to be an important factor in the development of nappy rash (see p. 307).

Previous history   In babies recurrent infection is uncommon, although it may sometimes occur following reinfection from the mother's nipples during breastfeeding or from inadequately sterilised bottle teats in bottle-fed babies.

Patients who experience recurrent infections should be referred to their doctor for further investigation.

Human immunodeficiency virus infection

Persistence of oral thrush and/or thrush of the nappy area after the neonatal period may be the first sign of HIV infection.

Medication

Antibiotics

Some drugs predispose to the development of thrush. For example, broad-spectrum antibiotic therapy can wipe out the normal bacterial flora, allowing the overgrowth of fungal infection. It would be useful to establish whether the patient has recently taken a course of antibiotics.

Immunosuppressives

Any drug that suppresses the immune system will reduce resistance to infection, and immunocompromised patients are more likely to get thrush. Cytotoxic therapy and steroids predispose to thrush. Patients using inhaled steroids for asthma are prone to oral thrush because steroid is deposited at the back of the throat during inhalation, especially if inhaler technique is poor. Rinsing the throat with water after using the inhaler may be helpful.

The pharmacist should identify any treatment already tried. In a patient with recurrent thrush it would be worth enquiring about previously prescribed therapy and its success.

When to refer
Recurrent infection
All except babies
Failed medication

Treatment timescale

Oral thrush should respond to treatment quickly. If the symptoms have not cleared up within 1 week, patients should see their doctor.

Management

Antifungal agents

Miconazole

The only specially formulated product currently available for sale OTC to treat oral thrush is miconazole gel. Preparations containing nystatin are also effective but are restricted to prescription-only status.

Miconazole gel is an orange-flavoured product, which should be applied to the plaques using a clean finger four times daily after food in adults and children over 6 years, and twice daily in younger children and infants. For young babies, the gel can be applied directly to the lesions using a cotton bud or the handle of a teaspoon. The gel should be retained in the mouth for as long as possible. Treatment should be continued for 2 clear days, after the symptoms have apparently gone, to ensure that all infection is eradicated.

Miconazole gel should not be recommended for patients taking anti-coagulants. There is evidence of an interaction with warfarin leading to an increase in bleeding time.

Practical points

Oral thrush and nappy rash

If a baby has oral thrush, the pharmacist should check whether nappy rash is also present. Where both oral thrush and candidal involvement in nappy rash occur, both should be treated at the same time. An antifungal cream containing miconazole or clotrimazole can be used for the nappy area.

Breastfeeding

Where the mother is breastfeeding, a small amount of miconazole gel applied to the nipples will eradicate any fungus present. For bottle-fed babies, particular care should be taken to sterilise bottles and teats.

Oral thrush in practice

Case 1

Helen Jones, a young mother brings her daughter, Jane, to see you. Mrs Jones wants you to recommend something for Jane's mouth that has white patches on the tongue and inside the cheeks. Jane is 8 years old and is not currently taking any medicines. She has not recently had any antibiotics or other prescribed medicines. Jane does not have any other symptoms.

The pharmacist's view

Jane should be referred to her doctor, since thrush is rare in children other than infants. There is no apparent precipitating factor such as recent antibiotic therapy and Jane should see her doctor for further investigation.

The doctor's view

Helen Jones should be advised to take Jane to the doctor. The description is certainly suggestive of oral thrush. If there were any doubt as to the diagnosis, a swab could be taken for laboratory examination. If Jane did have thrush, then treatment such as miconazole oral gel or nystatin oral suspension might be prescribed. Treatment is enhanced by cleaning the white plaques off with a cotton bud prior to application.

The next concern would be to determine a precipitating cause. General enquiries about Jane's health would be necessary. The doctor would be in a good position to know of previous medical history including any transfusions and family history. A general physical examination would be carried out, looking, in particular, for signs of anaemia, any rashes or bruising, enlargement of lymph nodes (glands), enlargement of abdominal organs (e.g. liver or spleen) or any other masses. The doctor would be looking for signs of a malignancy such as leukaemia or lymphoma. Almost certainly blood tests would be arranged. The doctor would also make an assessment of any HIV risk factors and counsel Helen and Jane accordingly before initiating any further action.

Case 2

A young mother asks for something to treat her baby son's mouth. You look inside the baby's mouth and see white patches on the tongue and inside the cheeks. The baby is 8 weeks old and has had the patches for 2 days: at first his mother thought they were milk curds. He had some antibiotic syrup last week for a chest infection and finished it yesterday. The baby is not taking any other medicines and his mother has not given him anything to treat the symptoms yet. He has no other symptoms.

The pharmacist's view

You could recommend the use of miconazole oral gel for this baby. He has a thrush infection following antibiotic therapy that should respond well to the imidazole antifungal. His mother should use 2.5 mL of gel twice daily after feeds, applying it to the inside of the mouth and tongue. Treatment should be continued for 2 days after the problem has cleared up. If the symptoms have not gone after 1 week, the baby should be seen by the doctor.

The doctor's view

Oral thrush seems the most likely diagnosis. It would be reasonable for the pharmacist to institute treatment in view of the baby's age alone, although in this case antibiotic treatment is an additional precipitating factor. If there were any doubt as to the diagnosis, his mother could seek the advice of the health visitor. It might be useful to ask the mother whether or not she was breastfeeding in case any gel needed applying to the nipples. When applying the gel to the mouth, the plaques should be scraped off, if possible, to increase the effectiveness of the treatment.

Insomnia

Difficulty sleeping

It is estimated that over 8 million people in the United Kingdom have problems sleeping. Temporary insomnia is common and can often be managed by the pharmacist. The key to restoring appropriate sleep patterns is advice on sleep hygiene (bedtime routines). Over the counter (OTC) products to aid sleep (the antihistamines *diphenhydramine* and *promethazine*) can help during the transition period and can also be useful in periodic and transient sleep problems. These products are advertised direct to the public and pharmacists sometimes report difficulties in declining sales for continued use. An initial focus on sleep hygiene and careful explanation that antihistamines are for short-term use are therefore important.

What you need to know
Age
Symptoms
Difficulty falling asleep
Waking during the night
Early morning waking
Poor sleep quality
Snoring, sleep apnoea, restless legs
Duration
Previous history
Previous episodes
Contributory factors
Shift working, being away from home
Current sleep hygiene
Medication

Significance of questions and answers

Age

In elderly people, the total duration of sleep is shorter and there is less deep (stage 4) sleep. Nocturnal waking is more likely because sleep is generally more shallow. However, people may still feel that they need

Symptoms in the Pharmacy: A Guide to the Management of Common Illness, Seventh Edition. Alison Blenkinsopp, Paul Paxton and John Blenkinsopp.
© 2014 John Wiley & Sons, Ltd. Published 2014 by John Wiley & Sons, Ltd.

more sleep and wish to take a medicine to help them sleep. Elderly people may nap during the day and this reduces their sleep need at night even further.

Many babies, toddlers and infants have poor sleep patterns, which understandably can cause anxiety to parents. In these situations, referral to the health visitor or doctor can be helpful. There are also some helpful self-help books and pamphlets available.

Symptoms

It is important to distinguish between the different types of sleep problems:

Difficulty in falling asleep (possibly a symptom of anxiety)

Early morning waking (possibly a symptom of depression)

Waking during the night, and poor sleep quality (further questioning needed to understand why). Sleep may be disturbed by snoring, sleep apnoea or restless legs. All of these can be associated with increased cardiovascular risk. Referral to the GP is necessary. Both snoring and sleep apnoea are amenable to treatment. Restless legs are more difficult to manage, but the GP needs to check for other cardiovascular disease (CVD) risk factors.

Sleep may also be disturbed by underlying physical conditions: heart disease; chronic obstructive pulmonary disease (COPD) or asthma; neurological disease (Alzheimer's, Parkinson's); overactive thyroid; joint or muscle pains; urinary symptoms or chronic pain (NHS choices). Any of these conditions requires referral to the GP.

Depression is an important cause of insomnia. Early morning waking is a classic symptom of depression. Here the patient may describe no problems in getting to sleep but waking in the early hours and not being able to get back to sleep. This pattern requires referral to the doctor for further investigation.

The onset of symptoms of bipolar disorder may be associated with lack of sleep. It is possible that insufficient sleep may actually trigger an episode of mania in bipolar disorder.

Anxiety can also cause insomnia. This is usually associated with difficulty in getting off to sleep because of an overactive mind. This is something that many people experience, particularly before an important occasion, for example, an examination. If, however, this occurs as a more regular pattern, referral to the general practitioner (GP) should be offered.

Duration

Sleep disorders are classified as follows:

Transient (days)

Short term (up to 3 weeks)
Chronic (longer than 3 weeks)
All chronic cases should be referred to the doctor

Previous history

Ask whether this is the first time problems in sleeping have occurred or whether there is a previous history. Where there is a previous history, it is helpful to know what treatments have been tried. It is also useful to be aware of a history of depression or anxiety or some other mental health problem.

Contributory factors

1 Shift work with changing shifts is a classic cause of sleep problems. Those who work away from home may experience difficulty in getting a good night's sleep because of the combination of travelling and staying in unfamiliar places.

2 Alcohol – while one or two drinks can help by decreasing sleep latency (the length of time taken to fall asleep), the sleep cycle is disturbed by heavy or continuous alcohol consumption. Tolerance to the sedative properties of alcohol develops after 3–4 days. Insomnia may be related to alcohol dependence.

3 Life changes can cause disrupted sleep, for example, change or loss of job, moving house, bereavement, loss or separation or the change of life (i.e. menopause).

4 Other stressful life events might include examinations, job interviews, celebrations (e.g. Christmas) and relationship difficulties.

5 Obesity can be associated with sleep apnoea and snoring, both of which can interrupt sleeping.

Current sleep hygiene

It is worth asking about the factors known to contribute to effective sleep hygiene (see 'Practical points' below).

Medication

Some drugs can cause or contribute to insomnia, including decongestants, selective serotonin reuptake inhibitors (SSRIs) and serotonin/noradrenaline reuptake inhibitors (SNRIs), monoamine oxidase inhibitors, *methylphenidate*, corticosteroids, appetite suppressants and *phenytoin* and *theophylline*. Medical problems can be associated with insomnia through pain (e.g. angina, arthritis, cancer and gastro-oesophageal reflux) or breathing difficulties (e.g. heart failure, chronic obstructive airways disease and asthma). Other medical conditions such as hyperthyroidism and Parkinson's disease can also cause insomnia.

Treatment timescale

There should be an improvement within days: refer after 1 week if the problem is not resolved.

Management

Antihistamines (diphenhydramine and promethazine)

Antihistamines reduce sleep latency and also reduce nocturnal waking. They should be taken 20–30 min before bedtime and can be recommended for adults and children over 16 years. Tolerance to their effects can develop and they should not be used for longer than 7–10 consecutive nights. *Diphenhydramine* has a shorter half-life than *promethazine* (5–8 h compared with 8–12 h). Following a 50 mg dose of *diphenhydramine* there is significant drowsiness for 3–6 h. These antihistamines have anticholinergic side effects, including dry mouth and throat, constipation, blurred vision and tinnitus. These effects will be enhanced if the patient is taking another drug with anticholinergic effects (e.g. tricyclic antidepressants and phenothiazines) but patients taking these drugs would be better referred anyway. Prostatic hypertrophy and closed-angle glaucoma are contraindications to the use of *diphenhydramine* and *promethazine*. *Diphenhydramine* and *promethazine* should not be recommended for pregnant or breastfeeding women.

Benzodiazepines

Despite the UK Committee on Safety of Medicines (CSM) statement on the use of benzodiazepines, recommending that these drugs are for short-term use only and should not be used for longer than 2–4 weeks, pharmacists are well aware that some patients continue to be on them for long periods of time. Research shows that success rates in weaning patients off benzodiazepines can be high. This is an area where pharmacists and doctors can work together and discussions with local doctors can initiate this process.

Complementary therapies

Some patients prefer alternative treatments for insomnia, perceiving them as more natural. Herbal remedies have been traditionally used for insomnia, with valerian and hops being the most commonly used ingredients. They are not recommended for pregnant or breastfeeding women. In studies, side effects have been mild and transient and with no differences from placebo. Evidence on the efficacy of valerian and hops in sleep disorders is inconclusive.

Aromatherapy

Lavender oil has been shown to induce a sense of relaxation, as has camomile. One or two drops of the essential oil sprinkled on a pillow or three or four drops in a warm (not hot) bath can be recommended.

Melatonin

Melatonin is currently available only as prescription-only medicine in the United Kingdom; however, it is widely used in the United States to treat insomnia. *Melatonin* is produced by the body's pineal gland during darkness and is thought to regulate sleep. Studies have shown that *melatonin* levels are lower in the elderly. Supplementation with *melatonin* can raise levels and help to restore the sleep pattern. *Melatonin* has a short half-life (2–3 h) and is subject to first-pass metabolism. Sublingual, controlled release products are therefore popular in the United States.

St John's wort (hypericum)

St John's wort (SJW), a herbal remedy, is commonly used in the self-treatment of depression and pharmacists will encounter people who come into the pharmacy to buy it and those who seek the pharmacist's opinion about whether to take it or not. In a study among people with depression, one in three had tried SJW.

A systematic review and meta-analysis found that overall the evidence relating to SJW is inconsistent and complex. In mild-to-moderate depression, SJW preparations and standard antidepressants appear to show similar effects. In major depression, SJW preparations had only small benefits over placebo; in older studies in patients with mild-to-moderate depression, *Hypericum perforatum* preparations appear to be of more benefit than placebo. Pharmacists should bear in mind that there is heterogeneity not only among the trials and their results but also among the different manufacturers' products tested. Products may differ considerably in their pharmaceutical quality and cannot be considered equally effective. Lack of standardisation of the amount of active ingredient is an issue and preparations are not standardised.

Pharmacists will make their own decisions about whether they will recommend SJW, and they need to be prepared to answer requests for advice about its use and to be aware of the emerging evidence. SJW is an inducer of drug-metabolising enzymes and there are some important drug interactions (see the *British National Formulary* for a full current listing). The CSM has advised that SJW should not be taken with other medicines. Pharmacists are an important source of information for patients about possible interactions.

Nasal plasters for snoring

These adhesive nasal strips work by opening the nostrils wider and enabling the body to become accustomed to breathing through the nose rather than through the mouth. A plaster is applied each night for up to 1 week to retrain the breathing process. The strips have been suggested for use in night-time nasal congestion during pregnancy.

Practical points
Sleep hygiene

Key points are as follows:

> Establish a regular bedtime and waking time
> Consciously create a relaxation period before bedtime
> No meals just before bedtime
> No naps during the daytime
> No caffeine after early afternoon
> Reduce extraneous noise (use earplugs if necessary)
> Get up if you can't sleep – go back to bed when you feel 'sleepy, tired'
> Restrict alcohol intake to 1–2 units a day or less
> Restrict nicotine intake immediately before bedtime

Exercise

There is evidence that regular exercise is beneficial in reducing depressive symptoms. A recent Cochrane review concluded that exercise seems to improve depressive symptoms when compared with no treatment or a control intervention and commented that in the more robustly designed studies the positive effects of exercise were smaller.

The Mental Health Foundation has run a campaign encouraging exercise in people with depression. Their website (www.mentalhealth .org.uk) gives free access to podcasts and booklets aimed at both professionals and patients.

Alternatives to medication are important especially as there is evidence that antidepressants are overall not beneficial in mild depression.

Bathing

A warm bath 1–2 h (not immediately) before bedtime can help induce sleep.

Using heat
An electric blanket can help sleep by relaxing the muscles and increasing the brain temperature. The effect is not needed throughout the night, only in inducing sleep. Using a timer to switch off the blanket after 1 or 2 h is sensible.

Caffeine
The stimulant effect of caffeine in coffee, tea and cola drinks is considerable. Avoiding caffeine in the late afternoon and evening is a sensible advice.

Insomnia in practice

Case 1
Chris Jenkins, a 20-year-old student, comes into the pharmacy requesting some tablets to help him sleep. He says that he has had problems sleeping ever since he returned from Indonesia 10 days ago. He says that he cannot get off to sleep because he does not feel tired. When he eventually does fall asleep, he sleeps fitfully and finds it difficult to get up in the morning. He has never suffered from insomnia before. He is otherwise well, is not taking any medicines and does not have any other problems or difficulties.

The pharmacist's view
Long-haul travel can result in disruption of the sleep pattern and some people are more affected by it than are others. It would be reasonable to recommend that Chris take an antihistamine *(diphenhydramine* or *promethazine)* for 4–5 days until the problem resolves. An alternative would be one of the herbal products to aid sleep. He should find that his normal sleep pattern is re-established within 1 week.

The doctor's view
This is quite likely to be a short-term problem due to his recent travelling. A very short course of antihistamines may re-establish a better pattern. Many people who complain of insomnia do not always admit to other problems in their lives. It is therefore important to be alert to this possibility. If his insomnia does not resolve quickly, or if the pharmacist were to notice that Chris seemed low or anxious, a referral would be appropriate.

Case 2
Maureen Thomas, aged about 50 years, comes in asking for something to help her sleep. She says she has seen an advertisement for some tablets that will help. Maureen explains that her sleep has been bad ever since she had her children, but over the last week it has got worse.

She says she has had problems in getting off to sleep and recently has been waking early and not getting back to sleep. She says that she has had some worries at work and her Mum has been unwell . . . 'but that's all, no more than usual. I've had to put up with a lot worse and managed! I just need a few days' good sleep and I'll be OK.' Otherwise she reveals that she is not on any other medication and has never troubled anyone before with her sleeping problem.

The pharmacist's view

This patient is experiencing a number of sources of stress and difficulty that are likely to be contributing to her sleep problems. In addition to having trouble getting to sleep, she is also waking early and unable to get back to sleep, indicating that the sleep disturbance is extensive. Early waking can also be a symptom of depression. It would be best for her to see the doctor and this will need a careful, persuasive explanation from the pharmacist. It would also be useful to talk about sleep hygiene to see if there are any practical actions that she could take to alleviate the problem. While the use of an antihistamine or herbal medicine for a few days would not be harmful, it may prevent her from seeking advice from the doctor. Therefore it would be better not to recommend a medicine on this occasion.

The doctor's view

Ideally, this woman should be advised to make an appointment to see her doctor. It is possible that she would be reluctant to do so, as she gives the impression that she thinks she should be able to cope and should not have to trouble anyone else with her problems. If the pharmacist could persuade her that it is completely acceptable to seek advice from her doctor, this would be the best course of action. She may be depressed and it would be helpful for a doctor to make a full assessment. This would include how she is feeling, how her life is being affected and what other symptoms she may have. It may be that she is also concerned by changes associated with the menopause.

Just the ability to talk to a good, attentive, accepting listener can be very beneficial. She may benefit from seeing a counsellor or a cognitive–behaviour therapist which the GP could arrange. She may benefit from an exercise programme and a change in her diet. A Mediterranean diet is believed to be beneficial, whereas processed food is less so. It is thought that having a diet with adequate essential fatty acids, for example, omega 3 and omega 6 complex, and foods containing sufficient vitamins (B_1, B_3, B_6, B_{12}, C and folic acid) and trace elements (zinc, magnesium and selenium) are necessary for good mental health. She might benefit from an assessment from a nutritionist. If she were to have moderate or severe depression then most doctors would offer her antidepressants.

Case 3

A man whom you do not recognise as a regular customer asks to speak with you. He tells you that he has been feeling rather stressed lately in his job. (He is an estate agent and works locally.) He says he is having trouble sleeping and feels that things are getting on top of him. He is not getting much exercise these days – he used to play football and go training regularly but since a knee injury he has given it up. He thinks he might be depressed but does not want to see his doctor because he does not want to end up on antidepressants. He read an article in the paper yesterday about SJW and would like to try it. He asks what you think and if it's safe. He is not taking any medicines.

The pharmacist's view

This is not an uncommon query. If someone just asks to buy SJW, I'd sell it to them after checking about other medication and asking whether they wanted to discuss anything. But if they ask for my view or advice, I would discuss it with them. I find that some people don't want to see the doctor even when they think they're depressed. In this case it's because of a dislike of the idea of taking antidepressants. Although there is evidence that they work, especially in severe depression, it's not so clear-cut for mild-to-moderate depression. Cognitive therapy would be another option. There's good evidence to support it but its availability varies. Also some people want to try to manage their depression themselves rather than get into the formal health system.

I would take this man to a quiet part of the pharmacy.

If he decided to try SJW, I would explain that it could take 3–4 weeks to work. I would tell him that it does have some sedative effect and that taking it at night could be helpful.

If it were a woman of childbearing age, I would always ask whether she was on the pill, because SJW interacts with the oral contraceptive pill and makes it less effective. If she still wanted to take SJW, I would give some advice about using extra contraceptive protection.

The doctor's view

The evidence on the effectiveness of SJW is variable. Some trials show benefit and others no benefit when compared to placebo.

The pharmacist could suggest that he goes to see his GP anyway whether he takes the SJW or not, and it could be pointed out that it would be his choice whether to take antidepressants.

If this man were to come to his GP, which would be very reasonable, it would be important to hear more about how he is being affected by his problem, that is, what it is like for him, what is the impact on his life, how he feels, etc. It would be useful to hear about his understanding of the problems and how he thinks he can be helped, and whether he would be prepared to see a counsellor. The GP would need to do a risk assessment and check whether he is feeling suicidal and, if so, whether he has specific plans as to how he might kill himself. Once an initial assessment has been made, it can often be useful to delay starting medication or making a referral at the first consultation and instead offer to review him in the next few days or week to see how he is. Just the fact of coming to see the GP, being listened to and taken seriously can be helpful, and the problem may be viewed in a different or better light on subsequent follow-up. In his case, it probably would be best to advise a non-pharmacological approach. Even if he were to take SJW or an antidepressant, the conditions triggering his depression are likely to be still there when he stops the medication. He could be referred for brief intervention counselling/therapy or cognitive–behavioural therapy if he were in agreement.

Another way to help him could be to enable him to get back to some exercise as this is known to improve depression. When he presented at the pharmacy he mentioned that he was unable to play football because of a knee injury. It might be really helpful to have this reassessed by the GP. Perhaps a referral to an orthopaedic surgeon or physiotherapist might be useful. It sounds as though a return to exercise could help him deal with some of his stress. It might be that he could try swimming as another form of exercise.

The customer's view

It was useful to know more about whether SJW works or not. The pharmacist made me feel as though it was my choice and told me that if I went to the doctor, I could say that I didn't want antidepressants. I decided to try SJW and some swimming for a few weeks and see how it goes.

Prevention of Heart Disease

Prevention of heart disease

This chapter is different from the others in this book, which are primarily concerned with responding to a symptom. Here the pharmacist is assessing risk and advising on prevention. The development of cardiovascular disease (CVD) is largely asymptomatic up to the point where an 'event' (such as a heart attack or stroke) occurs. Pharmacists can make interventions (primary prevention) to prevent the development of CVD while assisting people who are largely symptom free but at increased risk of developing heart disease in the future. Here the individual is not a patient because he or she does not have any disease or condition. Once a person has experienced an event and has ongoing disease, the prevention of subsequent events is termed secondary prevention.

CVD can be subdivided into stroke and coronary heart disease (CHD). CHD occurs because of narrowing and/or blockage of the coronary arteries. It may be sufficient to cause myocardial ischaemia – ischaemic heart disease (IHD) – and can be present without symptoms. CHD may remain asymptomatic until it manifests as angina, myocardial infarction (MI), sudden death or cardiac dysfunction (such as arrhythmias or cardiac failure). Some patients may therefore suffer consequences of myocardial ischaemia without any history of warning symptoms.

CHD is a leading cause of mortality and morbidity in the United Kingdom. Despite a fall in CHD mortality in recent years, it remains the most common cause of death in the United Kingdom. In 2010, CHD accounted for nearly 1 in 5 male deaths and 1 in 10 female deaths, making a total of nearly 80 000 deaths. The prevalence of angina in the United Kingdom is uncertain, but has been estimated for 65–74 year olds at 6–16% for men and 3–10% for women.

Preventing CHD is a national priority. The National Service Framework (NSF) for CHD in England set out a 10-year plan in 2000 to ensure the best care, in terms of prevention, diagnosis and treatment. The NSF also set the government target of cutting mortality from heart disease by 40% in people less than 75 years by 2010. This target was reached 5 years ahead of schedule. A national programme of screening for CVD risk (NHS Health Checks) was introduced in England in

Symptoms in the Pharmacy: A Guide to the Management of Common Illness, Seventh Edition.
Alison Blenkinsopp, Paul Paxton and John Blenkinsopp.
© 2014 John Wiley & Sons, Ltd. Published 2014 by John Wiley & Sons, Ltd.

2010 with the intention of including all individuals aged between 40 and 74 years. Community pharmacies provide screening in some areas as part of local arrangements. Risk is scored using an algorithm based on current clinical guidance.

The causes of CVD are multifactorial and are often termed 'risk factors'. The summation of these risk factors will provide an assessment of absolute CV risk, which should be the starting point for discussions with patients, and a reduction in absolute risk should be the goal of interventions.

What you need to know

Age, gender
  Ethnic origin
  Family history of CHD
  Smoking history
  Waist circumference/body mass index
  Diet
  Physical activity
  Alcohol intake
  Medical history (blood pressure, diabetes and cholesterol/lipid profile)
  Medication

Significance of questions and answers

Assessment of an individual's risk of developing CHD involves the summation of both modifiable and non-modifiable risk factors for developing the disease. Non-modifiable risk factors include age, gender, ethnic origin and family history of CHD. These risk factors cannot be altered. Interventions to reduce absolute CHD risk are focused on modifiable risk factors.

Age and gender
With age, the risk of developing CHD increases. Around 80% of people who die from heart disease are aged 65 years or over. It is commoner in men than in women. (The lifetime risk of developing it at age 40 years is one in two for men and one in three for women.) Postmenopausal women have a CV risk similar to that of men.

Ethnic origin
Heart disease in the United Kingdom is commoner in Afro-Caribbean people and those from the Asian subcontinent (Bangladesh, India, Pakistan and Sri Lanka).

Family history of CHD

Risk of developing CHD increases if an individual has a close relative (father, mother, brother or sister) with the disease. A family history of premature CHD (i.e. a father or brother who had a coronary event before the age of 55 years, or a mother or sister before the age of 65 years) is an even stronger indicator of risk.

Smoking history

Currently in the United Kingdom, 21% of men and 20% of women smoke. Smoking tobacco has been shown to increase the risk of MI. This effect is related to the number of cigarettes smoked; heavy smokers (more than 20 per day) increase their risk of MI by two- to fourfold over non-smokers. No level of smoking has been demonstrated to be safe. Those who have recently stopped smoking remain at a higher risk for as long as 5 years after stopping, but the risk begins to decline within a few months of stopping.

Waist circumference/body mass index

Obesity is associated with an increased risk of stroke, CHD, type 2 diabetes, hypertension and dyslipidaemia, that is, raised total cholesterol (TC), high low-density lipoprotein (LDL) cholesterol and high triglyceride levels. Abdominal obesity (apple-shaped body) is particularly significant, and waist circumference may be a better predictor of susceptibility to CHD than body mass index (BMI). A waist circumference of more than 94 cm in men or 80 cm in women is associated with a relatively increased risk of CHD. Waist circumference may be a better way of assessing risk, especially in the Asian population compared to BMI.

BMI is calculated by dividing an individual's weight (kilogrammes) by height (metre) squared. The normal range of BMI is between 18.5 and 25 kg/m^2. Overweight is defined as a BMI >25 kg/m^2 and obesity is defined as a BMI >30 kg/m^2.

Men in the United Kingdom increase their risk of CHD by 10% with every 1 kg/m^2 increase in BMI above 22 kg/m^2. Waist circumference >94 cm in men and 80 cm in women identifies a CHD risk equivalent to that of a BMI >25 kg/m^2. For a circumference >102 cm in men and 88 cm in women the risk is equivalent to that of a BMI >30 kg/m^2.

In 2011, about 47% of men and 33% of women in the United Kingdom were overweight and an additional 24% of men and 26% of women were obese. Overweight and obesity increase with age. Overweight and obesity are increasing. The percentage of adults who are obese has roughly doubled since the mid-1980s. Frequent fluctuations in weight are also associated with an increased risk of developing CHD.

Physical activity

Regular aerobic exercise has been proved to assist weight loss and reduce blood pressure. Physical inactivity is associated with an increased incidence of developing hypertension (a CHD risk factor).

Alcohol intake

Drinking more than 21 units of alcohol per week is associated with an increase in blood pressure, which can be reversed if the intake is reduced. Alcohol can affect most parts of the body and, in addition to causing liver damage, can cause infertility, skin damage, heart damage, cancer and strokes. Many accidents, episodes of violence and risk-taking behaviour, for example, unprotected sex, are associated with alcohol. Excess alcohol in those under the age of 20 years can damage the brain while it is still developing. A small amount of alcohol (1 unit per day) may help slightly reduce CHD risk but this would not be a reason for a non-drinker to start alcohol. Maximum drinking limits are 3–4 units per day for men and 2–3 units per day for women. Most experts advise at least two alcohol-free days each week. For information on the number of units of alcohol in different drinks, see http://www.breheny.com/www.homeoffice.gov.uk/knowyourlimits/stay_safe/index.html.

Medical history (hypertension, diabetes and cholesterol/lipid profile)

Raised blood pressure (>140/90 mm Hg) has been shown to be a risk factor for the development of stroke and CHD. Diastolic pressures of 90–109 mm Hg are found in about 20% of the middle-aged adult population. In younger people the prevalence is lower, and in elderly people it is higher. Current estimates suggest that in the United Kingdom around 40% of men and women have raised blood pressure. In addition, undertreated hypertension is common, with up to half of all people with diagnosed hypertension not reaching recommended targets.

Contributing factors to hypertension should be identified. These include obesity, excessive alcohol intake (3 units/day), high salt intake and physical inactivity.

Diabetes

Developing diabetes has the equivalent effect on increasing an individual's CHD risk as having a heart attack. It increases CHD mortality by two to three times in men and four to six times in women. Eighty per cent of type 2 diabetics (the commonest type of diabetes, by a ratio of 9:1) are obese. This has led to the coining of the term 'diabesity', which cleverly combines the two conditions. Patients with type 2 diabetes have a two- to fourfold increased risk of, and a fourfold increase in, mortality from CHD. Intensive glycemic control has a more modest effect on reducing macrovascular than microvascular complications. This is because the development of CVD is multifactorial, and hyperglycaemia is only one of many risk factors.

Epidemiological data suggest that a glycosylated haemoglobin (HbA1c) level of 7% or less is reasonable to avoid or minimise the complications associated with type 2 diabetes. Studies have shown that there is an increased risk of CV mortality even before the onset of type 2 diabetes.

Many studies, including the Framingham Heart Study, have clearly established that high TC levels are associated with increased risk of developing CHD. CHD is caused when the blood vessels to the heart (the coronary arteries) become narrowed by a gradual build-up of fatty material within their walls – a condition called atherosclerosis. Atheroma develops when LDL cholesterol is oxidised and is taken up by cells in the coronary artery walls where the narrowing process begins. On the other hand, high-density lipoprotein (HDL) cholesterol removes cholesterol from the circulation and appears to protect against CHD. So the ratio of HDL to LDL is important. The goal is to have a low level of LDL (>3 mmol/L) and a high level of HDL (>1 mmol/L).

As a general rule, the higher the TC level, the greater is the risk to health. A TC level of <5 mmol/L is often a target aimed for. However, more than half of adults in the United Kingdom have a TC level above this figure. Increasing importance is being placed on LDL rather than TC; from long-term epidemiological studies and intervention studies with statins, it is clear that reductions in LDL levels correlate closely with reduction in CHD risk. If someone has an absolute level of risk that justifies treatment, reducing the LDL will reduce that risk, whatever their starting level of cholesterol.

The level of LDL cholesterol in the blood tends to rise, and HDL falls, with the amount of saturated fat that is eaten. On the other hand, unsaturated fats have a good effect as they tend to lower LDL levels. A high level of triglycerides also increases the risk of CHD and stroke.

Medication

A full medication history is important as some medicines can affect CHD risk either positively or negatively. The potential contribution of over the counter (OTC) medicines should also be considered. Medications with a positive effect on CHD risk will be considered later in the chapter. Factors predisposing to CV toxicity include existing heart disease, uncorrected electrolyte abnormalities and poor renal function.

Sympathomimetic drugs such as *adrenaline, noradrenaline, dobutamine, dopamine* and *phenylephrine* can all cause systemic hypertension and precipitate heart failure. Other commonly prescribed medicines with CV side effects include *thyroxine,* tricyclic antidepressants and triptans.

Managing heart disease risk in the pharmacy

The modifiable risk factors for CHD are generally accepted as smoking, cholesterol/lipid imbalance, hypertension, poor diet, obesity, excessive alcohol intake, physical inactivity and inadequate diabetes control. A recent literature review demonstrated the contribution of community pharmacy-based services to the reduction of risk behaviours and risk factors for CHD. The evidence supports the wider provision of smoking cessation and lipid management through community pharmacies. Both primary and secondary prevention of CHD involve similar interventions.

Smoking cessation and nicotine replacement therapy

In recent years smoking cessation has become an increasingly important focus for the National Health Service (NHS) and the United Kingdom can now boast a world-leading smoking cessation service. Nonetheless, there are still around 13 million tobacco users in the United Kingdom and their cost to the NHS is £1.7 billion per year.

Research suggests that around 70% of smokers would like to give up, but only 2–3% of smokers manage to quit using willpower alone. Nicotine replacement therapy (NRT) is an effective aid to smoking cessation for those smoking more than 10 cigarettes a day. Smokers are about twice as likely to stop long-term smoking when prescribed NRT and are up to six times more likely to succeed when NRT and behavioural support are combined. The current National Institute for Health and Clinical Excellence (NICE) guidelines recommend varenicline (POM) or NRT for smokers who commit to a target stop date.

Smoking cessation – tips for customers about quitting

- Set a quit date, prepare for it and stick to it
- Get support and advice from friends, family and health professionals
- Consider NRT for the first few weeks
- Avoid situations where you will find it difficult not to smoke
- Change your routine to distract yourself from times and places you associate with smoking
- Stop completely if you can, rather than cut down
- Get rid of all cigarettes, lighters and ashtrays before your quit date
- Ask people not to smoke around you and tell everyone you are quitting
- Keep busy, especially when cravings start
- Reward yourself for not smoking
- Calculate how much money you will save and plan how you will now spend it

A range of NRT products are available. They vary in the ease and frequency of use, the speed of nicotine release and the amount of behavioural replacement provided. There are no conclusive studies to show that one formulation is any more effective than another at achieving cessation. All products will increase the chances of success if used correctly.

Nicotine replacement therapy – formulation options

Patches

Discreet – easy to wear and forget about, but watch for skin irritation
Continuous nicotine release – suitable for regular smokers
16-h patch (removed at night) – reduced insomnia
24-h patch – good for early morning cravings
Three strengths – allows a step-down reduction programme

Gum

Flexible regimen – controls cravings as they occur
Various flavours – allows customer preference
Various strengths – allows step-down reduction programme
Chewed slowly – to release nicotine and then 'park' gum between cheek and gum

Nasal spray

Fast-acting – helpful for highly dependent smokers
Local side effects (sore throat and rhinitis) – usually pass after first few days

Sublingual tablet

Discrete – placed under tongue and dissolves over 20 min
Dose variation – one or two (2 mg) tablets may be used per hour
Sublingual – sucking or chewing the tablet will reduce its effectiveness

Inhalator

Cigarette substitute – useful for smokers who miss hand-to-mouth action
Reduce usage over time – the recommended period is 12 weeks

Lozenge

Various strengths – allows step-down reduction programme
Highest strength (4 mg) – good for smokers who start within 30 min of waking
Sucked until taste is strong – lozenge then 'parked' between cheek and gum

Licensed indications for OTC nicotine replacement therapy

NRT can be recommended for adults and children aged 12 years or over, for pregnant women and those who are breastfeeding.

Some NRT products are licensed to aid smoking reduction with the eventual aim of smoking cessation ('reduce to quit'). The smoker should attempt to quit when he or she is ready – but not later than 6 months after reducing the cigarette consumption. Young people (aged 12–18 years) should attempt 'reduce to quit' only after consulting a health care professional.

Positive messages for new non-smokers

• Giving up smoking reduces the risk of developing smoking-related illness
• Eight hours after quitting, nicotine and carbon monoxide levels in the blood are reduced by half and oxygen levels return to normal
• After 24 h, carbon monoxide is eliminated
• After 48 h, nicotine is eliminated
• After 3 days, breathing becomes easier
• After 2–12 weeks, circulation is improved and smokers' coughs start to get better
• After 6 months, lung efficiency will have improved by 5–10%
• After 5 years, the risk of having a heart attack is half of that of a smoker
• After 10 years, the risk of heart attack is the same as that of a non-smoker
• After 10–15 years, the risk of developing lung cancer is only slightly greater than that of a non-smoker
• Research has shown that people who stop smoking before the age of 35 years survive about as well as lifelong non-smokers

Weight management

Being overweight increases the chance of having a heart attack. This is in part because obese individuals are more likely to have high blood pressure, diabetes and high blood fats. Less fat, sugar and alcohol in the diet is helpful for weight control. In order to achieve a healthy body weight, it is also important to build regular, moderate exercise into a daily routine.

Pharmacy staff should counsel customers whose BMI is >25 kg/m^2 on an appropriate plan for weight loss. A 3-month programme of weight reduction should aim for a 5- to 10-kg weight loss over 3 months or 0.5 kg per week (combining diet, exercise and behavioural strategies; see Table 1 for benefits of weight loss). In some areas, community pharmacies are commissioned to provide a weight management service.

Table 1 Benefits of 5- to 10-kg weight loss.

Condition	Health benefit
Mortality	20–25% fall in overall mortality
	30–40% fall in diabetes-related deaths
	40–50% fall in obesity-related cancer deaths
Blood pressure	10 mm Hg fall in diastolic and systolic pressures
Diabetes	Up to a 50% fall in fasting blood glucose
	Reduces risk of developing diabetes by over 50%
Lipids	Fall of 10% TC, 15% LDL and 30% triglycerides
	Increase of 8% HDL

Pharmacy staff can give advice on a healthy diet. The recommended calorie intake should be between 1200 and 1600 kcal per day. People should be advised to moderate fat intake by eating less fatty meat, fatty cheese, full-cream milk, fried food, lard, etc. and to reduce the amount of sugar. They should consider eating more vegetables, fruit, cereals, wholegrain bread, poultry, fish, rice, skimmed or semi-skimmed milk, grilled food, lean meat, pasta, etc.

If the customer does fry food, suggest choosing a vegetable oil high in polyunsaturates ('good fats'), such as sunflower or rapeseed oil. Suggest considering a low-fat spread that contains plant stanol esters. Such plant stanol-containing supplements have been shown to reduce cholesterol levels and may be useful adjuncts in lowering cholesterol levels. Reducing cholesterol levels is possible through dietary manipulation. However, the magnitude of such reductions is modest, even with strict adherence to a diet plan. In addition, many patients will find it hard to sustain a strict dietary regimen.

Physical inactivity is an important contributor to CHD. CV benefits of regular physical activity include reduced blood pressure and less likelihood of obesity, which help to reduce the risk of developing CHD. At least 30 min of steady activity for 5 or more days a week is recommended. This time can be accumulated during the day in periods of 10 min or more. Walking, jogging, swimming, cycling and dancing are all excellent choices. Remember to advise patients to start slowly and gradually build up their exercise.

OTC Orlistat

Orlistat 60 mg capsules are available OTC for individuals aged 18 and over with a BMI of 28 kg/m² or greater, to be used in conjunction with a reduced calorie diet that is low in fat and with exercise. Orlistat inhibits gastric lipases.

The amount of weight loss achieved with Orlistat varies. In 1-year clinical trials, between 35% and 55% of subjects achieved a 5% or greater decrease in body mass, although not all of this mass was necessarily fat. Between 16% and 25% achieved at least a 10% decrease in body mass. After Orlistat was stopped, a significant number of subjects regained weight – up to 35% of the weight they had lost.

What you need to know
Age and body mass index
Previous medical history
Medication
Current diet and physical activity

Significance of questions and answers

Age and body mass index

Those aged under 18 years cannot be treated with OTC Orlistat. Requests for Orlistat may be made by individuals who believe they need to lose weight but whose BMI is lower than 28 and pharmacy teams will need to handle these sensitively.

Previous medical history

Weight loss is likely to lead to improvements in metabolic control in diabetes, and to lower blood pressure in hypertension.

Medication

Some medicines may need an adjustment in dosage as a result of weight loss; these are discussed in the management section.

Current diet and physical activity

Control of dietary fat content is critical to successful use of Orlistat. Exploring current fat intake and helping the patient to assess the extent of the change needed is essential. Regular physical activity is also a key to weight management and the pharmacist needs to know the current amount of exercise taken.

Treatment timescale

If the patient has been unable to lose weight after 12 weeks of treatment, they should be referred to their general practitioner (GP) or nurse.

Management

Orlistat is taken at a dose of 60 mg three times daily immediately before, during or up to 1 h after meals. If a meal is missed or does not contain fat, the Orlistat should not be taken. While taking it, the patient's diet should be mildly hypocaloric and with approximately 30% of calories from fat (e.g. in a 1,800 kcal/day diet, this equates to <60 g of fat). A lower fat diet will not only aid weight loss but will also reduce gastrointestinal (GI) side effects (see below). The daily intake of fat should be spread throughout the day. A realistic target for weight loss is 0.5 kg to 1 kg (1–2 lb) a week for adults. Some pharmacists offer to monitor the patient's weight to help maintain motivation. Treatment can be continued for up to 6 months.

Contraindications

Patients with chronic malabsorption syndrome, those with cholestasis (bile flow from the liver is blocked) and pregnant or breastfeeding women should not take OTC Orlistat.

Side effects

The main side effects of Orlistat are GI related. Side effects are most severe when beginning therapy, and in trials they decreased in frequency with time, with nearly half of the side effects lasting less than a week, but some persisting for over 6 months. Because Orlistat's main effect is to prevent dietary fat from being absorbed, the fat is excreted unchanged in the faeces and so the stool may become oily or loose (steatorrhoea). Increased flatulence is also common. Bowel movements may become frequent or urgent, and cases of faecal incontinence have been seen in clinical trials. To minimise these effects, foods with high fat content should be avoided; the manufacturer advises consumers to follow a low-fat, reduced-calorie diet.

Patients should be advised to wear dark trousers and take a change of clothes with them to work. Oily stools and flatulence can be controlled by reducing the dietary fat content to somewhere in the region of 15 g per meal, and it has been suggested that the decrease in side effects over time may be associated with long-term compliance with a low-fat diet.

Referral to the GP

The doses of some medicines may need to be adjusted if the patient loses weight. Weight loss is likely to lead to improvements in metabolic control in diabetes and to lower blood pressure in hypertension. Doses of diabetic and antihypertensive medication may therefore need to be changed. Other medicines where the patient needs to check with their GP before starting Orlistat are amiodarone, oral anticoagulants (including warfarin), acarbose, ciclosporin and levothyroxine. There is an increased risk of convulsions when Orlistat is given with antiepileptics. Patients with kidney disease should consult their GP before using Orlistat.

Cautions

Absorption of fat-soluble vitamins and other fat-soluble nutrients is inhibited by the use of Orlistat. A multivitamin tablet containing vitamins A, D, E, K and β-carotene should be taken once a day, at least 2 h before or after taking the drug.

There is no clinical evidence of a drug interaction between Orlistat and oral contraceptives but if a woman taking Orlistat has severe diarrhoea, they should be advised to use an additional contraception method.

OTC simvastatin

Simvastatin has 'P' status at a dose of 10 mg and aims to reduce the risk of a first major coronary event (i.e. non-fatal MI and CHD deaths) in people who are likely to be at moderate risk of CHD.

Men aged 55 years and above are likely to be at moderate risk of CHD (approximately 10–15% 10-year risk of a first major coronary event). In addition, men aged 45–54 years and women aged 55 years and above are likely to be at moderate risk of CHD if they have one or more of the following risk factors:

- Family history of CHD in a first-degree relative (parent or sibling); CHD in male first-degree relative below 55 years or female first-degree relative below 65 years
- Smoker (is currently or has been a smoker in the last 5 years)
- Overweight (BMI >25 kg/m^2) or truncal obesity (waist 40 in or 102 cm in men and 35 in or 88 cm in women)
- Of South Asian ethnic origin

OTC *simvastatin* should be taken as part of a programme of actions designed to reduce the risk of CHD. People aged over 70 years should start OTC *simvastatin* following advice from their doctor. These include cessation of smoking, eating a healthy diet, weight loss and regular exercise. *Simvastatin* treatment can be initiated simultaneously with diet, exercise and smoking cessation.

In an essentially normal population, it is reasonable to use the lowest effective dose to achieve the proportionately greatest benefit. The rare adverse events (e.g. muscular pain) associated with statin use are dose-related and linked in many cases to drug–drug interactions that increase statin effects. The risk of such events with *simvastatin* 10 mg is very low and therefore the risk-to-benefit ratio for the self-medicating individual is favourable.

Pharmacists and their staff should encourage customers to read the patient information leaflet carefully, paying particular attention to the section on side effects. Research with the general public suggests that their understanding of the frequency of adverse events is at variance with statutory definitions. For example, the European Union (EU) definition of a rare adverse event would suggest a frequency of between 0.01% and 0.1%. When Berry et al. (*Lancet* 2002; 359: 853–854).

There is a possibility of rare but important side effects – liver disease, myopathy (unexplained generalised muscle pain, tenderness or weakness, e.g. muscle pain not associated with flu, unaccustomed exercise or recent strain or injury) and allergic reactions.

If taken regularly, *simvastatin* 10 mg will reduce an individual's LDL cholesterol by 27% on average. The relationship between *simvastatin* dose and LDL cholesterol reduction is log-linear in nature: a doubling of dose from 10 to 20 mg increases the relative reduction of LDL cholesterol from around 27% to 32%, and doubling the dose again to 40 mg produces a further 5% improvement.

In addition, the absolute reduction of LDL cholesterol achievable with 10-mg *simvastatin,* if sustained, will produce around 30% relative reduction in CHD risk. This will result in a worthwhile absolute risk reduction in those at moderate risk and if the individual also modifies other risk behaviours (such as stopping smoking, weight reduction and regular exercise), the benefits will be considerable.

Aspirin 75 mg

Low-dose *aspirin* tablets may be sold as a P medicine in packs of up to 100 tablets. They are currently licensed for the secondary prevention of thrombotic strokes, transient ischaemic attacks (TIAs or 'ministrokes'), heart attacks or unstable angina.

Low-dose *aspirin* is recommended by the *BNF,* for primary prevention of vascular events, as antiplatelet therapy in patients who have an estimated 10-year CHD risk greater than or equal to 15%. Patients with hypertension should have their blood pressure controlled to minimise the risk of antiplatelet therapy contributing to the risk of cerebrovascular bleeding. Patients should be assessed for contraindications to *aspirin* therapy and patients at increased risk of GI bleeding may require cover with a gastroprotective agent. There is no compelling evidence to currently support the use of *aspirin* in low-risk subjects, such as middle-aged males with no other risk factors.

Preventing heart disease in practice

Case 1

A man who looks as if he is in his mid-50s asks to speak to the pharmacist. He says, 'I've been wondering if I should take them junior *aspirins.* A few of the lads at the snooker club are on them – and they say it can stop you having a heart attack?' He asks what you think and if it is true that the *aspirin* tablets can prevent heart attacks. He does not appear to be overweight.

The pharmacist's view

I would first ask this man why he thinks he might need *aspirin*. That will give me an idea of how he has assessed his risk and it will be a good starting point. I would need to assess this man's risk of heart disease by asking about his family history, smoking, diet, physical activity and medication (looking particularly for diabetes and hypertension). On the basis of this assessment, I would decide whether he needed to be referred to the GP. If he were a smoker, I would prioritise that and discuss his readiness to quit. Then I would decide what to do next.

The doctor's view

I would agree with the pharmacist about checking his overall risk factors, his understanding of these factors and the areas he needs to work on. *Aspirin* is mainly used for secondary CHD prevention but if the 10-year risk for CHD is 15% or more, then it can be used for primary prevention. If he hasn't had a blood pressure or cholesterol test in the last year or so, then it would make sense for this to be done. Some pharmacies provide this service. In most GP surgeries further assessment and information can be gleaned from seeing the practice nurse. The most important aspect of advice is to cover all the risk factors and not just focus on one area. A follow-up review is often helpful to see how lifestyle has changed and what difficulties have been experienced.

Case 2

A woman in her 40s comes in asking for some patches to help her give up cigarettes. The pharmacist finds out that she is a heavy smoker, 20–30 per day, and has smoked for 25 years. She knows that she is overweight and struggles to keep it down. She managed to stop smoking for about 3 months once, but put on weight. She has a family history of diabetes and two of her grandparents died of heart attack in their seventies. Her uncle who is 60 years has angina. She saw her GP about 1 year ago who told her that her cholesterol level was mildly raised at 6 and her blood pressure was borderline. She was supposed to go back for a review but has not done so yet.

The pharmacist's view

I would ask this woman to tell me about her previous attempt to quit, including whether she used NRT that can be bought OTC; in many parts of the United Kingdom, pharmacies are part of local NHS smoking cessation services and can provide treatment. Many people are concerned that they will put on weight when they stop smoking and I would talk with her about this. The health benefits of stopping smoking far outweigh any additional risk from being overweight, and discussing the figures can get this point across. Talking about what happened after she stopped smoking last time including her diet and eating patterns might provide some ideas about minimising weight gain this time.

The doctor's view

It is very encouraging that she wants to do something about her smoking, especially as she has several risk factors for CHD. I think the pharmacist is in a good position to counsel and perhaps advise an appropriate NRT. It would be useful to ascertain how she managed to stop last time and the reasons for starting cigarettes again. The pharmacist is also in a position to offer advice about her weight and find out about her level of physical exercise. It would also be helpful to suggest a review at her GP's surgery to follow up her blood pressure and cholesterol. It is likely that the GP would want to do some blood tests: fasting lipid profile, fasting blood glucose, electrolytes and renal function and liver profile. In addition, a urine test checking for proteinuria and glycosuria would be useful and, possibly, an electrocardiogram. If after three readings she remained hypertensive, medication such as an angiotensin-converting enzyme inhibitor, or calcium channel blocker if African or Caribbean ethnicity, may be advised. Of course, if she were able to lose weight and increase exercise, this would also help to lower her blood pressure.

Appendix: Summary of Symptoms for Direct Referral

Chest
Chest pain
Shortness of breath
Wheezing
Swollen ankles
Blood in sputum
Palpitations
Persistent cough
Whooping cough
Croup
Sputum mucoid, coloured

Gut
Difficulty with swallowing
Blood in vomit
Bloody diarrhoea
Vomiting with constipation
Weight loss
Sustained alteration in bowel habit

Eye
Painful red eye
Loss of vision
Double vision

Ear
Pain
Discharge
Deafness
Irritation
Tinnitus
Vertigo

Symptoms in the Pharmacy: A Guide to the Management of Common Illness, Seventh Edition. Alison Blenkinsopp, Paul Paxton and John Blenkinsopp.
© 2014 John Wiley & Sons, Ltd. Published 2014 by John Wiley & Sons, Ltd.

Genitourinary
Difficulty in passing urine
Blood in urine
Abdominal/loin/back pain with cystitis
Temperature with cystitis
Urethral discharge
Vaginal discharge
Vaginal bleeding in pregnancy

Other
Neck stiffness/rigidity with temperature
Vomiting (persistent)
Non-blanching skin rash (purpura)

Index

abdominal pain 125
accidents 14
aciclovir 169–70
acne 153
  considerations
    affected areas 154
    age 153–4
    duration 154–5
    medication 155
    severity 154
  management 155
    antibacterials 157
    benzoyl peroxide 155–6
    diet 157
    hygiene 158
    make-up 158
    nicotinamide 156
    sunlight 157
  referral 155
  treatment timescale 155
acrivastine 26
  allergic rhinitis (hay fever) 57
  cautions, side-effects and interactions 58
acupressure wristbands for motion sickness
    101
acupuncture 217, 240
acute laryngotracheitis (croup) 35
acute otitis media (AOM) 21
alcohol
  cautions, side-effects and interactions 26
  heart disease 346
  heartburn 81
  nausea and vomiting 97
alcometasone 147
alginates 79
allergic rhinitis (hay fever) 53
  case examples 60–1
  considerations
    age 53–4
    duration 54
    history 55
    symptoms 54–5
  danger symptoms 55
    earache and facial pain 56
    purulent conjunctivitis 56
    wheezing 55–6
  management 57
    antihistamines 57–8
    antihistamines, topical 59–60
    decongestants 58–9
    steroid nasal sprays 59

medication 56
referral 56
treatment timescale 57
aluminium salt antacids 90
alverine citrate 127
amantadine 29–30
ampicillin 48
anaesthetics, local 74, 135
analgesics, topical 215
analgesics for sore throat 49
angina, atypical 87–8
angiotensin-converting enzyme (ACE)
    inhibitors in coughing 37
anogenital warts 173
antacids 79, 89–91
  cautions, side-effects and interactions 91
antibiotics in colds and flu 30
anticholingeric agents motion sickness
    100
antidiarrhoeals 128
anti-emetics 97
antihistamines
  allergic rhinitis (hay fever) 57–8
  cautions, side-effects and interactions
    26–7, 58
  coughs 40
  insomnia 334
  motion sickness 99–100
anti-inflammatory agents, topical 216–17
antipruritics 148
antiseptics 136
antispasmotics 126–7
antivirals in colds and flu 29–30
anxiety and chest pain 63
aphthous ulcers 69
  types 70
aromatherapy 335
ASMETHOD mnemonic for consultation
    10–13
aspirin 31
  cautions, side-effects and interactions
    201–2
  dysmenorrhoea (period pains) 239
  headache 201–2
  heart disease prevention 355
  nausea and vomiting 97
  sore throat 49
asthma 22, 36
  shortness of breath 63
  wheezing 64
astringents 136

Symptoms in the Pharmacy: A Guide to the Management of Common Illness, Seventh Edition.
Alison Blenkinsopp, Paul Paxton and John Blenkinsopp.
© 2014 John Wiley & Sons, Ltd. Published 2014 by John Wiley & Sons, Ltd.

athlete's foot 159
  case examples 164–6
  considerations
    appearance 159
    duration 159
    history 160
    location 160
    medication 160
    severity 160
  management 161
    azoles 161
    footwear 163
    fungal nail infections 164
    griseofulvin 162
    hydrocortisone 162–3
    hygiene 163
    ringworm 163–4
    terbinafine 161–2
    tolnaftate 162
    undecanoates 162
  referral 161
  treatment timetable 161
atorvastatin 32
azelastine 59–60
azithromycin 227, 230
azoles 161

back pain 212–13
  pregnancy 263–4
  prevention 218–19
barbiturates
  cautions, side-effects and interactions 26
beclometasone 46
  nasal spray 59
Behçet's syndrome 70, 71
benign prostatic hyperplasia (BPH) 269
  considerations
    age 269
    duration 270
    history 270
    medication 270
    symptoms 269–70
  lifestyle advice 272–3
  management 271
    tamulosin 271–2
  referral 270
  treatment timescale 271
benzocaine
  mouth ulcers 74
  sore throat 49, 50
benzodiazepines 334
  cautions, side-effects and interactions 26
benzoyl peroxide 155–6
benzydamine mouthwash 73
benzydamine spray 49
bifonazole 161
bisacodyl 105
bismuth salts 136
bisoprolol 31
bloating 125
blood
  altered 133
  in stool 103
  in urine 227
  vomiting 96–7
body mass index (BMI) 345
bowel cancer 103

breath, shortness of
  cardiac causes
    heart failure 63
  other causes
    hyperventilation syndrome 63–4
  respiratory causes
    asthma 63
    chronic bronchitis and emphysema
      (COPD) 63
bronchitis, chronic 36, 63
  sputum 64
bronchitis, wheezy 64
bruising 211
buclizine 203
budesonide 46
bulk-forming laxatives 106
bursitis 211–12

caffeine 203
  dysmenorrhoea (period pains) 239
calamine lotion 148
calcipotriol 188
calcium carbonate 90
cancer
  bowel cancer 103
  colorectal cancer 133–4
  oral cancer 70–1
candidiasis (thrush)
  oral 323
    age 323
    appearance 323–4
    case examples 325–7
    management 325
    medication 324
    referral 324
    treatment timescale 325
  throat 48
  vaginal 246
    age 246–7
    case examples 252–4
    duration 247
    history 248–9
    management 250–2
    medication 249–50
    symptoms 247–8
capsaicin/capsicum 216
carbimazole 47
cardiovascular conditions
  cardiac pain 62
  coughing 36
  heart failure 63
    sputum 65
    wheezing 64
cardiovascular disease (CVD) 343, 344
catarrh 21
cetrizine 26
  allergic rhinitis (hay fever) 57
  cautions, side-effects and interactions 58
cetylpyridinium 50
checkpoints for consultations 9
chest pain
  non-respiratory causes
    anxiety
    cardiac pain 62
    heartburn 62
  respiratory causes 62
chesty coughs 34–5

chickenpox (varicella) 298
children 297
  colic 303
    age 303
    feeding 303
    management 304–5
    mother smokes 304
    symptoms 303
  constipation 106–7
  head lice 313
    age 313
    case examples 317–18
    management 315–17
    medication 315
    signs of infection 314–15
  napkin (nappy) rash 307
    case examples 310–12
    duration 308
    management 309–10
    nature and location 307
    referral 309
    severity 307–8
    treatment timescale 309
  oral thrush 323
    age 323
    appearance 323–4
    case examples 325–7
    management 325
    medication 324
    referral 324
    treatment timescale 325
  rashes 297
    chickenpox (varicella) 298
    fifth disease 299–300
    German measles (rubella) 300
    management 301–2
    measles 298–9
    meningitis 300, 301
    non-blanching 300–1
    referral 301–2
    roseola infantum 299
  teething 306
  threadworms 319
    age 319
    appearance 320
    management 321–2
    medication 320
    referral 321
    signs of infection 319–20
chlamydial infection 226–7, 230
chlorhexidine gluconate mouthwash 73
chlorphenamine 26
  allergic rhinitis (hay fever) 58
  cautions, side-effects and interactions
    58
chondroitin 217
chronic bronchitis 36, 63
  sputum 64
chronic daily headache (CDH) 196
chronic obstructive pulmonary disease
    (COPD) 22, 63
cinnarizine 99–100
Clinical Knowledge Summaries (CKS) 8
clobetasone 147
clotrimazole 161
cluster headaches 196–7
coal tar 185

coconut, anise and ylang ylang spray
    316
codeine 39
  cautions, side-effects and interactions
    202–3
  headache 202–3
coeliac disease 72
cold sores (herpes labialis) 167
  considerations
    age 167–8
    duration 168
    history 169
    location 168
    medication 169
    precipitating factors 169
    symptoms and appearance 168
  management
    aciclovir and penciclovir 169–70
    eczema herpeticum 171
    hydrocolloid gel patch 170
    sunscreens 171
  referral 169
colds and flu 19
  case examples 30–2
  considerations
    age 19–20
    duration 20
    history 22
    medication, current 23
    symptoms 20–2
    treatment timescale 23
  differentiating between 22
  flu pandemic 29
  flu prevention 28–9
  management 23–4
    antibiotics 30
    antihistamines 25–7
    antivirals 29–30
    decongestants 24–5
    Echinacea 27
    practical considerations 27–9
    surgical face masks 30
    vitamin C 27
    zinc 27
  referral 23
colic 303
  age 303
  feeding 303
  management 304–5
  mother smokes 304
  symptoms 303
colorectal cancer 133–4
Community Pharmacy Contractual
    Framework (CPCF) 7
conjunctivitis 56, 281–3
constipation 102
  case examples 107–11
  considerations
    associated symptoms 103
    blood in stool 103
    bowel cancer 103
    bowel habit 102–3
    diet 104
    medication 104, 105
  management 105
    bulk-forming laxatives 106
    children 106–7

constipation (*Continued*)
  elderly patients 107
  laxative abuse 107
  osmotic laxatives 106
  pregnancy 107
  stimulant laxatives 105
  pregnancy 263
  referral 104
  treatment timescale 105
consultation in the pharmacy
  see also patients in the pharmacy
  accidents and injuries 14
  checkpoints 9
  partnerships with other health service
    providers 15–16
  Patient Group Directions (PGDs) 15
  privacy 14–15
  risk assessment 13
  skills development 8–9
  structure
    ASMETHOD 10–13
    WHAM 9–10
  tips for successful consultation 3
contact lenses 284
contraception, emergency hormonal (EHC)
  255
contraceptive pill: headache 198
corneal ulcers 283
coronary heart disease (CHD) 343
corticosteroids, topical
  eczema and dermatitis 147–8
  mouth ulcers 73
coughing 33
  case examples 42–4
  colds and flu 20
  considerations
    age 33
    associated symptoms 35
    croup (acute laryngotracheitis) 35
    duration 34
    history 36
    medication, current 36–7
    productive coughs 34–5
    referral 37
    smoking 36
    tuberculosis (TB) 35
    unproductive coughs 34
    whooping cough (pertussis) 35
  management 38
    antihistamines 40
    demulcents 38, 39
    diabetes 41
    expectorants 38, 39–40
    fluid intake 42
    steam inhalation 41–2
    suppressants 38, 39
    sympathomimetics 40–1
    treatment timescale 38
counterirritants 136, 215–16
cromoglicate eye drops 59
crotamiton 148
croup (acute laryngotracheitis) 35
cryotherapy 175
cyclophosphamide 229
cystitis 225
  associated symptoms 227–8
  case examples 231–3

  considerations
    age 226
    gender 226
    duration 228
    history 228–9
    management 229
      azithromycin 230
      complementary therapies 230
      potassium and sodium citrate
        229–30
    medication 229
    pregnancy 226, 264
    referral 226, 229
    symptoms 226–7
    treatment timescale 229

dandruff 182
  considerations
    aggravating factors 183
    appearance 182
    history 183
    location 183
    medication 183
    severity 183
  management 184
    coal tar 185
    ketoconazole 184
    selenium sulphide 184
    zinc pyrithione 184
  referral 183
  treatment timescale 184
danger symptoms 13
decision making based upon patient
  descriptions 6
decongestants
  allergic rhinitis (hay fever) 58–9
  sympathomimetics 24–5
demulcents 38, 39
dequalinium 50
dermatitis *see* eczema and dermatitis
dextromethorphan 39
diabetes
  coughs 41
  heart disease 346–7
  sore throat 50
diarrhoea 112
  causes
    bacterial infections 114–15
    chronic diarrhoea 115–16
    irritable bowel syndrome (IBS) 116
    protozoan infections 115
    viral infections 114
  considerations
    age 112
    duration 113
    history 113
    recent travel abroad 113–14
    severity 113
    symptoms 113
  management
    case examples 119–23
    diphenoxyxylate/atropine
      (co-phenotrope) 118
    kaolin 118
    loperamide 118
    morphine 119
    oral rehydration therapy 117–18

practical points 119
  probiotics 119
referral 117
treatment timescale 117
diclofenac
  cautions, side-effects and interactions
    201
  dysmenorrhoea (period pains) 238
  headache 200–1
diet
  acne 157
  constipation 104
  indigestion 88
  irritable bowel syndrome (IBS) 128–9
digoxin
  nausea and vomiting 97
dimethicone 315–16
dimeticone 90–1
diphenhydramine 26
  allergic rhinitis (hay fever) 57–8
  cautions, side-effects and interactions
    58
  coughs 40
  insomnia 334
diphenoxyxylate/atropine (co-phenotrope)
  118
dithranol 188
docusate sodium 105
domperidone 91–2
doxycycline
  nausea and vomiting 97
doxylamine 203
dry coughs 34
duct tape 175
duodenal ulcer 86
dysmenorrhoea (period pains) 234
  case examples 241–2
  considerations
    age 234
    history 235
    nature of pain and timing 235–6
  management 238
    aspirin 239
    caffeine 239
    hyoscine 239
    non-drug treatments 239–40
    NSAIDs 238
    paracetamol 239
  medication 237
  other symptoms 236
    premenstrual syndrome (PMS)
      236–7
  referral 237–8
  treatment timescale 238
dyspepsia see indigestion
dysphagia 47, 77
dysuria 248

ear problems 289
  case examples 293–4
  otitis externa (OE) 290–1
  otitis media 291–3
  wax 289–90
earache
  allergic rhinitis (hay fever) 56
  colds and flu 21
Echinacea 27

eczema and dermatitis 143
  case examples 148–52
  considerations
    age/distribution 143–4
    aggravating factors 145
    history 144–5
    medication 145
    occupation/contact 144
  management 146
    advice 147
    antipruritics 148
    emollients 146–7
    topical corticosteroids 147–8
  referral 145
  treatment timescale 146
eczema herpeticum 171
elderly patients and constipation 107
emergency hormonal contraception (EHC)
  255
  case examples 259–62
  considerations
    age 255
    necessity 255–6
  management 257–9
  referral 257
  treatment timescale 257
emollients 146–7
emphysema 63
endometriosis 235–6
ephedrine 24–5
  cautions, side-effects and interactions 25
Epsom salts 106
Epstein–Barr virus 48
erythema multiforme 71
erytherma infectosum 299–300
eucalyptus 42
evening primrose oil 237
expectorants 38, 39–40
eyes
  allergic rhinitis 55
  conjunctivitis 56
  painful 281
    case examples 286–8
    conjunctivitis 281–3
    considerations 285
    contact lenses 284
    corneal ulcers 283
    dry eyes 284–5
    glaucoma 284
    iritis 283
    management 285–6
    referral 285
    uveitis 283

face, pain in 56
face masks 30
famotidine 79–80, 91
fever in colds and flu 20, 22
feverfew 205
fibromyalgia 212
fifth disease 299–300
fish oils 240
flu see colds and flu
flurbiprofen lozenges 49
fluticasone nasal spray 59
formaldehyde 175
fungal nail infections 164

gallstones 87
gargles 50
gastric ulcer 86–7
gastroenteritis 96
gastrointestinal tract problems
    constipation 102
        associated symptoms 103
        blood in stool 103
        bowel cancer 103
        bowel habit 102–3
        case examples 107–11
        diet 104
        management 105–7
        medication 104, 105
        referral 104
        treatment timescale 105
    coughing 36
    diarrhoea 112
        age 112
        case examples 119–23
        causes 114–16
        duration 113
        history 113
        management 117–19
        recent travel abroad 113–14
        referral 117
        severity 113
        symptoms 113
        treatment timescale 117
    haemorrhoids 132
        case examples 137–9
        duration and history 132–3
        management 135–7
        medication 134–5
        referral 135
        symptoms 133–4
        treatment timescale 135
    heartburn 76
        age 76
        case examples 81–4
        management 79–81
        referral 78
        symptoms/associated factors 77–8
        treatment timescale 78
    indigestion (dyspepsia) 85
        age 86
        atypical angina 87–8
        case examples 92–4
        diet 88
        duration/history 86
        gallstones 87
        gastro-oesophageal reflux 87
        irritable bowel syndrome (IBS) 87
        management 89–92
        medication 88–9
        more serious disorders 88
        pain/associated symptoms 86
        referral 89
        smoking 88
        symptoms 86
        treatment timescale 89
        ulcer 86–7
    irritable bowel syndrome (IBS) 124
        age 124
        aggravating factors 126
        case examples 129–31
        duration 125

        history 125
        management 126–9
        medication 126
        referral 126
        symptoms 125
        treatment timescale 126
    motion sickness 98
        age 98
        history 98
        management 99–101
        medication 99
        mode of travel and journey length 99
    mouth ulcers 69
        age 69
        case examples 74–5
        duration 70
        history 71
        management 72–4
        medication 72
        nature of ulcers 69–70
        oral cancer 70–1
        other symptoms 71–2
        referral 72
        treatment timescale 72
    nausea and vomiting 95
        age 95–6
        alcohol intake 97
        associated symptoms 96–7
        duration 96
        history 97
        management 97
        medication 97
        pregnancy 96
gastro-oesophageal reflux 87
gastro-oesophageal reflux disease (GORD) 77
German measles (rubella) 300
giardiasis 113–14
ginger for motion sickness 100–1
glandular fever 48
glaucoma 284
glipizide 32
glucosamine 217
glue ear 292–3
gluteraldehyde 175
glycerine suppositories 106
griseofulvin 162
guaifenesin (guaiphenesin) 38, 40

H₂ antagonists 79–80
    indigestion (dyspepsia) 91
haemorrhoids 132
    case examples 137–9
    considerations
        duration and history 132–3
        medication 134–5
    management 135
        antiseptics 136
        astringents 136
        counterirritants 136
        hygiene 137
        laxatives 136
        local anaesthetics 135
        self-diagnosis 137
        shark liver oil/live yeast 136
        skin protectors 135–6
        topical steroids 136

pregnancy 134, 263
referral 135
symptoms 133
    bleeding 133–4
    bowel habit 134
    constipation 134
    irritation 133
    pain 133
    treatment timescale 135
hair loss 274
    gender 274
    history and duration 274–5
    location and extent 275
    management 276–7
    medication 275
    referral 276
    treatment timescale 276
hay fever see allergic rhinitis
head injury 211
head lice 313
    age 313
    case examples 317–18
    management 315
        coconut, anise and ylang ylang spray
            316
        dimethicone 315–16
        isopropyl myristate/cyclomethicone
            315–16
        malathion 316–17
        wet combing 316
    medication 315
    signs of infection 314–15
headache 193
    colds and flu 20, 21
    considerations
        age 193–4
        associated symptoms 195
        duration 194
        frequency and timing of symptoms
            194–5
        history 195
        nature and site of pain 194
    management
        aspirin 201–2
        buclizine 203
        caffeine 203
        case examples 205–9
        codeine 202–3
        diclofenac 200–1
        doxylamine 203
        feverfew 205
        ibuprofen 200–1
        paracetamol 199–200
        sumatriptan 203–4
    medication 198
        contraceptive pill 198
    precipitating factors 197
    pregnancy 264
    recent eye test 198
    recent trauma or injury 197
    referral 199
    treatment timescale 199
    types 195–7
heart disease prevention 343–4
    age 344
    alcohol intake 346
    case examples 356–7

ethnic origin 344
    family history 345
    managing risk 348
        age 352
        cautions, side-effects and interactions
            353–4
        management 352–3
        medication 352
        referral 353
        smoking cessation 348–50
        weight management 350–2
    medical history 346
        diabetes 346–7
        medication 347
        physical activity 346
        smoking 345
        waist circumference/body mass index
            (BMI) 345
heart see cardiovascular conditions
heartburn 62, 76
    case examples 81–4
    considerations
        age 76
    management 79
        alginates 79
        antacids 79
        clothing 81
        eating habits 81
        H_2 antagonists 79–80
        obesity 81
        other aggravating factors 81
        posture 81
        proton pump inhibitors (PPIs) 80
    pregnancy 264
    referral 78
    symptoms/associated factors 77
        dysphagia 77
        medication, current 78
        pregnancy 78
        regurgitation 77–8
        severe pain 77
    treatment timescale 78
Helicobacter pylori infections 87
heparinoid 217
herpes labialis see cold sores
herpetiform ulcers 69, 70
hoarseness 47
hyaluronidase 217
hydrocolloid gel patch 170
hydrocortisone
    athlete's foot 162–3
    eczema and dermatitis 147
    haemorrhoids 136
    mouth ulcers 73
hyoscine
    butylbromide 127
    dysmenorrhoea (period pains)
        239
    hydrobromide 100
hyperventilation syndrome 63–4

ibuprofen
    cautions, side-effects and interactions
        201
    dysmenorrhoea (period pains) 238
    headache 200–1
    sore throat 49

indigestion (dyspepsia) 85
  case examples 92–4
  considerations
    age 86
    atypical angina 87–8
    diet 88
    duration/history 86
    gallstones 87
    gastro-oesophageal reflux 87
    irritable bowel syndrome (IBS) 87
    medication 88–9
    more serious disorders 88
    pain/associated symptoms 86
    smoking 88
    symptoms 86
    ulcer 86–7
  management 89
    antacids 89–91
    domperidone 91–2
    H₂ antagonists 91
  referral 89
  treatment timescale 89
influenza see colds and flu
information gathering from patients 4–6
injuries 14
insomnia 331
  age 331–2
  case examples 337–40
  contributory factors 333
  duration 332–3
  history 333
  management 334–7
    antihistamines 334
    benzodiazepines 334
    complementary therapies 335–6
  medication 333
  referral 334
  symptoms 332
  treatment timescale 334
iritis 283
irritable bowel syndrome (IBS) 87, 124
  case examples 129–31
  considerations
    age 124
    aggravating factors 126
    duration 125
    history 125
    medication 126
    symptoms 125
  diarrhoea 116
  management
    antidiarrhoeals 128
    antispasmotics 126–7
    bulking agents 128
    complementary therapies 129
    diet 128–9
  referral 126
  treatment timescale 126
irritation in pregnancy 265
isopropyl myristate/cyclomethicone
    315–16
ispaghula husk 128

joints, painful 212

kaolin 118
Karposi's varicelliform eruption 171

ketoconazole 161, 184
Koplik spots 298

lactitol 106
lactulose 106
laryngotracheitis, acute (croup) 35
laxatives 136
  abuse 102, 107
  bulk-forming 106
  osmotic 106
  stimulant 105
lidocaine
  mouth ulcers 74
  sore troat 49
listening to patients symptom description
    5–6
local anaesthetics 74
loose coughs 34–5
loperamide 118, 128
loratadine 26
  allergic rhinitis (hay fever) 57
  cautions, side-effects and interactions 58
lozenges 50
lungs
  pulmonary embolus 62
  pulmonary oedema 65

macrogol 106
magnesium salt antacids 90
magnesium sulphate 106
Malassezia furfur 182
malathion 180, 316–17
measles 298–9
measles, mumps, rubella (MMR) vaccine
    298
mebendazole 321
mebeverine hydrochloride 127
meclozine 99–100
MEDLINE 8
melatonin 335
meningitis 300
  symptoms 301
menorrhagia 243
  age 243
  management 244
    tranexamic acid 244–5
  referral 244
  symptoms 244
  treatment timescale 244
men's health
  benign prostatic hyperplasia (BPH) 269
    age 269
    duration 270
    history 270
    lifestyle advice 272–3
    management 271–2
    medication 270
    referral 270
    symptoms 269–70
    treatment timescale 271
  hair loss 274
    history and duration 274–5
    location and extent 275
    management 276–7
    medication 275
    referral 276
    treatment timescale 276

menstrual cycle 243
menthol 42, 136, 216
metformin 32
methyl salicyclate 215
miconazole 161
migraine headaches 194, 195
  diagnostic pointers 196
minoxidil lotion 276–7
Mittelschmertz 235
monoamine oxidase inhibitors (MAOIs)
  cautions, side-effects and interactions 25
morning sickness 265
morphine 119
motion sickness 98
  considerations
    age 98
    history 98
    medication 99
    mode of travel and journey length 99
  management 99
    alternative approaches 100–1
    anticholingeric agents 100
    antihistamines 99–100
    treatment summary 101
mouth ulcers 69
  case examples 74–5
  considerations
    age 69
    duration 70
    history 71
    medication 72
    nature of ulcers 69–70
    oral cancer 70–1
    other symptoms 71–2
  management 72–3
    chlorhexidine gluconate mouthwash
      73
    local anaesthetics 74
    local analgesics 73
    other treatments 74
    topical corticosteroids 73
  referral 72
  treatment timescale 72
mouthwashes 49, 50
muscle pain 211
musculoskeletal problems 210
  case examples 219–21
    age 210
    symptoms and history 210–14
  management 214–15
    acupuncture 217
    analgesics, topical 215
    anti-inflammatory agents, topical
      216–17
    counterirritants and rubefacients
      215–16
    first-aid treatment 217–18
    glucosamine and chondroitin 217
    heat 217
    heparinoid and hyaluronidase 217
    prevention 218–19
  medication 214
  referral 214
  treatment timescale 214
  types
    back pain 212–13
    bruising 211

bursitis 211–12
fibromyalgia 212
head injury 211
joints, painful 212
muscle pain 211
repetitive strain disorder 213
shoulder, frozen 212
sprains and strains 211
whiplash injuries 213
myalgia 62

nail infections, fungal 164
named products, patient requests for 3–4
  response 4
napkin (nappy) rash 307
  case examples 310–12
  duration 308
  management 309–10
  nature and location 307
  referral 309
  severity 307–8
  treatment timescale 309
naproxen
  dysmenorrhoea (period pains) 238
nasal sprays vs. drops 28
nausea and vomiting 95
  considerations
    age 95–6
    alcohol intake 97
    associated symptoms 96–7
    duration 96
    history 97
    medication 97
    pregnancy 96
  management 97
  pregnancy 264–5
NHS Choices 8
nicotinamide 156
nicotinates 216
nicotine replacement therapy (NRT)
  348–50
nits 314
non-steroidal anti-inflammatory drugs
  (NSAIDs)
  indigestion 88
  nausea and vomiting 97
norovirus 114
nose
  congestion 54
  itching 55
  runny/blocked 20
    antihistamines 25–6
  sneezing 55

obesity and heartburn 81
oedema 63
oesophagitis 77
omeprazole 80
onychomycosis 164
open questions 5
oral cancer 70–1
oral rehydration therapy 117–18
Orlistat 351–2
oseltamivir 29
osmotic laxatives 106
otitis externa (OE) 290–1
otitis media 291–3

outcomes 8
over the counter (OTC) medicines
  colds and flu 19
  patient requests for 3–4
    response 4
  preferred treatments 7–8

painful conditions
  headache 193
    age 193–4
    associated symptoms 195
    case examples 205–9
    duration 194
    frequency and timing of symptoms
      194–5
    history 195
    management 199–205
    medication 198
    nature and site of pain 194
    precipitating factors 197
    recent eye test 198
    recent trauma or injury 197
    referral 199
    treatment timescale 199
    types 195–7
  musculoskeletal problems 210
    age 210
    case examples 219–21
    management 214–19
    medication 214
    referral 214
    symptoms and history 210–14
    treatment timescale 214
pantoprazole 80
paracetamol 31
  cautions, side-effects and interactions
    200
  dysmenorrhoea (period pains) 239
  headache 199–200
  liver toxicity 200
  sore throat 49
pastilles 50
Patient Group Directions (PGDs) 15
patients in the pharmacy 1–2
  accidents and injuries 14
  consultation skills development 8–9
  consultation structure 9–13
  partnerships with other health service
    providers 15–16
  Patient Group Directions (PGDs) 15
  privacy 14–15
  requests for named products 3–4
    response 4
  risk assessment 13
  symptoms, responding to requests 4
    decision making 6
    information gathering 4–6
    outcomes 8
    treatment 6–8
  tips for successful consultation 3
  working in partnership with 2
pelvic inflammatory disease (PID) 227, 236
penciclovir 169–70
peppermint oil 127
peptic stricture 77–8
period pains *see* dysmenorrhoea

permethrin 180
pertussis (whooping cough) 35
pharmacy (P) medicine 7
phenol 136
phenothiazines
  cautions, side-effects and interactions 26,
    40
pholcodine 38, 39
phototherapy (PUVA) 188–9
piperazine 321–2
pleurisy 62
pneumonia: sputum 64–5
polyvinylpyrrilidone (PVP) 74
postnasal drip 35
posture and heartburn 81
potassium citrate 229–30
pregnancy
  common symptoms
    back pain 263–4
    constipation 263
    cystitis 264
    haemorrhoids 263
    headache 264
    heartburn 264
    irritation 265
    nausea and vomiting 264–5
    vaginal discharge 265
  constipation 107
  cystitis 226
  haemorrhoids 134
  heartburn 78
  nausea and vomiting 96
  vaginal thrush 248–9
premenstrual syndrome (PMS) 236–7
prescription-only medicine (POM) 7
privacy in the pharmacy 14–15
probiotics 119
productive coughs 34–5
promethazine 26, 99–100
  allergic rhinitis (hay fever) 57–8
  cautions, side-effects and interactions 58
  insomnia 334
proton pump inhibitors (PPIs) 80
pseudoephedrine 24–5
  cautions, side-effects and interactions 25
  coughs 40–1
psoriasis 186
  considerations
    appearance 186
    diagnosis 187
    medication 187
    psychological factors 186–7
  management 187–8
    calcipotriol 188
    dithranol 188
    tacalcitol 188
pulmonary embolus 62
pyridoxine 237, 240

questions, open 5

rabeprazole 80
ramipril 31
ranitidine 79–80, 91
red flag symptoms 13
regurgitation 77–8, 96

repetitive strain disorder 213
resorcinol 136
respiratory problems
  allergic rhinitis (hay fever) 53
    age 53–4
    case examples 60–1
    danger symptoms 55–6
    duration 54
    history 55
    management 57–60
    medication 56
    referral 56
    symptoms 54–5
    treatment timescale 57
  colds and flu 19
    age 19–20
    case examples 30–2
    duration 20
    history 22
    management 23–30
    medication, current 23
    referral 23
    symptoms 20–2
    treatment timscale 23
  coughs 33
    age 33
    associated symptoms 35
    case examples 42–4
    croup (acute laryngotracheitis) 35
    duration 34
    history 36
    management 38–42
    medication, current 36–7
    productive coughs 34–5
    referral 37
    smoking 36
    treatment timescale 38
    tuberculosis (TB) 35
    unproductive coughs 34
    whooping cough (pertussis) 35
  direct referral
    chest pain 62–4
    shortness of breath 63–4
    sputum 64–5
    wheezing 64
  sore throat 45
    age 45
    associated symptoms 46
    case examples 50–2
    duration 46
    history 46
    management 49–50
    medication, current 46–7
    referral 47–8
    severity 46
    smoking 46
    treatment timescale 49
Reye's syndrome 73
rhinitis, allergic see allergic rhinitis (hay
    fever)
rhinorrhoea 54
ringworm 163–4
risk assessment 13
roseola infantum 299
rubefacients 215–16
rubella (German measles) 300

salicyclic acid 174–5
scabies 178
  considerations
    age 178
    history 179
    medication 179
    symptoms 179
  management 180
    malathion 180
    permethrin 180
  referral 179
Scottish Inter-Collegiate Guideline
    Network (SIGN) 8
selenium sulphide 184
shark liver oil 136
shortness of breath see breath, shortness of
shoulder, frozen 212
simethicone 304
Simple Lictus 38, 39
simvastatin 31, 354–5
sinusitis 21, 35, 197
skin conditions
  acne 153
    affected areas 154
    age 153–4
    duration 154–5
    management 155–8
    medication 155
    referral 155
    severity 154
    treatment timescale 155
  athlete's foot 159
    appearance 159
    case examples 164–6
    duration 159
    history 160
    location 160
    management 161–4
    medication 160
    referral 161
    severity 160
    treatment timetable 161
  cold sores 167
    age 167–8
    duration 168
    history 169
    location 168
    management 169–71
    medication 169
    precipitating factors 169
    referral 169
    symptoms and appearance 168
  dandruff 182
    aggravating factors 183
    appearance 182
    history 183
    location 183
    management 184–5
    medication 183
    referral 183
    severity 183
    treatment timescale 184
  eczema/dermatitis 143
    age/distribution 143–4
    aggravating factors 145
    case examples 148–52

skin conditions (*Continued*)
  history 144–5
  management 146–8
  medication 145
  occupation/contact 144
  referral 145
  treatment timescale 146
psoriasis 186
  appearance 186
  diagnosis 187
  management 187–9
  medication 187
  psychological factors 186–7
scabies 178
  age 178
  history 179
  management 180–1
  medication 179
  referral 179
  symptoms 179
warts and verrucae 172
  age 172
  duration 172–3
  history 173
  location 173
  management 174–7
  medication 174
  referral 174
  treatment timescale 174
skin protectors 135–6
smoking
  cessation 348–50
  coughing 36
  heart disease 345
  heartburn 81
  indigestion 88
  sore throat 46
sneezing 55
  colds and flu 20
sodium bicarbonate 90
sodium citrate 229–30
sodium cromoglicate 57, 58, 59
sodium hyaluronate (SH) 74
sprains and strains 211
  first-aid treatment 217–18
sputum 64
  bronchitis 64
  cardiac causes 65
  haemoptysis 65
  pneumonia 64–5
St John's wort (hypericum) 335–6
steam inhalation 41–2
steroid nasal sprays 59
steroids, topical 136, 188
stimulant laxatives 105
subarachnoid heamorrhage (SAH) 194
sumatriptan 203–4
  cautions, side-effects and interactions
    204–5
summer colds 20
suppressants, cough 38, 39
surgical face masks 30
swimming pools and verrucae 176–7
sympathomimetics 24–5
  cautions, side-effects and interactions
    25
  coughs 40–1

symptoms
  for direct referral 359–60
  responding to patient requests 4
    decision making 6
    information gathering 4–6
    outcomes 8
    treatment 6–8

tacalcitol 188
tamulosin 271–2
teething 306
temperature raised in colds and flu 20, 22
temporal arteritis 197
tension headaches 194
terbinafine 161–2
theophylline for coughs 41
threadworms 248, 319
  age 319
  appearance 320
  management 321
    mebendazole 321
    piperazine 321–2
  medication 320
  referral 321
  signs of infection 319–20
throat, sore 45
  case examples 50–2
  colds and flu 21
  considerations
    age 45
    associated symptoms 46
    duration 46
    history 46
    medication, current 46–7
    severity 46
    smoking 46
  management 49
    diabetes 50
    lozenges and pastilles 50
    mouthwashes and sprays 49
    oral analgesics 49
  referral
    appearance 47–8
    dysphagia 47
    glandular fever 48
    hoarseness 47
    thrush (candiasis) 48
  treatment timescale 49
thrush (candidiasis)
  oral 323
    age 323
    appearance 323–4
    case examples 325–7
    management 325
    medication 324
    referral 324
    treatment timescale 325
  sore throat 48
  vaginal 246
    age 246–7
    case examples 252–4
    duration 247
    history 248–9
    management 250–2
    medication 249–50
    symptoms 247–8
tickly coughs 34

tight coughs 34
tolnaftate 162
topical corticosteroids for mouth ulcers 73
tracheitis 62
tranexamic acid 244–5
transcutaneous electrical nerve stimulations
    (TENS) 239–40
travel sickness *see* motion sickness 99
treatment decisions 6–7
    effectiveness of treatments 7–8
tuberculosis (TB) 35

ulcer, duodenal 86
ulcer, gastric 86–7
undecanoates 162
unproductive coughs 34
upper respiratory tract infections (URTIs)
    19
urinary tract infections (UTIs) 227–8
uveitis 283

vaginal discharge 227, 247–8
    pregnancy 265
varicella (chickenpox) 298
verrucae *see* warts and verrucae
vitamin C 27
vomiting *see* nausea and vomiting

waist circumference 345
warts and verrucae 172
    considerations
        age 172
        duration 172–3
        history 173
        location 173
        medication 174
    management 174
        cryotherapy 175
        duct tape 175
        formaldehyde 175
        gluteraldehyde 175
        salicyclic acid 174–5
    referral 174
    treatment timescale 174
weight management 350–2
wet combing 316
WHAM nmemonic for consultation 9–10
wheezing 55–6
    asthma 64
    bronchitis 64
    cardiac causes 64
whiplash injuries 213
whooping cough (pertussis) 35
Wolff–Parkinson–White syndrome 204
women's health
    cystitis 225
        age 226
        associated symptoms 227–8

case examples 231–3
duration 228
history 228–9
management 229–31
medication 229
pregnancy 226
referral 226, 229
symptoms 226–7
treatment timescale 229
dysmenorrhoea 234
    age 234
    case examples 241–2
    history 235
    management 238–41
    medication 237
    nature of pain and timing 235–6
    other symptoms 236–7
    referral 237–8
    treatment timescale 238
emergency hormonal contraception
    (EHC) 255
    age 255
    case examples 259–62
    management 257–9
    necessity 255–6
    referral 257
    treatment timescale 257
menorrhagia 243
    age 243
    management 244–5
    referral 244
    symptoms 244
    treatment timescale 244
pregnancy, common symptoms
    back pain 263–4
    constipation 263
    cystitis 264
    haemorrhoids 263
    headache 264
    heartburn 264
    irritation 265
    nausea and vomiting 264–5
    vaginal discharge 265
vaginal thrush 246
    age 246–7
    case examples 252–4
    duration 247
    history 248–9
    management 250–2
    medication 249–50
    symptoms 247–8

yeast 136
Yellow Card scheme 10

zanamivir 29
zinc 27
zinc pyrithione 184

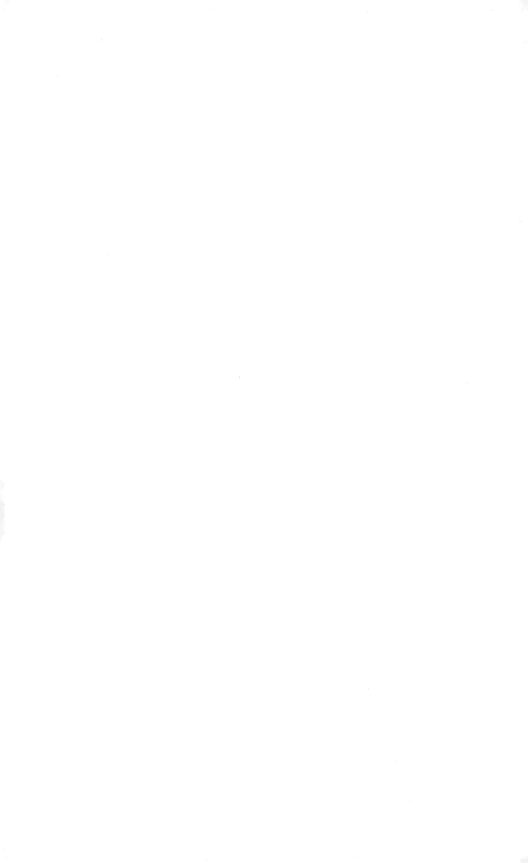